3-Dimensional Modeling in Cardiovascular Disease

3-Dimensional Modeling in Cardiovascular Disease

Edited by

EVAN M. ZAHN, MD
Proffesor of Pediatrics
Director
Guerin Family Congenital Heart Program
Smidt Heart Institute and the Department of Pediatrics
Cedars Sinai Medical Center
Los Angeles, CA, USA

ELSEVIER

Publisher: Dolores Meloni
Acquisition Editor: Robin R. Carter
Editorial Project Manager: Megan Ashdown
Production Project Manager: Sreejith Viswanathan
Cover Designer: Miles Hitchen

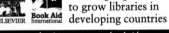

Working together
to grow libraries in
developing countries

www.elsevier.com • www.bookaid.org

List of Contributors

Darren Berman, MD
The Heart Centre
Nationwide Children's Hospital
Columbus, OH, United States

Ronny R. Buechel, MD
Senior Consultant
Department of Nuclear Medicine
University Hospital Zurich
Zurich, Switzerland

Jeffrey A. Feinstein, MD, MPH
Professor
Department of Pediatrics (Cardiology)
Stanford University
Stanford, CA, United States

Stefano Filippini, MS
Houston Methodist DeBakey Heart & Vascular Center
Houston, TX, United States

Biomedical Engineer
Cardiology
The Methodist Hospital
Houston, TX, United States

Reena Maria Ghosh, MD
Pediatric Cardiology Fellow
Department of Cardiology
Children's Hospital of Philadelphia
Philadelphia, PA, United States

Andreas A. Giannopoulos, MD, PhD
Deputy Attending Physician
Cardiac Imaging
Department of Nuclear Medicine
University Hospital Zurich
Zürich, Switzerland

Department of Cardiology
University Hospital Zurich
Zurich, Switzerland

Narutoshi Hibino, MD, PhD
Division of Cardiac Surgery
The University of Chicago Advocate Children's
    Hospital
Chicago, IL, United States

Assistant Professor of Surgery
Division of Cardiac Surgery
The University of Chicago Advocate Children's
    Hospital
Chicago, IL, United States

Nabil Hussein, MBChB (Hons)
Cardiovascular Surgery Research Fellow
Cardiovascular Surgery
The Hospital for Sick Children (Sickkids)
Toronto, ON, Canada

Cardiothoracic Resident
Cardiothoracic Surgery
Castle Hill Hospital
Cottingham, United Kingdom

Plasencia Jonathan, PhD
Research Scientist
Heart Center Research
Phoenix Children's Hospital
Phoenix, AZ, United States

Ryan Justin, PhD
Research Scientist
3D Innovations Lab
Rady Children's Hospital
San Diego, CA, United States

Damien Kenny, MD, FACC
Department of Congenital Heart Disease
Our Lady's Children's Hospital
Crumlin, Dublin, Ireland

Christopher Z. Lam, MD
Doctor
Diagnostic Imaging
Hospital for Sick Children
Toronto, ON, Canada

Stephen H. Little, MD
Houston Methodist DeBakey Heart & Vascular Center
Houston, TX, United States

Associate Professor
Cardiology
Houston Methodist Hospital
Houston, TX, United States

Alison L. Marsden, PhD
Associate Professor
Departments of Pediatrics (Cardiology) and
    Bioengineering
Stanford University
Stanford, CA, United States

Colin J. Mc Mahon, MD, FRCPI, FAAP, FACC
Department of Congenital Heart Disease
Our Lady's Children's Hospital
Crumlin, Dublin, Ireland

Dimitris Mitsouras, PhD
Department of Radiology and Biomedical Imaging
University of California, San Francisco
San Francisco, CA, United States

Associate Professor of Radiology
University of California, San Francisco
San Francisco, CA, United States

Associate Professor
Departments of Radiology and Biochemistry
Microbiology and Immunology
The University of Ottawa
Ottawa, ON, Canada

Associate Professor
Department of Biochemistry
Microbiology and Immunology
The University of Ottawa Faculty of Medicine
Ottawa, ON, Canada

Lucy L. Nam, BA
Division of Cardiac Surgery
Johns Hopkins Hospital
Baltimore, MD, United States

Medical Student
Johns Hopkins School of Medicine
Baltimore, MD, United States

Laura Olivieri, MD
Associate Professor of Pediatrics
George Washington University School of Medicine
Division of Cardiology
Children's National Health System
Washington, DC, United States

Ahmed Ouda, MD
Consultant Cardiac Surgeon
Cardiaovascular Surgery
Clinic for Heart and Vascular Surgery
University Hospital Zurich
Zurich, Switzerland

Francesca Plucinotta, MD
Department of Congenital Heart Disease
Gruppo San Donato
Milan, Italy

Stephen Pophal, MD
Professor
Pediatrics
University of Arizona
Phoenix Children's Hospital
Phoenix, AZ, United States

Silvia Schievano, MEng, PhD
UCL Institute of Cardiovascular Science & Great
    Ormond Street Hospital for Children
London, United Kingdom

Professor
Institute of Cardiovascular Science
UCL
London, United Kingdom

Elizabeth Silvestro, MSE
Department of Radiology
Children's Hospital of Philadelphia
Pennsylvania, United States

Sanjay Sinha, MD
Assistant Clinical Professor
Department of Pediatrics
Division of Cardiology
UCLA Mattel Children's Hospital/UC Irvine
Los Angeles/Orange, CA, United States

Andrew M. Taylor, MD
UCL Institute of Cardiovascular Science & Great
  Ormond Street Hospital for Children
London, United Kingdom

Divisional Director
Cardiac Unit
Great Ormond Street Hospital for Children
London, United Kingdom

Professor
Centre for Cardioavscular Imaging
UCL
London, United Kingdom

Israel Valverde, MD
Head of Unit
Pediatric Cardiology Unit & Cardiovascular
  Pathophysiology Group
Institute of Biomedicine of Seville (IBIS)
CIBER-CV
Hospital Virgen de Rocio/CSIC/University of Seville
Seville, Spain

Honorary Senior Lecturer
Division of Biomedical Engineering and Imaging
  Sciences
King's College London
London, United Kingdom

Locum Consultant
Department of Congenital Heart Disease
Evelina London Children's Hospital
Guy's and St Thomas NHS Foundation Trust
London, United Kingdom

Glen van Arsdell, MD
Chief of Congenital Cardiovascular Surgery
University of California Los Angeles Medical Center
Los Angeles, CA, United States

Marija Vukicevic, PhD
Research Scientist
Cardiology
Houston Methodist DeBakey Heart & Vascular Center
Houston, TX, United States

Assistant Professor of Cardiology Research
Cardiology
Weill Cornell Medicine
Houston, TX, United States

Kevin K. Whitehead, MD, PhD
Associate Professor of Medicine
Division of Cardiology
Department of Pediatrics
Children's Hospital of Philadelphia
Perelman School of Medicine at the University of
  Pennsylvania
Pennsylvania, United States

Shi-Joon Yoo, MD
Professor of Medical Imaging and Paediatrics
University of Toronto, Hospital for Sick Children
Toronto, Canada

Weiguang Yang, PhD
Research Associate
Department of Pediatrics (Cardiology)
Stanford University
Stanford, CA, United States

Foreword

Interest in the cardiovascular system has evolved over the last two millennia from a description of morbid anatomy to the application of sophisticated diagnosis and surgical/interventional techniques. In the foreword to Maude Abbott's landmark 1936 *Atlas of Congenital Heart Disease*, Dr. Paul D. White wrote she "[made] the subject one of such general and widespread interest that we no longer regard it with either disdain or awe as a mystery for the autopsy table alone to discover and to solve!" In the seventy-some years that followed, dedicated clinicians and surgeons have revolutionized the management of the infant and child with congenital heart disease, where today there are more adults with congenital heart disease than children. This revolution and management has in no small part been due to a better understanding of the complex relationships in cardiovascular structure *(in vivo)*, which has been advanced with the development of MR and CT imaging, and the ability to volume-render the image in three-dimensional (3-D) space. However, this technology had been limited to the 2-D representation of the anatomy, requiring the mental reconstruction of the 3-D image. What started in the 1960s by Ivan Sutherland with the creation of 3-D digital representations using specialized computer software has now involved as the foundation for the creation of physical models of cardiovascular anatomy. As such there is now a need for a book which reviews the fundamentals of 3-D modeling and its application to cardiovascular science. Such a book should not only be meant for those working in the field of 3-D modeling, but for all those who daily deal with the challenges of managing cardiovascular disorders from cardiology trainees to surgeons, interventionalists, and medical educators.

Dr. Evan Zahn has invited experts in the field to detail contemporary aspects of modeling in this book, *3-Dimensional Modeling in Cardiovascular Disease*. He and his coauthors are to be commended for their efforts in addressing this burgeoning field. The book is composed of 13 chapters starting with the evolution of 3-D modeling in cardiovascular disease, technical aspects of creating a 3-D model, its personalized role in the planning of congenital and acquired a cardiac surgery and case examples, through its application in interventional procedures and bioprinting.

Dr. Zahn and coauthors have produced a much needed book at a time when advances in imaging and their direct application to patient care are at a tipping point. The text will act as a reference for those caring for patients with cardiovascular disease, allowing an understanding of the many aspects of 3-D modeling today, and for the future.

Lee Benson, MD, The Hospital for Sick Children
Toronto, Canada, August 25, 2019

Introduction

Cardiac imaging has guided diagnosis, treatment, and improved patient outcomes in the field of cardiovascular medicine for over 50 years. Until recently, the cardiac practitioner was charged with comprehensive understanding of complex three-dimensional anatomy based on a compilation of two-dimensional renderings. Whether it be a simple chest X-ray, cineangiogram, echocardiogram, cardiac CT, or MRI, viewing of a patient's cardiac anatomy had remained constrained to a two-dimensional screen or piece of paper. However, that is ancient history …

Nearly 40 years ago, in 1981, Hideo Lodama of Nagoya Municipal Industrial Research Institute published a report on a functional rapid prototyping system utilizing photopolymer technology,[1] quickly followed by Charles Hull's patented stereolithography technology. Hull is widely credited as the father of modern day 3D printing. 3D printing technology or rapid prototyping is based upon the concept of additive manufacturing; that is, building structures by depositing materials layer by layer as opposed to standard manufacturing techniques that typically rely on manipulating raw materials (molding, cutting, etc.). Consequently, 3D printing has the ability to create remarkably complex structures using a wide variety of materials in a relatively short period of time. First adopted by the manufacturing industry to produce product prototypes and components, 3D printing quickly found its way into selected surgical subspecialties. In 1990, the first report(s) of medical rapid prototyping described a model of cranial bone anatomy created based upon CT source data.[2] This report was followed by numerous descriptions of similar models and manufactured implants of bony structures over the next several years. With further advances in medical imaging technology (particularly CT, MRI, and echocardiography) along with remarkable advances in computer hardware and 3D image processing software, medical rapid prototyping expanded to the cardiac sciences. As early as 2007, we began to see reports describing the utility of 3D printing in the design of new mechanical support devices and percutaneous valves.[3,4] Subsequently, the use of 3D printing in cardiovascular disease has been described in hundreds of papers and is on the cusp of becoming a mainstream tool in both acquired and congenital heart disease.

The timing, therefore, is ideal to gather an international group of experts in this emerging field to provide a comprehensive up-to-date text examining the most relevant aspects of 3D modeling in cardiovascular disease today.

Chapters 1 and 2 introduce the most common computational and physical 3D modeling methodologies and provide a comprehensive look at the techniques and global technologies currently used to generate cardiovascular 3D models.

In Chapters 3−8, we turn our attention to the clinical utility of these technologies in a wide variety of clinical settings including congenital and acquired heart surgery, congenital and structural interventional cardiology, and the role of 3D modeling in the treatment of advanced heart failure.

In Chapter 9, we examine current real world issues surrounding 3D modeling including the challenges associated with using these models as a standard clinical tool. A practical focus on image acquisition challenges, creating and maintaining a 3D laboratory, and the time and costs associated with this technology are all discussed.

Maintaining that real-world theme, Chapter 10 attempts to examine the data surrounding this novel technology and provides a guide on how to critically evaluate the current and future literature on the subject.

Our final two Chapters 12 and 13 provide a glimpse into the near future of personalized medicine as they discuss the evolving clinical use of computational modeling to guide complex surgical interventions and the evolution and current state of the art of 3D bioprinting. When reading these last two chapters one cannot help but be excited about what the future of cardiovascular medicine will look like as we tap into the ultimate potential of this ground-breaking technology.

REFERENCES

1. H. Kodama, "A scheme for three-dimensional display by automatic fabrication of three-dimensional model," IEICE Trans Electron, vol. J64-C, No. 4, pp. 237–241.
2. Mankovich NJ, Cheeseman AM, Stoker NG. The display of three-dimensional anatomy with stereolithographic models. *J Digit Imaging*. 1990;3:200–203.
3. Noecker AM, Chen JF, Zhou Q, et al. Development of patient-specific three-dimensional pediatric cardiac models. *Am Soc Artif Intern Organs J*. 2006;52:349–353.
4. Schievano S, Migliavacca F, Coats L, et al. Percutaneous pulmonary valve implantation based on rapid prototyping of right ventricular outflow tract and pulmonary trunk from MR data. *Radiology*. 2007;242:490–497.

Contents

CHAPTER 1

The Evolution of 3D Modeling in Cardiac Disease

SILVIA SCHIEVANO, MENG, PHD • ANDREW M. TAYLOR, MD

INTRODUCTION

Biomedical engineering is the application of engineering principles and methods to the medical field. It combines the design and problem-solving skills of engineering with medical and biological sciences, to help improve patient healthcare and the quality of life of individuals. As a relatively new discipline, much of the work in biomedical engineering consists of research and development, covering an array of techniques and fields, including three-dimensional (3D) modeling, the process of developing a simplified representation of a complex object/system in three dimensions. In general, the aim of 3D modeling is to replicate the behavior of the system it represents, using actual, known properties of the system itself and its components. A model can take on a diversity of forms—it can be physical, mathematical, statistical, animal, etc.—and can serve a wide variety of roles, including deepening understanding, contextualizing data, tracing chains of causation, facilitating experimental design to make predictions and inspiring new theories. To achieve these goals, models are required to bring together information of different kinds, from multiple fields and spanning a range of length scales.

The application of 3D modeling to medicine and the human body originated from the fields of engineering and physics. When computers became available to industry and university researchers in the 1970s, computational models came to play an increasingly central role in various branches of engineering, especially in the structural, aerospace, mechanical, electromagnetic, fluid dynamics, chemical, control, and electrical domains. The validations necessary to bring confidence to the modeling calculations were established, and development of extensive algorithm took place. During this period, a new technique called finite element (FE) analysis was first implemented for the aerospace industry and rapidly became the most widely accepted modeling framework to analyze complex structures.

The earliest computer programs for medicine and biology were coded to investigate the mechanics of cell–cell interactions. Researchers quickly realized that they could modify the properties of the virtual cells in their models and the rules that governed their interactions at will, and that by doing so they could test hypotheses, understand the features that gave rise to particular outcomes and perform almost any type of virtual experiment. Over time, the algorithms they used improved and became more reliable, stronger connections were forged between models and real-world experiments, and modeling ultimately entered mainstream biology. Even though many of those early studies were rudimentary by current standards, they were instrumental in defining the field of 3D modeling in biology and medicine.

In the same years, modeling was introduced in cardiovascular research for simple, two-dimensional (2D), computational simulations of cardiac mechanics and electrophysiology. In the decades that followed, advancements within medical imaging technology, together with computer power, boosted the evolution from generic, simplified models to current highly detailed, complex, individualized, 3D heart models that faithfully represent the anatomy and features of a specific subject. Nowadays, 3D modeling is a common tool used in all areas of cardiovascular medicine and research to answer different questions ranging from clinical image segmentation and diagnosis to quantification of anatomical structure and physiological responses of the cardiac system under normal, diseased, and surgically altered states; from patient risk stratification to interventional and surgical planning; and from engineering device design to education and communication. In particular, thanks to the most recent efforts in multidisciplinary collaborations, patient-specific cardiovascular 3D modeling is emerging from decades of academic research and is beginning to transition to

3-Dimensional Modeling in Cardiovascular Disease. https://doi.org/10.1016/B978-0-323-65391-6.00001-6

impact clinical treatment, directly via marketed devices and indirectly by improving our understanding of the underlying mechanisms of cardiovascular pathophysiology within specific clinical contexts.

In the pages that follow, we present a brief overview of the most common computational and physical 3D modeling methodologies that have evolved in the past decades to help solve clinical cardiac problems and ultimately answer the question: what is the best treatment for my patient? We aim to highlight the most significant advances of these techniques relevant to clinical decision-making, surgical planning, education, and overall pathophysiological understanding of the cardiovascular system, with examples in congenital (CHD) and structural, acquired (AHD) heart diseases.

3D ANATOMICAL MODELS (FIG. 1.1)

Interpretation of 3D anatomical information and complex spatial relationships has always been an integral part of medicine, and has become even more important with the development of advanced medical imaging

techniques. Detailed 3D anatomical models have been widely demonstrated to allow better understanding of complex cardiovascular morphology and spatial arrangement of the different structures, potentially enhancing decision-making and preoperative planning, improving communication within the multidisciplinary team and with patients/parents, and for educational purposes as will be further demonstrated within subsequent chapters.[1-5]

The creation of any 3D cardiac model, either computational or physical, requires as a first step, the reconstruction of the anatomy of the heart and vessels. Early 3D models of cardiac anatomy, still in use for specific applications, were based on simple geometrical shapes, like truncated concentric spheroids/ellipsoids for the ventricles[6-8] and cylinders or pipes for the arteries,[9] both for in silico and in vitro experiments. In the 70–80s, more realistic anatomical models were established from measurements taken on explanted hearts/vessels, biplane cineangiography[10,11] and 2D ultrasound[12] or by manually segmenting histological slices,[13,14] still with a low level of anatomical detail

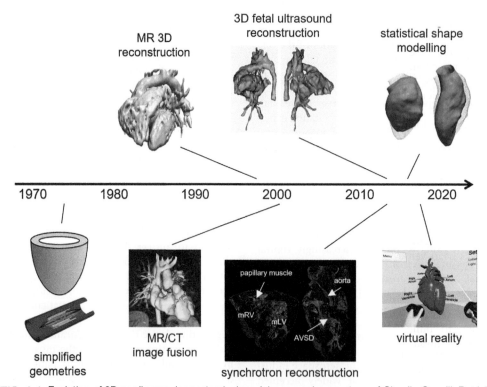

FIG. 1.1 Evolution of 3D cardiovascular anatomical models: examples courtesy of Claudio Capelli, Patricia Garcia-Canadilla, Jan Bruse, and Endrit Pajaziti. *AVSD*, atrioventricular septal defect; *mLV*, morphologically left ventricle; *mRV*, morphologically right ventricle.

due to the lengthy manual process and poor quality of the data used to build them. Over the last 20 years, the evolution of medical imaging technology, capable of providing 3D structural and functional information of cardiac tissue, has provided the possibility of building realistic, patient-specific 3D cardiac models, from in vivo[15−17] and high-resolution ex vivo[18−21] data. Routinely acquired clinical 3D magnetic resonance (MR), computed tomography (CT), echocardiography, and rotational angiographic imaging data from patients can be postprocessed to create 3D models.

Statistical Shape Models

Progress in medical image processing techniques and ever-growing availability of patient image databases, paired with an increase in computational power and deep learning algorithms, has driven the development of computational cardiac atlases, the latest advancement in 3D anatomy analysis.[22−25] Statistical shape models (SSM) are assembled by averaging several 3D image datasets from a population of subjects, thus allowing the description of an average, mean anatomical 3D shape and of the shape variability around the mean.[26] Using the mean shape and its principal modes of variation, descriptive or predictive statistical models of shape can be built to explore associations between 3D shape features and external (e.g., functional) parameters,[23] to examine particular characteristics of a population of anatomies,[27−29] and to discover unexpected patterns.[30,31] Outliers could be detected automatically and followed-up more closely. Clustering techniques could uncover previously unknown shape subgroups or morphological patterns, and subsequent classification techniques could explore if any of these subgroups is at a higher risk of following a certain pathologic pathway. Regression and correlation of distinct anatomical shape features with clinical or functional parameters could identify potential biomarkers for adverse events.[31]

Early SSMs in cardiac research described the variability of 2D heart ventricle shape contours based on a few subjects,[32] but with the advancement of 3D image modalities, current SSMs range from elaborate 3D models of the whole heart,[33] including thousands of subjects,[34,35] to projects such as the Cardiac Atlas Project[31] aiming to build exhaustive image databases including large amounts of patient clinical data for population-based studies. Other more clinically oriented examples include the initial work of Remme et al. in 2004,[36] who compared the shape of the left ventricle (LV) of healthy versus diabetic subjects, finding significant regional shape feature differences.

The focus for SSM research that followed has been predominantly on ventricular shape and motion analysis in different patient populations such as women with preeclampsia for risk assessment,[37] adults who were born preterm,[38] patients suffering from pulmonary hypertension by combining SSM with machine learning techniques to predict outcomes.[39] In the latter, authors described how 3D right ventricle (RV) motion parameters obtained via SSM significantly improved survival prediction, independent of conventional risk factors. In the field of CHD, Farrar et al. analyzed ventricular shapes and wall motion of adult single ventricle patients and compared them with a cardiac atlas of a healthy control population to derive shape z-scores as a measure of shape abnormality.[40]

SSMs based on nonparametric currents-based approaches, predominantly applied to analyze brain structures[41] were introduced to the CHD field by Mansi et al.[42−44] The authors studied the shape of the LV and RV from a population of Tetralogy of Fallot patients and established correlations between distinct shape features of the ventricles and clinically relevant parameters such as regurgitation fractions. Furthermore, they created a growth model that predicted ventricular shape changes based on changes in body surface area.[44] Most SSM cardiovascular work to date has focused on ventricular shape, with other cardiac structures rarely considered, until 2016 when Bruse and colleagues adopted nonparametric SSMs to study the aortic arch morphology of repaired aortic coarctation and hypoplastic left heart syndrome patients after palliation, compared to normal subjects.[45−47] Surgically modified aortic vessel often present challenging anatomy and a wide range of shape variations that despite successful repair may have long-term consequences impacting the long-term hemodynamics and function of the cardiovascular system.

Finally, an innovative application of SSM is in the design of new devices and treatments, especially for CHD, as SSMs can define more relevant target anatomical subgroups for the new technologies. An example[48] is the study of the geometric variability in extracardiac conduit vascular grafts connecting inferior vena cava and pulmonary arteries in the single ventricle population. Many cavopulmonary assist devices are being developed to provide support to these patients' deficient circulation; taking into account more realistic conduit shape information may prove useful to provide more accurate device design specifications, both in geometry and hemodynamic requirements.

Cardiovascular SSM can provide a powerful platform in research, clinical, and treatment design[49]: shape biomarkers and undiscovered disease patterns could assist clinicians in decision-making and risk stratification, especially in complex heart disease. Large databases of cardiovascular atlases could allow for comparison of any new patient with individuals with similar clinical history to detect similarities, appealing in rare diseases. Subgroup anatomical models could allow for more effective population-specific approaches for device design and treatment development, particularly in CHD.

Extended Reality Models

For many years, extended reality technologies have promised to clinicians the ability to overcome the limitations of visualizing 3D anatomical models on 2D flat screens that can greatly influence the 3D image perception and interpretation.[50] However, only recently, advances in high-resolution display technology and miniaturization of components have enabled a new class of head mounted display devices to make this a reality. These devices, now relatively low-cost and user friendly, create the perception of depth for high-quality clinical data 3D models through stereoscopy, with response times that are fast enough for clinical use.

Extended reality ranges from fully immersive, curated digital experiences in virtual reality (VR) to unobtrusive annotations within easy access of the operator in augmented reality (AR).[51] It encompasses 2D annotations on real-time video, 3D models, and true interference-based animated holograms. VR fully replaces the wearer's visual and auditory fields as the user interacts within a completely synthetic environment. Conversely, AR allows the wearer to see their native environment while placing 2D or 3D images within it through an annotated "window on the world." These AR applications minimally interfere with the normal field of vision, providing useful information only when called upon by the user. In the medical setting, contextually relevant graphics, reference data, or vital information is presented alongside (rather than in place of) the physical surroundings. In the cardiovascular fields, this translates to physicians being able to view, measure, and manipulate real-time stereoscopic images of a patient's heart during medical procedures—while still being able to clearly see the operating room environment—giving physicians complete, real-time, visual control of both the virtual images and the real physical world.

Several applications have been explored for extended reality technology in medicine including procedural planning, intraprocedural visualization, rehabilitation, patient point of care, emergency response, telemedicine, and education.[52,53]

The first cardiovascular research studies presented the use of extended reality versus traditional medical image readouts for interpretation of heart and vasculature: (1) in pulmonary atresia cases with major aortopulmonary collateral arteries, showing significantly reduced time in VR compared to traditional display[54]; (2) in standard catheterization laboratory procedures, creating real-time 3D digital holograms from rotational angiography, echocardiography, electroanatomic mapping[55–60] where AR empowers the interventional cardiologists and electrophysiologists to visualize patient-specific 3D cardiac geometry with real-time catheter locations, with the additional advantage of direct control of the display without breaking sterility; and (3) in surgical cases, for preoperative planning.[61,62]

Extended reality provides a wide range of possibilities for educational and training applications.[63,64] Some applications leverage the immersion that VR enables to simulate the entire operating environment alongside the educational materials. Another class of applications brings existing medical simulations from tablets and mobile phones to VR as the next platform that trainees will have access to. Other applications allow multiple wearers to interact and discuss with each other while viewing the same educational material in a natural environment.

COMPUTATIONAL MECHANISTIC MODELS (FIG. 1.2)

Although anatomical models can provide data-driven, observational, or phenomenological insight into relationships between shape and function, mechanistic modeling[65] has been widely applied in the biomedical engineering community to provide mechanistic insight into various phenomena. In a computational model, patient data—age, gender, diagnosis, anatomy, measurements from various instruments and systems, etc.—are merged with mathematical equations that govern the physical process being modeled, and other external data—material properties, tissue structure, biophysics models, etc.—obtained from a variety of sources such as experimental results, clinical studies and the literature, to provide information on organ function.

Computational models allow quantitative, mathematical analysis and prediction of cardiac biomechanical, biochemical, and electrophysiological function based on physical laws. These models can help to form and test novel hypotheses, potentially yielding insight into underlying disease mechanisms, novel associations between shape and function, and development of new surgical procedures, devices, and other

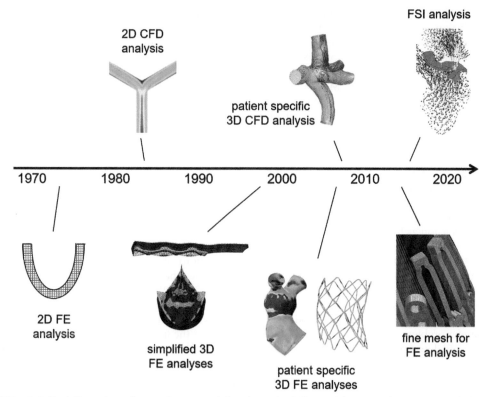

FIG. 1.2 Evolution of cardiovascular computational mechanistic models: examples courtesy of Emilie Sauvage, Claudio Capelli, Giorgia Bosi, and Benedetta Biffi.

therapies.[65] The biggest advantage of computational modeling is the possibility to alter certain geometric and/or functional boundary conditions, while controlling for others. This allows untangling the effect of changing one single parameter on the behavior of the entire system. For example, and according to the model purpose, preoperative physiologic data need to be extracted and the model modified to incorporate, test, and predict the outcome of a specific operative plan. Overall, results can be visualized and quantified to provide relevant physiologic data or derived information. The amount of complexity and heterogeneity of the model parameters may increase the accuracy of a given model, however, at the expense of incurring complicated validation processes and time/costs. A compromise is often required, as complex models are not always the answer, but rather simple models may already provide a good proxy of what is happening in reality. However, the introduction of sophisticated patient-specific models over the past 15 years has undoubtedly accelerated the transition from basic research to clinical application of this type of modeling.[66–69]

Predictive personalized medicine postulates that the use of 3D models that integrate patient-specific medical imaging (as well as other measurements) to simulate and quantify physiologic and pathophysiologic function of the cardiovascular system will ultimately result in personalizing and optimizing treatment, ultimately improving an individual patient's outcome. Patient-specific computational modeling has received increasing attention from regulatory agencies. The European Commission has heavily sponsored the Virtual Physiological Human (VPH) initiative, since 2006, with the major goal of simulating individualized and predictive healthcare, and has more recently funded the development of a "roadmap" to describe the route by which in silico techniques of computer simulation will be introduced into clinical trials (Avicenna). In the United States, the National Institutes of Health (NIH) announced in 2007 a funding opportunity for "Predictive Multiscale Models of the Physiome in Health and Disease" followed in 2009 by the National Institute of Biomedical Imaging and Bioengineering challenge grant "Toward the Virtual Patient" to stimulate the design of realistic computational models to make predictions about clinical outcomes. The US Food and Drug Administration (FDA) in 2013 released a new report entitled "Paving the Way for Personalized Medicine: FDA's Role in a New Era of Medical Product Development" and has created the Medical Device Innovation Consortium with the main goal of assessing new methods, approaches, and standards to enhance the quality and performance of medical devices and improve the timeline of availability of these products to patients.

Computational mechanistic simulations can focus on structures and their interactions (FE), and hemodynamics and fluid flow, with (fluid—structure interaction, FSI) and without (computational fluid dynamics, CFD) solid interaction as further described later.

Finite Element Modeling

The main purpose of FE analyses is to define the relationship between force and deformation, stress, and strain, as these relationships define how a structure deforms under a given force. The essence of FE modeling is to take a complex problem whose solution may be difficult to obtain, and decompose it into small, finite pieces (elements). The elements are assembled together and connected by nodes. The forces and deformations of each element (local approximate solution) affect the behavior of each adjacent element through the connecting nodes. The behavior of the overall structure (global approximate solution) is represented by the displacement of these elements and their material properties. FE models are based on three key inputs: geometry, material properties, and boundary conditions. Output is the detailed visualization of the distribution and location of stresses and deformations on structures, thus enabling construction, refinement, and optimization of entire designs before prototypes are manufactured, substantially decreasing production development time and costs. This method is applicable to a wide range of physical and engineering problems and is employed in many industrial fields to understand the complex behavior of assemblies, explore some concepts for new designs, and simulate manufacturing processes.

FE modeling entered the cardiovascular field at the beginning of the 1970s, with initial efforts focused on ventricular mechanics,[70–77] in particular on the LV, for the determination of the stress distributions in the myocardial wall during the cardiac cycle in normal hearts. The researchers advocated that the real future of FE cardiac models was for regional analyses, particularly for the inverse, in vivo quantification of the regional myocardial properties, as from the viewpoint

of clinical applications, local muscle dysfunction that initiates various cardiac problems should be investigated with highest priority.[73] They presented indeed the first FE analysis of myocardial diastolic stress and strain relationships in the intact heart and bioprosthetic valve tissue studies.

Although the FE method had been routinely used in industrial engineering to understand the complex behavior of mechanical parts, explore concepts for new designs, and simulate manufacturing processes for decades, applications of this methodology to study cardiovascular devices, balloons, valve prostheses, metallic stents—rather than the biological tissue—appeared only in 1980s, with one precursor study[78] and subsequently others, focusing on bioprosthetic valves[79–82] to quantify leaflet stresses under various pressure-loading conditions. Angioplasty balloons were thoroughly explored in the following years as well as their interaction with plaque treated vessels.[83–86] We reported the first use of the FE approach to study the mechanical behavior of a pediatric device[87] when we reported our analysis of the stent frame of the first percutaneous pulmonary valve (Melody TPV, Medtronic, USA) as well as its interaction with a patient-specific implantation site.[67]

Patient-specific models of cardiovascular mechanics can play an important role in the development of medical devices. The design and assessment require inputs from the clinical problem that the device needs to tackle and the intended function of the device itself. The 3D morphology of the implantation site, along with its dynamic, the anatomic variability between different individuals, the forces the body exerts on the device under a range of pathophysiologic conditions, the mechanical performance of the device when subject to cyclic in vivo forces, and the biological and mechanical impact of the device on the body are all aspects that influence the device design. Therefore, realistic biomechanical models based on medical imaging could provide invaluable data on the environment where devices are to be working and the effect of the devices on physiologic function.[66]

Computational Fluid Dynamics

CFD is a specialist area of mechanics that utilizes physical properties such as velocity, pressure, temperature, density, and viscosity, and different computational techniques to examine and quantify fluid flow behavior and patterns. The mathematical description for CFD analysis is provided by the Navier—Stokes equations on the conservation law of fluid's physical properties (mass, momentum, and energy), which are stable constants within a closed system—what comes in, must go out. CFD is capable of providing valuable hemodynamics parameters, useful in the clinical assessment of heart performance, the diagnosis of heart dysfunction, and the comparison between different treatments.[88]

A PubMed search of "computational fluid dynamics" and "cardiovascular" lists a paper on the mitral valve as the earliest study using CFD.[89] A number of CFD applications have followed focusing on issues ranging from thromboembolic potential of the mechanical caged-ball prosthesis created by Starr and Edwards,[90] to the analysis of blood flow in arterial bifurcations[91] to the assessment of LV ejection using CFD techniques[92], to a number of other applications[92a,b], including in vivo data[92c] and 3D models.[92d-f]

Over 20 years ago, CFD simulations based on in vitro tests showed how 3D modeling could provide insight into local hemodynamics in the total cavopulmonary connection of Fontan patients.[93–95] These studies showed that the abrupt geometrical change created by the surgically reconstructed anatomy led to important energy loss, which could be minimized, however, by optimizing the geometrical connection. Computational results led to changes in surgical practice, the first example of computer modeling influencing clinical treatment in CHD.

Significantly advanced CFD methodologies for cardiovascular simulations have subsequently been developed, demonstrated by the first successful clinical trial and subsequent FDA approval in 2014 of a simulation platform, HeartFlow, Inc. which uses patient CT images and CFD analysis-based fractional flow reserve to evaluate the risk of coronary artery disease in clinically stable symptomatic patients, noninvasively.[69,96,97]

Fluid—Structure Interaction

The addition of fluid within the solid structure—FSI—allows accurate analysis of the flow within the body analyzed and requires special methods to allow coupling of these two elements together: two theoretical formulations are usually adopted for powerful FSI techniques—the arbitrary Lagrangian Eulerian and the immersed boundary methods. FSI simulations are becoming more and more important for engineering purposes, as well as in biomedical engineering, as coupling of fluid flow and tissue mechanics are obviously vital to the human body as well as many other physical phenomena. One obvious example is blood circulation in compliant vessels, and the heart dynamics in the cardiovascular system, where pumping of blood from the heart is the result of large deformations produced by the myocardium and valve leaflets, and the subsequent pulsatile hemodynamic loads produced

during the cardiac cycle. Not surprisingly, the use of FSI cardiac models for clinical evaluation as well as for the assessment of medical devices is a topic of active investigation.

The first cardiovascular studies to utilize FSI methodologies quantified the effect of distensibility (compliance) of the wall of the carotid artery bifurcation on the local flow field, and were able to determine the mechanical stresses placed upon that arterial wall.[98,99] Subsequently, evidence was presented in the late 1990s that low shear stress in human coronary vessels promotes atherosclerosis,[100] and that FSI was useful for aneurysmal artery assessment.[101,102] Additional complexity was added to FSI models developed to study a wide variety of cardiac disease states including ventricular pathophysiology related to myocardial infarction, dilated cardiomyopathy, hypertrophic cardiomyopathy, hypoplastic left heart syndrome, and tetralogy of Fallot.[88,103–105] A final area of great interest involving FSI modeling is related to the testing of various valves and devices. Here, FSI can be utilized to assess the hemodynamics and mechanical properties of healthy and diseased valves, as well as support device designs thereby helping to expedite and augment product development.[106–110] The most advanced FSI models now incorporate realistic image-based ventricular and atrial geometries, leaflet kinematics, and valves structural response[111a,b], as well as biological models of platelet activation, thereby assisting in the development of newer optimized treatment strategies for both the mitral and aortic valves.

Most recently, patient-specific FSI models of the cardiovascular system that can simulate healthy or diseased states coupled with valvar structural response and intraventricular hemodynamics in a realistic model during the entire cardiac cycle are being actively pursued.[111] These models would not only enhance our basic understanding of the functional morphology of these structures, but also allow quantification of clinically relevant results and a better understanding of the implications of medical, surgical and interventional therapies, with the ultimate goal of supporting a complex clinical decision-making process, providing improved insights into surgical planning and ultimately resulting in improved clinical outcomes.

PHYSICAL MODELS—3D PRINTING (FIG. 1.3)

Most of the 3D modeling techniques described so far, despite indisputably powerful in many cardiovascular applications, convey information on a flat computer screen subjected to interpretation. True 3D representation of cardiovascular structures can be achieved by

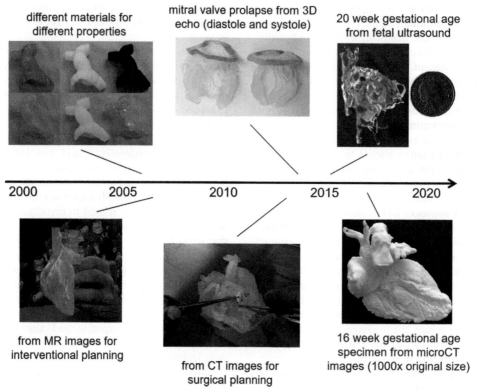

FIG. 1.3 Evolution of 3D printed cardiovascular models: examples courtesy of Marija Vukicevic, Giuliano Giusti, Claudio Capelli, Andrew Cook, and Aadam Akhtar.

creating tangible, physical models, hard copies of computational anatomical models that can provide both visual and tactile information of 3D cardiac structures, thus enhancing the experience of displaying 3D anatomy on a 2D screen.

In 1984, Charles Hull filed a patent for an "apparatus for production of three-dimensional objects by stereolithography."[112] Hull's apparatus was the World's first 3D printer, a mechanical system and process whereby solid objects were created by "printing" successive layers of material to replicate a shape modeled in a computer. Since then, the adoption of 3D printing across industry has been widespread including within the healthcare sector. Clinicians and surgeons have been using scan data to build 3D representations of patients' organs for decades. The first clinical application of 3D printing in cardiovascular medicine dates back to 1999[113] when solid anatomical biomodels were manufactured from 15 patients with cerebral aneurysms and one patient with a cerebral arteriovenous malformation from CT and/or MR angiograms. These

biomodels were successfully used for patient education, diagnosis, operative planning, and surgical navigation, with the only reported disadvantage at that time being cost and manufacturing time. The following year, the first intracardiac application was reported[114] when stereolithography was successfully used to create high precision, true-to-scale biomodels of the mitral valve using 3D echocardiographic datasets. This study showed for the first time the feasibility and potential of 3D printing to provide accurate detailed models of intracardiac anatomy and pathology in a clinical setting, and was soon followed by studies describing 3D modeling of aortic aneurysms,[115,116] aortic valve,[117] vasculature,[118] structural heart disease,[119–121] and scaffold fabrication for tissue engineering[122] among others.

A few years later, 3D printing technology made its appearance in CHD.[123–128] Despite improved results in the treatment of CHD, the surgical and interventional catheterization planning often remains difficult and is associated with major limitations, particularly in cases with complex anatomy, structural arrangements, and reoperations. 3D printing was first described in six patients with pulmonary atresia/ventricular septal defect and major aortopulmonary collateral arteries,[123] with the surgeons using the models for preoperative and intraoperative planning. Of the major aortopulmonary collateral arteries identified during surgery and conventional angiography, 96% and 93%, respectively, were accurately represented by the models. The surgeons reported the models very useful in visualizing the vascular anatomy, communicating complex imaging data, and as intraoperative reference. Subsequent publications described the use of physical models as an adjunct to treating patients with aberrant subclavian artery,[125] percutaneous pulmonary valve implantation,[126] heart transplantation,[127] and a wide variety of complex congenital surgical procedures.[128]

In less than 15 years, clinical use of rapid prototyping in cardiovascular disease has grown exponentially, and, although 3D printed heart models remain static, the unique interactivity and a hands-on experience they offer make their clinical and educational use valuable.[129–131] By allowing both anatomic and clinical information to be conveyed in a visual and tactile form, 3D printed models can be used in three main broad areas:

- clinical practice and research: to elucidate the complex anatomy and structure arrangement in both acquired and congenital heart disease; clarify the aims and limitations of corrective surgery and catheter-based procedures; practice challenging procedures; assess the likelihood of success/failure; select appropriate equipment and devices; and design novel devices, catheterizations treatments and surgical procedures. Rigid and compliant models can be printed for experimental bench investigations, to validate computational studies, test cardiovascular implants, and use the data for calibration and therapeutic procedures.[129–132]
- education and public engagement: physical models can nowadays be created from any patient who has undergone advanced cardiac imaging, thereby overcoming the reliance in education on the inherently limited supply of autopsy specimens available, as well as the moral and ethical issues surrounding their continued use. The same model can be printed an infinite number of times, at low costs and present no conservation/storage issues, thus scaling up massively the potential delivery of cardiovascular and surgical training.[133] Fetal and infant heart specimens can be reproduced at larger scales allowing appreciation of the cardiac microstructure.

- patients and parents' communication: doctor–patient interaction is crucial for patient adherence and satisfaction, but often challenging given the complexity of heart disease, the need for multiple surgeries, and the continuous follow-up requirements as well through delicate transition phases for CHD patients.[134] 3D rapid prototyping models during medical consultations can aid the communication process and improve patient experience and engagement.[135,136]

Ultimately, by allowing clinicians and patients to better understand the complex 3D anatomy inherent to heart diseases, 3D printing technology may serve to enhance the overall level of care provided to both adults and children with variety of cardiovascular disease.

DISCUSSION

With the rise of computers, ever-growing computational power, and manufacturing technologies, 3D modeling has become a commonly applied tool for solving complex problems and generating solutions in many modern engineering fields. The merits of 3D modeling are in developing new system designs and improved, optimized solutions, resulting in enhanced efficiency and lower production costs. Conversely, in the biomedical field, 3D modeling is still in its infancy, primarily due to the tremendous complexity of the human body. Additionally, there is a lack of large-scale validation studies, along with an absence of strong regulatory guidelines and legislation, which have been in place in other engineering fields for decades.

Despite major advances in overall understanding of the underlying mechanisms of cardiovascular disease and of the bioengineering modeling methodologies, the clinical decision-making process is still currently based on consensus opinion of experts, and is supported by empirical retrospective or prospective data from cohorts of patients with similar conditions. This methodology might not reflect an individual subject and do not allow making accurate, individualized outcome predictions in response to a variety of therapeutic options.

In response to these unmet needs, 3D modeling holds promises in multiple cardiovascular disease applications. Simulations can be used to augment clinical imaging, and support clinical decisions in surgical planning and device placement. Modeling can also provide a quantitative means to elucidate the relationship between hemodynamics and biological processes such as thrombosis, growth and remodeling, and mechanobiology. However, it must be noted that, now, without a critical mass of evidence and data from controlled randomized trials, most of these general benefits remain anecdotal.

As highlighted in the studies reviewed here, in many areas, research directions have now begun to move away from mere technical demonstration of tools and case studies, toward higher impact clinical applications and larger clinical studies.[137] It is becoming more apparent that if modeling tools are to become commonplace in the clinic, well-powered clinical trials demonstrating impact on patient outcomes from clinical use of 3D modeling are essential. The first FDA-cleared simulation platform (Heartflow) for cardiovascular modeling to support cardiologists in the decision-making process for coronary intervention represents a culmination of decades of basic research. This platform uses patient-specific anatomy derived from CT images and a number of nonpersonalized parameters to objectively measure coronary blood flow. Heartflow FFRCT followed standard regulatory pathways for medical device approval. Ongoing activities at the FDA indicate foresight about 3D modeling to improve the effectiveness of the product development process and to support regulatory decision-making, as computational modeling can play a key role in receiving FDA clearance or approval for medical devices.[138]

Currently, there is much discussion on the benefits of precision medicine: the integrative approach to disease prevention and treatment that considers an individual's particular characteristics and offers clinical advice based on the predictive response of the individual patient rather than the traditional approach based on the response of an average patient.[139] In this context, patient-specific 3D modeling, that can transform clinical therapies from those intended for an average patient to those designed for an individual patient, has significant appeal, particularly in CHD. Compared to adult patients with AHD, patients with CHD typically present a wide range of different anatomies and conditions, that are sometimes unique and extremely complex, and that change as a child grows; not only these patients are born with different anatomy and physiology, but they also undergo multiple operations over their lifetime to fix the disease, and the modified cardiac structures grow with time. Therefore, in CHD, concepts such as "one size fits all" do not work. The development of tools and devices designed for children lags a decade behind device development for adults, as the pediatric market is far smaller, making it difficult for companies to invest in research and development expenses for these devices. It is standard practice for industry to

develop treatment solutions tested in relatively constant, average conditions that can be replicated in vivo in animal models or in vitro with bench testing. It is, however, not sustainable for companies to develop relevant in vivo or experimental tests for the huge range of anatomical variations routinely encountered in pediatric practice, both in time and costs. These fundamental differences warrant a patient-specific approach, which can be highly facilitated by 3D modeling.

Finally, individual decision-making in cardiovascular disease is the basis of planning for complex treatments and surgeries. Many examples are reported in the literature demonstrating that better preoperative planning shortens intraoperative time, which, in turn, has significant impact on complication rate, blood loss, postoperative length of stay, etc. Therefore, detailed knowledge of an individual patient's 3D anatomy is a prerequisite before embarking on any individual surgical procedure. The advance of 3D printing and AR/VR technologies, coupled with innovative devices, surgical tools, and operating systems, will ultimately deliver a patient avatar for cardiologists/cardiovascular surgeons to navigate with unprecedented precision and an adequate real-time response.[140] Of course, there are challenges ahead and many problems to solve, especially as the organ of interest is the heart, with complex moving anatomy that changes shape and size in time with the cardiac cycle. Nevertheless, the potential of 3D modeling has paved the way for a clinical revolution, reviving an intellectual enthusiasm comparable to the one that established anatomy as a medical science and initiated modern medicine and surgery 500 years ago.

In conclusion, with recent advances in cardiovascular imaging, modeling methodologies, and increased availability of computing power to solve complex analyses, 3D cardiovascular modeling is now poised to gain greater clinical acceptance than ever before. Closer interactions between academic research organizations in biomedical and bioengineering sciences, clinicians, regulatory agencies, policymakers, and industry, in addition to dedicated cross-disciplinary training, will be crucial to fully bridge the gap between basic science and daily clinical practice and firmly establish 3D modeling as a vital tool potentially providing immense clinical benefit for patients.

REFERENCES

1. Marks Jr SC. The role of three-dimensional information in health care and medical education: the implications for anatomy and dissection. *Clin Anat.* 2000;13: 448−452.

2. Huk T. Who benefits from learning with 3D models? The case of spatial ability. *J Comput Assist Learn.* 2006;22: 392–404.

3. Guillot A, Champely S, Batier C, Thiriet P, Collet C. Relationship between spatial abilities, mental rotation and functional anatomy learning. *Adv Health Sci Educ Theory Pract.* 2007;12:491–507.

4. Khalil MK, Mansour MM, Wilhite DR. Evaluation of cognitive loads imposed by traditional paper-based and innovative computer-based instructional strategies. *J Vet Med Educ.* 2010;37:353–357.

5. Fredieu JR, Kerbo J, Herron M, Klatte R, Cooke M. Anatomical models: a digital revolution. *Med Sci Edu.* 2015;25(2):183–194.

6. Ghista D, Sandler H. An analytic elastic-viscoelastic model for the shape and the forces in the left ventricle. *J Biomech.* 1969;2:35–47.

7. Dieudonne JM. The left ventricle as confocal spheroids. *Bull Math Biophys.* 1969;31:433–439.

8. Nielsen PM, Le Grice IJ, Smaill BH, Hunter PJ. Mathematical model of geometry and fibrous structure of the heart. *Am J Physiol.* 1991;260(4 Pt 2):H1365–H1378.

9. Lassaline JV, Moon BC. A computational fluid dynamics simulation study of coronary blood flow affected by graft placement. *Interact Cardiovasc Thorac Surg.* 2014;19(1): 16–20.

10. Chang SK, Chow CK. The reconstruction of the three dimensional objects from two orthogonal projections and its application to cardiac cineangiography. *IEEE Trans Comput.* 1973;22:18–25.

11. Yettram AL, Vinson CA. Geometric modelling of the human left ventricle. *J Biomech Eng.* 1979;101:221–223.

12. Geiser EA, Lupkiewicz SM, Christie LG, et al. A framework for three-dimensional time-varying reconstruction of the human left ventricle: sources of error and estimation of their magnitude. *Comput Biomed Res.* 1980;13:225–241.

13. Janicki JS, Weber KT, Gochman RF, Shroff S, Geheb FJ. Three-dimensional myocardial and ventricular shape: a surface representation. *Am J Physiol.* 1981;241:Hl–Hll. Heart Circ Physiol 10.

14. Mclean MR, Prothero J. Coordinated three-dimendimensional reconstruction from serial sections at macroscopic and microscopic levels of resolution; the human heart. *Anat Rec.* 1987;219:434–439.

15. O'Brien JP, Srichai MB, Hecht EM, Kim DC, Jacobs JE. Anatomy of the heart at multidetector CT: what the radiologist needs to know. *Radiographics.* 2007;27(6): 1569–1582.

16. Valsangiacomo Buechel ER, Grosse-Wortmann L, Fratz S, et al. Indications for cardiovascular magnetic resonance in children with congenital and acquired heart disease: an expert consensus paper of the Imaging Working Group of the AEPC and the Cardiovascular Magnetic Resonance Section of the EACVI. *Eur Heart J Cardiovasc Imaging.* 2015;16(3):281–297.

17. Bhat V, Belaval V, Gadabanahalli K, Raj V, Shah S. Illustrated imaging essay on congenital heart diseases: multimodality approach Part III: cyanotic heart diseases and complex congenital anomalies. *J Clin Diagn Res.* 2016; 10(7):TE01–TE10.

18. Badea CT, Wetzel AW, Mistry N, Pomerantz S, Nave D, Johnson GA. Left ventricle volume measurements in cardiac micro-CT. The impact of radiation dose and contrast agent. *Comput Med Imag Graph.* 2008;32(3): 239–250.

19. Gonzalez-Tendero A, Zhang C, Balicevic V, et al. Whole heart detailed and quantitative anatomy, myofibre structure and vasculature from X-ray phase-contrast synchrotron radiation-based micro computed tomography. *Eur Heart J Cardiovasc Imaging.* 2017;18(7):732–741.

20. Stephenson RS, Atkinson A, Kottas P, et al. High resolution 3-Dimensional imaging of the human cardiac conduction system from microanatomy to mathematical modeling. *Sci Rep.* 2017;7(1):7188.

21. Garcia-Canadilla P, Dejea H, Bonnin A, et al. Complex congenital heart disease associated with disordered myocardial architecture in a midtrimester human fetus. *Circ Cardiovasc Imaging.* 2018;11(10):e007753.

22. Frangi AF, Rueckert D, Schnabel JA, Niessen WJ. Automatic construction of multiple-object three-dimensional statistical shape models: application to cardiac modeling. *IEEE Trans Med Imaging.* 2002;21(9): 1151–1166.

23. Lamata P, Casero R, Carapella V, et al. Images as drivers of progress in cardiac computational modelling. *Prog Biophys Mol Biol.* 2014;115:198–212.

24. Bruse JL, McLeod K, Biglino G, et al. Modeling of Congenital Hearts Alliance (MOCHA) Collaborative Group. A statistical shape modelling framework to extract 3D shape biomarkers from medical imaging data: assessing arch morphology of repaired coarctation of the aorta. *BMC Med Imaging.* 2016;16(1):40.

25. Biglino G, Capelli C, Bruse J, Bosi GM, Taylor AM, Schievano S. Computational modelling for congenital heart disease: how far are we from clinical translation? *Heart.* 2017;103:98–103.

26. Young AA, Frangi AF. Computational cardiac atlases: from patient to population and back. *Exp Physiol.* 2009; 94:578–596.

27. Lötjönen J, Kivistö S, Koikkalainen J, Smutek D, Lauerma K. Statistical shape model of atria, ventricles and epicardium from short- and long-axis MR images. *Med Image Anal.* 2004;8(3):371–386.

28. Faghih Roohi S, Aghaeizadeh Zoroofi R. 4D statistical shape modeling of the left ventricle in cardiac MR images. *Int J Comput Assist Radiol Surg.* 2013;8(3): 335–351.

29. Lekadir K, Keenan NG, Pennell DJ, Yang GZ. An interlandmark approach to 4-D shape extraction and interpretation: application to myocardial motion assessment in MRI. *IEEE Trans Med Imaging.* 2011;30(1):52–68.

30. Izenman AJ. *Modern Multivariate Statistical Techniques — Regression, Classification, and Manifold Learning.* Springer Science+Business Media LLC; 2008.

31. Fonseca CG, Backhaus M, Bluemke DA, et al. The Cardiac Atlas Project–an imaging database for computational

modeling and statistical atlases of the heart. *Bioinforma Oxf Engl.* 2011;27:2288−2295.

32. Cootes T, Hill A, Taylor C, Haslam J. Use of active shape models for locating structures in medical images. *Image Vis Comput.* 1994;12:355−365.

33. Lorenz C, von Berg J. A comprehensive shape model of the heart. *Med Image Anal.* 2006;10:657−670.

34. Medrano-Gracia P, Cowan BR, Bluemke DA, et al. Large scale left ventricular shape atlas using automated model fitting to contours. In: Ourselin S, Rueckert D, Smith N, eds. *Functional Imaging and Modeling of the Heart*. Berlin Heidelberg: Springer; 2013:433−441.

35. Bai W, Shi W, de Marvao A, et al. A bi-ventricular cardiac atlas built from 1000+ high resolution MR images of healthy subjects and an analysis of shape and motion. *Med Image Anal.* 2015;26(1):133−145.

36. Remme E, Young A, Augenstein K, Cowan B, Hunter P. Extraction and quantification of left ventricular deformation modes. *IEEE Trans Biomed Eng.* 2014;51(11):1923−1931.

37. Lamata P, Lazdam M, Ashcroft A, Lewandowski AJ, Leeson P, Smith N. Computational mesh as a descriptor of left ventricular shape for clinical diagnosis. In: *Computing in Cardiology Conference (CinC)*. 2013:571−574.

38. Lewandowski AJ, Augustine D, Lamata P, et al. Preterm heart in adult life cardiovascular magnetic resonance reveals distinct differences in left ventricular mass, geometry, and function. *Circulation.* 2013;127:197−206.

39. Dawes TJW, de Marvao A, Shi W, et al. Machine learning of three-dimensional right ventricular motion enables outcome prediction in pulmonary hypertension: a cardiac MR imaging study. *Radiology.* 2017;283(2):381−390.

40. Farrar G, Suinesiaputra A, Gilbert K, et al. Atlas-based ventricular shape analysis for understanding congenital heart disease. *Prog Pediatr Cardiol.* 2016;43:61−69.

41. Durrleman S, Pennec X, Trouvé A, Ayache N. Measuring brain variability via sulcal lines registration: a diffeomorphic approach. *Med Image Comput Comput Assist Interv.* 2007;10:675−682.

42. MacLeod RS, Stinstra JG, Lew S, et al. Subject-specific, multiscale simulation of electrophysiology: a software pipeline for image-based models and application examples. *Philos Trans R Soc Math Phys Eng Sci.* 2009;367:2293−2310.

43. Mansi T, Durrleman S, Bernhardt B, et al. A statistical model of right ventricle in tetralogy of Fallot for prediction of remodelling and therapy planning. In: Yang G-Z, Hawkes D, Rueckert D, Noble A, Taylor C, eds. *Medical Image Computing and Computer-Assisted Intervention − MICCAI 2009*, Springer Berlin Heidelberg; 214−221.

44. Mansi T, Voigt I, Leonardi B, et al. A statistical model for quantification and prediction of cardiac remodelling: application to tetralogy of Fallot. *IEEE Trans Med Imaging.* 2011;30:1605−1616.

45. Bruse JL, Khushnood A, McLeod K, et al. Modeling of Congenital Hearts Alliance Collaborative Group. How

successful is successful? Aortic arch shape after successful aortic coarctation repair correlates with left ventricular function. *J Thorac Cardiovasc Surg.* 2017;153(2):418−427.

46. Bruse JL, Cervi E, McLeod K, et al. Modeling of congenital hearts alliance (MOCHA) collaborative group. Looks do matter! Aortic arch shape after hypoplastic left heart syndrome palliation correlates with cavopulmonary outcomes. *Ann Thorac Surg.* 2017;103(2):645−654.

47. Sophocleous F, Biffi B, Milano EG, et al. Aortic morphological variability in patients with bicuspid aortic valve and aortic coarctation. *Eur J Cardiothorac Surg.* 2019;55(4):704−713.

48. Bruse JL, Giusti G, Baker C, et al. Statistical shape modeling for cavopulmonary assist device development: variability of vascular graft geometry and implications for hemodynamics. *J Med Dev.* 2017;11(2).

49. Richardson JE, Ash JS, Sittig DF, et al. Multiple perspectives on the meaning of clinical decision support. *AMIA Annu Symp Proc.* 2010:1427−1431.

50. Silva JN, Southworth MK, Raptis C, Silva J. Emerging applications of virtual reality in cardiovascular medicine. *JACC Basic Transl Sci.* 2018;3(3):420−430.

51. Milgram P, Kishino FA. Taxonomy of mixed reality visual-displays. *Ieice T Inf Syst.* 1994;E77d:1321−1329.

52. Giuseppe R, Wiederhold BK. The new dawn of virtual reality in health care: medical simulation and experiential interface. *ARCTT.* 2015;3.

53. Jang J, Tschabrunn CM, Barkagan M, Anter E, Menze B, Nezafat R. Three-dimensional holographic visualization of high-resolution myocardial scar on HoloLens. *PLoS One.* 2018;13(10):e0205188.

54. Chan F, Aguirre S, Bauser-Heaton H, Hanley F, Perry S. Head tracked stereoscopic pre-surgical evaluation of major aortopulmonary collateral arteries in the newborns. In: *Radiological Society of North America 2013 Scientific Assembly and Annual Meeting; Chicago, Illinois.*

55. Bruckheimer E, Rotschild C, Dagan T. Computer-generated real-time digital holography: first time use in clinical medical imaging. *Eur Heart J Cardiovasc Imaging.* 2016;17:845−849.

56. Bruckheimer E, Rotschild C. Holography for imaging in structural heart disease. *EuroIntervention.* 2016;12(Suppl X):X81−X84.

57. Currie ME, McLeod AJ, Moore JT, et al. Augmented reality system for ultrasound guidance of transcatheter aortic valve implantation. *Innov Technol Tech Cardiothorac Vasc Surg.* 2016;11(1):31−39.

58. Silva JN, Southworth MK, Dalal A, Van Hare GF, Silva JR. Improving visualization and interaction during transcatheter ablation using an augmented reality system: first-in-human experience (abstr). *Circulation.* 2017;136.

59. Kuhlemann I, Kleemann M, Jauer P, Schweikard A, Ernst F. Towards X-ray free endovascular interventions−using HoloLens for on-line holographic visualisation. *Healthc Technol Lett.* 2017;4(5):184.

60. Tandon A, Burkhardt BEU, Batsis M, et al. Vinus venosus defects: anatomic variants and transcatheter closure

feasibility using virtual reality planning. *JACC Cardiovasc Imaging*. 2018. Epub ahead of print.

61. Ong CS, Krishnan A, Huang CY, et al. Role of virtual reality in congenital heart disease. *Congenit Heart Dis*. 2018;13(3):357−361.

62. Mendez A, Hussain T, Hosseinpour AR, Valverde I. Virtual reality for preoperative planning in large ventricular septal defects. *Eur Heart J*. 2018. Epub ahead of print.

63. Stanford Children's Health, Stanford LPCsH, Lucile Packard Children's Hospital Stanford pioneers use of VR for patient care, education and experience. http://www.stanfordchildrens.org/en/about/news/releases/2017/virtual-reality-program.

64. Case Western Reserve, Cleveland Clinic. Case Western Reserve, Cleveland Clinic collaborate with Microsoft on 'earth-shattering' mixed-reality technology for education. http://case.edu/hololens/.

65. Frangi AF, Taylor ZA, Gooya A. Precision Imaging: more descriptive, predictive and integrative imaging. *Med Image Anal*. 2016;33:27−32.

66. Taylor CA, Figueroa CA. Patient-specific modeling of cardiovascular mechanics. *Annu Rev Biomed Eng*. 2009;11:109−134.

67. Schievano S, Taylor AM, Capelli C, et al. Patient specific finite element analysis results in more accurate prediction of stent fractures: application to percutaneous pulmonary valve implantation. *J Biomech*. 2010;43(4):687−693.

68. Hsia TY, Cosentino D, Corsini C, Pennati G, Dubini G, Migliavacca F. Modeling of Congenital Hearts Alliance (MOCHA) Investigators. Use of mathematical modeling to compare and predict hemodynamic effects between hybrid and surgical Norwood palliations for hypoplastic left heart syndrome. *Circulation*. 2011;124(11 Suppl):S204−S210.

69. Fairbairn TA, Nieman K, Akasaka T, et al. Real-world clinical utility and impact on clinical decision-making of coronary computed tomography angiography-derived fractional flow reserve: lessons from the ADVANCE Registry. *Eur Heart J*. 2018;39(41):3701−3711.

70. Pao YC, Ritman EL, Wood EH. Finite-element analysis of left ventricular myocardial stresses. *J Biomech*. 1974;7(6):469−477.

71. Janz RF, Grimm AF. Finite-element model for the mechanical behavior of the left ventricle. Prediction of deformation in the potassium-arrested rat heart. *Circ Res*. 1972;30(2):244−252.

72. Janz RF, Grimm AF. Deformation of the diastolic left ventricle. Nonlinear elastic effects. *Biophys J*. 1973;13(7):689−704.

73. Heethaar RM, Pao YC, Ritman EL. Computer aspects of three-dimensional finite element analysis of stresses and strains in the intact heart. *Comput Biomed Res*. 1977;10(3):271−285.

74. Ghista DN, Hamid MS. Finite element stress analysis of the human left ventricle whose irregular shape is developed from single plane cineangiocardiogram. *Comput Progr Biomed*. 1977;7(3):219−231.

75. Ritman EL, Heethaar RM, Robb RA, Pao YC. Finite element analysis of myocardial diastolic stress and strain relationships in the intact heart. *Eur J Cardiol*. 1978;7(Suppl):105−119.

76. McPherson DD, Skorton DJ, Kodiyalam S, et al. Finite element analysis of myocardial diastolic function using three-dimensional echocardiographic reconstructions: application of a new method for study of acute ischemia in dogs. *Circ Res*. 1987;60(5):674−682.

77. Watanabe T, Ohtake T, Kosaka N, Momose T, Nishikawa J, Iio M. Computer simulation of ventricular wall motion using the finite element method. *Radiat Med*. 1988;6(4):165−170.

78. Rossow MP, Gould PL, Clark RE. A simple method for estimating stresses in natural and prosthetic heart valves. *Biomater Med Devices Artif Organs*. 1978;6(4):277−290.

79. Hamid MS, Sabbah HN, Stein PD. Computer-assisted methods for design optimization of cardiac bioprosthetic valves. *Henry Ford Hosp Med J*. 1984;32(3):178−181.

80. Sabbah HN, Hamid MS, Stein PD. Estimation of mechanical stresses on closed cusps of porcine bioprosthetic valves: effects of stiffening, focal calcium and focal thinning. *Am J Cardiol*. 1985;55(8):1091−1096.

81. Hamid MS, Sabbah HN, Stein PD. Influence of stent height upon stresses on the cusps of closed bioprosthetic valves. *J Biomech*. 1986;19(9):759−769.

82. Black MM, Howard IC, Huang X, Patterson EA. A three-dimensional analysis of a bioprosthetic heart valve. *J Biomech*. 1991;24(9):793−801.

83. Young S, Pincus G, Hwang NH. Dynamic evaluation of the viscoelastic properties of a biomedical polymer (biomer). *Biomater Med Devices Artif Organs*. 1977;5(3):233−254.

84. Lee RT, Loree HM, Cheng GC, Lieberman EH, Jaramillo N, Schoen FJ. Computational structural analysis based on intravascular ultrasound imaging before in vitro angioplasty: prediction of plaque fracture locations. *J Am Coll Cardiol*. 1993;21(3):777−782.

85. Oh S, Kleinberger M, McElhaney JH. Finite-element analysis of balloon angioplasty. *Med Biol Eng Comput*. 1994;32(4 Suppl):S108−S114.

86. Rogers C, Tseng DY, Squire JC, Edelman ER. Coronary balloons/stents − balloon-artery interactions during stent placement: a finite element analysis approach to pressure, compliance, and stent design as contributors to vascular injury. *Circ Res*. 1999;84(4):378−383.

87. Schievano S, Petrini L, Migliavacca F, et al. Finite element analysis of stent deployment: understanding stent fracture in percutaneous pulmonary valve implantation. *J Interv Cardiol*. 2007;20(6):546−554.

88. Doost SN, Ghista D, Su B, Zhong L, Morsi YS. Heart blood flow simulation: a perspective review. *Biomed Eng Online*. 2016;15(1):101.

89. McQueen DM, Peskin CS, Yellin EL. Fluid dynamics of the mitral valve: physiological aspects of a mathematical model. *Am J Physiol*. 1982;242:H1095−H1110.

90. Tansley GD, Mazumdar J, Noye BJ, Craig IH, Thalassoudis K. Assessment of haemolytic and thromboembolic potentials—from CFD studies of Starr—Edwards cardiac valve prostheses. *Australas Phys Eng Sci Med*. 1989; 12:121—127.

91. Xu XY, Collins MW. A review of the numerical analysis of blood flow in arterial bifurcations. *Proc Inst Mech Eng [H]*. 1990;204:205—216.

92. Georgiadis JG, Wang M, Pasipoularides A. Computational fluid dynamics of left ventricular ejection. *Ann Biomed Eng*. 1992;20:81—97.

92a. Satcher Jr RL, Bussolari SR, Gimbrone Jr MA, Dewey Jr CF. The distribution of fluid forces on model arterial endothelium using computational fluid dynamics. *J Biomech Eng*. 1992;114:309—316.

92b. Taylor CA, Hughes TJR, Zarins CK. Finite element modeling of blood flow in arteries. *Comput Methods Appl Mech Eng*. 1998;158:155—196.

92c. Moore JA, Rutt BK, Karlik SJ, Yin K, Ethier CR. Computational blood flow modeling based on in vivo measurements. *Ann Biomed Eng*. 1999;27:627—640.

92d. Lopez-Perez A, Sebastian R, Ferrero JM. Three-dimensional cardiac computational modelling: methods, features and applications. *Biomed Eng Online*. 2015;14:35.

92e. Laszlo K. Three-dimensional modelling and three-dimensional printing in pediatric and congenital cardiac surgery. *Transl Pediatr*. 2018;7(2):129—138.

92f. Shim EB, Yeo JY, Ko HJ, et al. Numerical analysis of the three-dimensional blood flow in the Korean artificial heart. *Artif Organs*. 2003;27(1):49—60.

93. Van Haesdonck JM, Mertens L, Sizaire R, et al. Comparison by computerized numeric modeling of energy losses in different Fontan connections. *Circulation*. 1995;92(9 Suppl):II322—I326.

94. Dubini G, de Leval MR, Pietrabissa R, Montevecchi FM, Fumero R. A numerical fluid mechanical study of repaired congenital heart defects. Application to the total cavopulmonary connection. *J Biomech*. 1996;29: 111—121.

95. Migliavacca F, de Leval MR, Dubini G, Pietrabissa R. A computational pulsatile model of the bidirectional cavopulmonary anastomosis: the influence of pulmonary forward flow. *J Biomech Eng*. 1996;118:520—528.

96. Taylor CA, Fonte TA, Min JK. Computational fluid dynamics applied to cardiac computed tomography for noninvasive quantification of fractional flow reserve: scientific basis. *J Am Coll Cardiol*. 2013;61(22):2233—2241.

97. Leipsic J, Weir-McCall J, Blanke P. FFR$_{CT}$ for complex coronary artery disease treatment planning: new opportunities. *Interv Cardiol*. 2018;13(3):126—128.

98. Perktold K, Rappitsch G. Computer simulation of local blood flow and vessel mechanics in a compliant carotid artery bifurcation model. *J Biomech*. 1995;28:845—856.

99. Milner JS, Moore JA, Rutt BK, Steinman DA. Hemodynamics of human carotid artery bifurcations: computational studies with models reconstructed from magnetic resonance imaging of normal subjects. *J Vasc Surg*. 1998;28(1):143—156.

100. Krams R, Wentzel JJ, Oomen JAF, et al. Evaluation of endothelial shear stress and 3D geometry as factors determining the development of atherosclerosis and remodeling in human coronary arteries in vivo. Combining 3D reconstruction from angiography and IVUS (ANGUS) with computational fluid dynamics. *Arterioscler Thromb Vasc Biol*. 1997;17(10):2061—2065.

101. Torii R, Oshima M, Kobayashi T, Takagi K, Tezduyar TE. Fluid—structure interaction modeling of a patient-specific cerebral aneurysm: influence of structural modeling. *Comput Mech*. 2008;43:151—159.

102. Sharzehee M, Khalafvand SS, Han HC. Fluid—structure interaction modeling of aneurysmal arteries under steady-state and pulsatile blood flow: a stability analysis. *Comput Methods Biomech Biomed Eng*. 2018;21(3):219—231.

103. Lemmon JD, Yoganathan AP. Three-dimensional computational model of left heart diastolic function with fluid—structure interaction. *J Biomech Eng*. 2000;122(2): 109—117.

104. Yang C, Tang D, Haber I, Geva T, Del Nido PJ. In vivo MRI-based 3D FSI RV/LV models for human right ventricle and patch design for potential computer-aided surgery optimization. *Comput Struct*. 2007;85(11—14): 988—997.

105. Tang D, Yang C, Geva T, Del Nido PJ. Image-based patient-specific ventricle models with fluid—structure interaction for cardiac function assessment and surgical design optimization. *Prog Pediatr Cardiol*. 2010; 30(1—2):51—62.

106. Luraghi G, Wu W, De Castilla H, et al. Numerical approach to study the behavior of an artificial ventricle: fluid—structure interaction followed by fluid dynamics with moving boundaries. *Artif Organs*. 2018;42(10): E315—E324.

107. De Hart J, Peters GW, Schreurs PJ, Baaijens FP. A two-dimensional fluid—structure interaction model of the aortic valve [correction of value]. *J Biomech*. 2000;33(9): 1079—1088.

108. De Hart J, Peters GW, Schreurs PJ, Baaijens FP. A three-dimensional computational analysis of fluid—structure interaction in the aortic valve. *J Biomech*. 2003;36(1): 103—112.

109. Borazjani I. A review of fluid—structure interaction simulations of prosthetic heart valves. *J Long Term Eff Med Implant*. 2015;25(1—2):75—93.

110. Bahraseman HG, Languri EM, Yahyapourjalaly N, Espino DM. Fluid—structure interaction modeling of aortic valve stenosis at different heart rates. *Acta Bioeng Biomech*. 2016;18(3):11—20.

111. Dassault Systems. The Living Heart Project A Translational Research Initiative to Revolutionize Cardiovascular Science Through Realistic Simulation. https://www.3ds.com/products-services/simulia/solutions/life-sciences/the-living-heart-project/.

111a. Mao W, Caballero A, McKay R, Primiano C, Sun W. Fully-coupled fluid—structure interaction simulation of the aortic and mitral valves in a realistic 3D left ventricle model. *PLoS One*. 2017;12(9):e0184729.

111b. Feng L, Qi N, Gao H, et al. On the chordae structure and dynamic behaviour of the mitral valve. *IMA J Appl Math.* 2018;83(6):1066–1091.

112. Hull C. *Apparatus for Production of Three-dimensional Object by Stereolithography.* 1986. US Patent 4,575,330.

113. D'Urso PS, Thompson RG, Atkinson RL, et al. Cerebrovascular biomodelling: a technical note. *Surg Neurol.* 1999;52:490–500.

114. Binder TM, Moertl D, Mundigler G, et al. Stereolithographic biomodeling to create tangible hard copies of cardiac structures from echocardiographic data: in vitro and in vivo validation. *J Am Coll Cardiol.* 2000;35: 230–237.

115. Carmi D, Zegdi R, Grebe R, Fabiani JN. Three-dimensional modelling of thoracic aortic aneurysm: a case report [in French]. *Arch Mal Coeur Vaiss.* 2001;94: 277–281.

116. Kato K, Ishiguchi T, Maruyama K, Naganawa S, Ishigaki T. Accuracy of plastic replica of aortic aneurysm using 3D-CT data for transluminal stent-grafting: experimental and clinical evaluation. *J Comput Assist Tomogr.* 2001;25: 300–304.

117. Gilon D, Cape EG, Handschumacher MD, et al. Effect of three-dimensional valve shape on the hemodynamics of aortic stenosis: three-dimensional echocardiographic stereolithography and patient studies. *J Am Coll Cardiol.* 2002;40:1479–1486.

118. Knox K, Kerber CW, Singel SA, Bailey MJ, Imbesi SG. Rapid prototyping to create vascular replicas from CT scan data: making tools to teach, rehearse, and choose treatment strategies. *Cathet Cardiovasc Interv.* 2005;65: 47–53.

119. Weber S, Sodian R, Markert M, Reichart B, Daebritz S, Lueth TC. 3D printing of anatomical heart models for surgical planning in cardiac surgery. *Int J CARS.* 2007;2: 171–173.

120. Kim MS, Hansgen AR, Carroll JD. Use of rapid prototyping in the care of patients with structural heart disease. *Trends Cardiovasc Med.* 2008;18(6):210–216.

121. Kim MS, Hansgen AR, Wink O, Quaife RA, Carroll JD. Rapid prototyping: a new tool in understanding and treating structural heart disease. *Circulation.* 2008; 117(18):2388–2394.

122. Sodian R, Loebe M, Hein A, et al. Application of stereolithography for scaffold fabrication for tissue engineered heart valves. *Am Soc Artif Intern Organs J.* 2002;48:12–16.

123. Ngan EM, Rebeyka IM, Ross DB, et al. The rapid prototyping of anatomic models in pulmonary atresia. *J Thorac Cardiovasc Surg.* 2006;132(2):264–269.

124. Noecker AM, Chen JF, Zhou Q, et al. Development of patient-specific three-dimensional pediatric cardiac models. *Am Soc Artif Intern Organs J.* 2006;52(3): 349–353.

125. Sodian R, Weber S, Markert M, et al. Stereolithographic models for surgical planning in congenital heart surgery. *Ann Thorac Surg.* 2007;83:1854–1857.

126. Schievano S, Migliavacca F, Coats L, et al. Percutaneous pulmonary valve implantation based on rapid prototyping of right ventricular outflow tract and pulmonary trunk from MR data. *Radiology.* 2007;242:490–497.

127. Sodian R, Weber S, Markert M, et al. Pediatric cardiac transplantation: three-dimensional printing of anatomic models for surgical planning of heart transplantation in patients with univentricular heart. *J Thorac Cardiovasc Surg.* 2008;136(4):1098–1099.

128. Mottl-Link S, Hübler M, Kühne T, et al. Physical models aiding in complex congenital heart surgery. *Ann Thorac Surg.* 2008;86(1):273–277.

129. Milano EG, Capelli C, Wray J, et al. Current and future applications of 3D printing in congenital cardiology and cardiac surgery. *Br J Radiol.* 2018. Epub ahead of print.

130. Wang DD, Gheewala N, Shah R, et al. Three-dimensional printing for planning of structural heart interventions. *Interv Cardiol Clin.* 2018;7(3):415–423.

131. Grant EK, Olivieri L. The role of 3-D heart models in planning and executing interventional procedures. *Can J Cardiol.* 2017;33(9):1074–1081.

132. Vukicevic M, Mosadegh B, Min JK, Little SH. Cardiac 3D printing and its future directions. *JACC Cardiovasc Imaging.* 2017;10(2):171–184.

133. Yoo SJ, Spray T, Austin EH, Yun TJ, van Arsdell GS. Hands-on surgical training of congenital heart surgery using 3-dimensional print models. *J Thorac Cardiovasc Surg.* 2017;153:1530–1540.

134. Fuertes JN, Toporovsky A, Reyes M, Osborne JB. The physician-patient working alliance: theory, research, and future possibilities. *Patient Educ Counsel.* 2017;100: 610–615.

135. Biglino G, Capelli C, Koniordou D, et al. Use of 3D models of congenital heart disease as an education tool for cardiac nurses. *Congenit Heart Dis.* 2017;12(1): 113–118.a Biglino G, Capelli C, Wray J, et al. 3D-manufactured patient-specific models of congenital heart defects for communication in clinical practice: feasibility and acceptability. *BMJ Open.* 2015;5(4):e007165.

136. Biglino G, Koniordou D, Gasparini M, et al. Piloting the use of patient-specific cardiac models as a novel tool to facilitate communication during cinical consultations. *Pediatr Cardiol.* 2017;38(4):813–818.

137. Capelli C, Sauvage E, Giusti G, et al. Patient-specific simulations for planning treatment in congenital heart disease. *Interface Focus.* 2018;8(1):20170021.

138. FDA. *Reporting of Computational Modeling Studies in Medical Device Submissions;* 2016. https://www.fda.gov/downloads/medicaldevices/deviceregulationandguidance/guidancedocuments/ucm381813.pdf.

139. Gray RA, Pathmanathan P. Patient-specific cardiovascular computational modeling: diversity of personalization and challenges. *J Cardiovasc Transl Res.* 2018;11(2):80–88.

140. González D, Cueto E, Chinesta F. Computational patient avatars for surgery planning. *Ann Biomed Eng.* 2016; 44(1):35–45.

CHAPTER 2

The Technical Basics of Cardiac 3D Printing

DIMITRIS MITSOURAS, PHD • ANDREAS A. GIANNOPOULOS, MD, PHD

INTRODUCTION

The first additive manufacturing technology, stereolithography, was developed by Chuck Hull in the 1980s to enable engineers to rapidly produce prototypes. The technology was subsequently commercialized in 1987 by a then newly founded company, 3D Systems, which to date remains a major manufacturer of additive manufacturing equipment. A number of additive manufacturing technologies beyond stereolithography are available today and are collectively commonly referred to simply as "3D printing" technologies.

In one aspect, all 3D printing technologies still function in the same manner as the original stereolithography process in that a physical three-dimensional (3D) object is manufactured layer by layer, with each layer selectively solidified and adhered to the previously completed layer. In contrast, in terms of the particular method by which materials are "printed" and adhered to previous layers of material, a number of diverse techniques have been developed in the now 30-year history of 3D printing. Some of these technologies still employ the same physical process as stereolithography, namely, photopolymerization. Many 3D printers used for medical models today rely on the exact same technique with little change, and many more rely on recent technological advances that have significantly enhanced the versatility and speed of the technique with photopolymer-based 3D printers now able to produce physical objects containing millions of colors and different mechanical properties in different regions of a model, while others are able to print many medical models in less than an hour.

Concurrently, a number of other, very different technologies, such as powder bed fusion and material extrusion, have significantly expanded the types of materials from which physical objects can be printed beyond photopolymers. Many of those materials such as bioresorbable materials, metals, and synthetic polymers and those that are possible to impregnate with bioactive substances are highly relevant and are used and being developed for clinical applications. This chapter will review the technical aspects of those 3D printing technologies that are widely used in a present-day clinical environment. 3D printing technologies that are now emerging that lie between anatomic models printed for surgical planning and functional models that can replicate tissue characteristics will also be described. Finally, more forward-looking technologies, primarily aimed at "bioprinting" whole, living organs, which can perhaps be considered the ultimate goal of medical 3D printing, are outside the scope of this chapter, but will be reviewed in a subsequent chapter.

It is also important to recognize that 3D printing technologies are only one component of the (presently) highly technically demanding aspects of creating 3D-printed medical models. Potentially the most complex aspect today, particularly in the context of cardiovascular models, is how one can produce the computer model that the 3D printer will actualize, starting from a patient's clinical imaging studies.[1-5] This chapter will review the technical aspects of this often-, but ill-termed "DICOM to STL conversion process." It is also in this aspect of 3D printing in conjunction with 3D printing materials advances that fast-paced technological innovations for medical applications are taking place today. These innovations range from techniques to create, for example, models that consolidate relevant information from multiple imaging studies,[6-8] such as computed tomography (CT) plus ultrasound (US) or positron emission tomography (PET), or that have similar mechanical or functional properties as tissue,[9,10] or similar imaging signal characteristics as tissue when imaged with clinical imaging modalities.[11-14] Many of these advances are most relevant for, and indeed some are driven by the needs of cardiovascular

3-Dimensional Modeling in Cardiovascular Disease. https://doi.org/10.1016/B978-0-323-65391-6.00002-8

applications, where functional information is often required in addition to anatomic information for a model to be clinically useful.

The final technical aspect of 3D printing of medical models that is covered in this chapter concerns their quality and safety. As clinical uses of 3D printing continuously expand, it is paramount that models are created in an appropriate and safe manner.[6,15,16] Cardiovascular models pose a particularly difficult subset of medical 3D printing in that they most often require the interpretation of soft tissues depicted in imaging studies. The difficulty here arises from the often-limited contrast between soft tissues, which renders the process of interpreting their precise spatial extents, necessary to actualize an anatomic model, prone to significant operator error. Determining the extent of myocardium on CT is more difficult than for example interpreting the spatial extent of bone in CT, which benefits from an order of magnitude difference between the Hounsfield units of bone and surrounding tissues. Techniques to establish the reproducibility and accuracy of 3D printed models, thereby establishing their safety are actively being developed, as are quality assurance procedures to ensure the delivery of safe, consistent clinical services.[15,16] These techniques should be considered an integral and necessary component of a clinical 3D printing service.

The first medical applications of 3D printing were reported 25 years ago, as early as 1994.[17] However, despite the near-exponential growth of medical 3D printing in the last few years[15,18] and as the following sections will elucidate, it is important to recognize that most technology development in 3D printing to date has been geared to industrial applications, both in hardware as well as software. Thus, unfortunately, at present the clinical scientist or clinician needs to become familiar with various engineering concepts to be able to effectively utilize the technology in a clinical setting. It is nonetheless noteworthy that the well-informed clinician can impact change in their practice and better care for their patient[19,20] by mastering the concepts described in this chapter. Later, we build these concepts from the bottom up, describing the individual techniques first, and, building on this technical basis, bringing together a high-level view.

ADDITIVE MANUFACTURING TECHNOLOGIES FOR PRODUCING 3D-PRINTED MODELS

3D printers manufacture physical objects from their digital representations. These digital representations are typically stored in computer-aided design (CAD) files such as for example the Standard Tessellation Language (STL, also called a STereoLithography) file or an Additive Manufacturing file Format (AMF). Generating these files from patient imaging will be reviewed in the next section of this chapter. Given such a file, the initial step for a 3D printer to manufacture the object encoded in its digital representation is to "slice" the digital object in a user-selected or automatically selected orientation at a user-specified slice thickness (e.g., 0.1 mm). The slicing direction is the z, or equivalently layer axis of the printer.

Model Slicing

Selecting the slicing, or equivalently model orientation for 3D printing is, unfortunately, of paramount importance for a number of reasons. First, in all printing modalities it greatly affects printing time, typically rendering it advantageous to orient the object to yield the minimum number of slices, that is, orienting the object so that slices will span the shortest axis of the object (Fig. 2.1). Second, for printing modalities that do not completely surround the model being printed by support material, and that instead require that support scaffolds are printed along with the model (vat photopolymerization and often material extrusion, further described later), orientation selection may greatly affect the likelihood of successfully or accurately printing the model. This is because overhangs of models cannot be printed atop empty space. For example, the aortic arch cannot be printed if the supraaortic arteries are included in the model and a craniocaudal orientation is selected for the print—the entirety of the aortic arch is an overhanging feature throughout its surface area, other than in the two locations where the supraaortic vessels meet the aortic arch. Simply, once the printer has finished printing the supraaortic vessels and reaches the level of the aortic arch, there will not be any material on top of which to print the first layer of the arch, except in those locations where the supraaortic vessels arise from. Support material is thus required to be printed to support the model being printed in this scenario. The support material will be printed in the form of scaffolds from the first layer on top of the printer bed, all the way up to the level of the slices that intersect the entire surface of the aortic arch's most cranial aspect. For 3D printing modalities that require such scaffolding support structures to be printed, printer software typically automatically generates the scaffold for any given model orientation (Fig. 2.2). Nonetheless, judicious choice of orientation can reduce the probability that a given print will lead to overhangs that, for example,

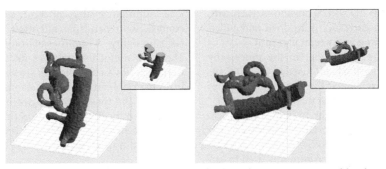

FIG. 2.1 Impact of slicing orientation on scan time of a hepatic artery aneurysm blood pool model. In orientation on left-hand panel, print time would be 4 h and 10 min; inset shows slice 708 of 1045 when 0.1-mm-thick layers are selected for the print. In orientation on right-hand panel, print time would be 3 h and 20 min; inset shows slice 655 of 826 for the same layer thickness.

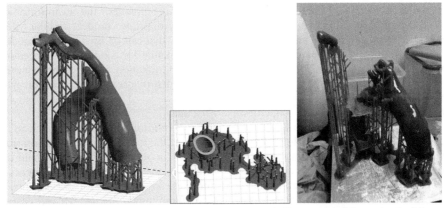

FIG. 2.2 Inappropriate support structure selection in printing a hollow model of the aorta. Avoiding printing supports in the internal (lumen) aspect of the model does not sufficiently support the material to be printed (arrow), leading to failure of the print.

geometrically deform during printing, or that entirely fail to print (Fig. 2.2).

Finally, slice orientation also affects the mechanical properties of the printed model, as the adhesion of material in one layer to the immediately prior layer printed is typically not as strong as it is for material within the layer. Different 3D printing modalities thus yield varying levels of anisotropic mechanical properties that primarily differ in the slice direction.[21,22] Depending on the functional requirements for the intended use of a given model, mechanical anisotropy can impact utility. For example, with most 3D printing modalities a hollow vessel model printed with a flexible material to allow simulation of the vessel wall compliance in the presence of pulsatile flow will likely benefit from selecting the layer direction along the length of the vessel rather than along the long axis of the vessel. This orientation will help achieve improved circumferential elastic modulus and tear strength.

Printing Technologies

The 3D printer creates a solid object from the slices of the digital model. In each of the slices, the object occupies some area in the form of a set of two-dimensional (2D) regions and does not occupy any other areas within the slice outside those regions. The printer then simply deposits, solidifies, or binds its raw material in the pattern of the 2D regions occupied by the object, at the preselected thickness of the slice, thereby printing one "layer" of the object. Each 3D printing process is designed so that solidification of one such layer will also bind or fuse it to the immediately previous layer, which will allow the printed layers of the object to remain in one piece after printing. This is equivalent to 3D imaging performed by multiple sequential, contiguous 2D slice acquisitions, each with a fixed slice thickness; each slice is acquired and added to the volume becoming an integral part of it.

3D printing technologies differ in the process by which each layer is solidified and fused to the previous layer. Recent efforts to standardize the terminology of the numerous processes by which this can be achieved[23] have unfortunately not yet caught on in the biomedical literature, leading to a lack of portable descriptions that are easy for the reader to interpret.[18] Here, we describe the processes from most to least commonly used in cardiovascular 3D printing, primarily adhering to the nomenclature set forth in the American Society for Testing and Machines (ASTM) standard F2792.[23] In this standard, there are seven major groups of 3D printing technologies, viz. vat photopolymerization, material jetting, material extrusion, binder jetting, powder bed fusion, sheet lamination, and direct energy deposition. The latter two of these modalities are not often used in the medical setting, and the interested reader is referred to other sources.[1]

If we were to list those features likely to be considered most important for 3D printing of cardiovascular models, we would likely choose material properties, so that we can simulate soft tissues as well as rigid components such as certain lesions; multiple colors so that we may convey the separation of tissues or vascular and cardiac territories, or to highlight anatomic abnormalities and pathologies; water tightness and overall model surface smoothness so that we might be able to simulate blood flow and endovascular procedures using standard instrumentation; and finally the ability to produce models that would resemble the patient anatomy in terms of their functional or imaging characteristics, so that for example the model can be used in lieu of the patient in the catheterization laboratory or in an ultrasound-guided procedure to simulate and test an intervention.

Unfortunately, none of the 3D printing modalities available today is capable of providing all these features. However, different modalities provide one or more of these features, rendering it important to determine the needs of a particular 3D printing service before committing to purchasing a 3D printer. Often, in a clinical 3D printing service, it is beneficial to own a printer that can produce most models encountered in the particular practice within the desired budget, and to use outside commercial printing services for those models that the particular printer cannot produce. We thus summarize the different technologies in this context, with particular attention to the strengths of each modality. A summary is provided in Table 2.1. The most useful technologies for anatomic and functional cardiovascular models are vat photopolymerization, material jetting, and material extrusion, and we thus describe these technologies in detail. Less detail is provided for those modalities that are presently less applicable in the cardiovascular arena, namely binder jetting and powder bed fusion.

Vat Photopolymerization

The original stereolithography, or, using standard nomenclature, vat photopolymerization process represents one of the more robust technologies for cardiovascular models. This is due a combination of its excellent resolution properties, the near-isotropic mechanical properties of printed models, and the types of materials available, that can be used to print models mimicking the vasculature for endovascular procedure simulation. The main limitation of the technology is its inability to print models that contain multiple colors and materials.

Process

The vat photopolymerization process involves the curing of the top (or bottom, for bottom-up printers) surface of a photosensitive liquid held in a vat, using a light source at a particular frequency. Typical frequencies are ultraviolet (UV) in the 355–405 nm wavelength range. The incident light causes the liquid to solidify by inducing polymerization and cross-linking of the monomers and oligomers it is composed of. The liquid is typically an epoxy- or acrylic-based photocurable resin, and the light source is either a laser or a digital light processing (DLP) microelectromechanical display device such as those found on digital projectors. The light source is in any case controlled so as to cure a layer of the liquid in the shape of the regions that the object occupies in the slice currently being printed. In the case of a laser-based system, the laser is traced in a raster fashion to cover the entire area of the regions occupied by the object in that slice using a galvanoscanner mirror system. In a DLP system, an image in the shape of all the regions in the slice is instead projected instantaneously. Once the object layer is cured sufficiently to be structurally stable, but not fully so, so that the layer may remain in a semi-reacted state for the following layer to also be able to bond to it, the model is either raised from (for

TABLE 2.1
Relevant 3D Printing Modalities for Cardiovascular Models and Their Relative Strengths and Weaknesses.

Technology	Model (Material Cost for Typical Model)	Model-Specific Pros	Model-Specific Cons
Vat Photo-polymerization Printer cost: $$-$$$$ *Pros:* Easy to site and operate; sufficient for ~50–70% of CV models; high resolution. *Cons:* Limited to single-material models; "off-label" to achieve tissue properties.	Vascular ($)	- Smooth, accurate, watertight models without much postprocessing required. - Ideal for endovascular models (no supports required in lumen) as well as blood pool models.	- Fixed material mechanical properties, with some "off-label" control possible via mixing materials or inserting additives. - Single-material models (cannot, e.g., print rigid calcifications in flexible vessel wall model)
	Cardiac ($$)	- Suited for smoother models (e.g., soothed cardiac muscle) without many small protrusions.	- Single color models. - Increasing detail (e.g., chordae tendinae, valves) difficult to print due to support strut needs and postprocessing to remove them (access for strut removal may require cutting model open). - Lower material strength.
	Devices ($$)	- Only short-term biocompatible material available, suited for surgical tools and guides	
Material jetting Printer cost: $$$$-$$$$$ *Pros:* Can print ~95% of CV models; built-in ability to print realistic tissue mechanical properties; high resolution. *Cons:* Cost; extensive siting requirements; effort to operate and maintain.	Vascular ($$$$)	- Simple to print multimaterial multicolor models, e.g., flexible clear vessel wall with rigid white calcifications, or different colors for arterial versus venous sides. - Complex metamaterial designs (see text) allow closely matching anisotropic tissue mechanical properties. - Complex model designs allow distinct CT/MR imaging characteristics for different anatomic entities (e.g., tumor vs. tissue). - Low print failure rate regardless of model complexity.	- High print failure rate in postprocessing due to wax-like support material that is difficult to remove from lumen of hollow tissues. - Time consuming to remove support material without damaging model. - Available through expensive, specialized commercial printing services.
	Cardiac ($$$$$)	- *Same as vascular.* - Control of material mechanical properties renders it ideal for quick creation of surgical simulation models that roughly feel like tissue.	- *Same as vascular.*
	Devices ($$$$)	- Only short term biocompatible material available, suited for surgical tools and guides	- Lower material strength.
Binder jetting Printer cost: $$$ *Pros:* Easy to print and interpret anatomic models. Only printer with ("off-label") ability to print realistic X-ray attenuation properties.	Vascular ($$)	- Multicolor, ideal for anatomic component separation. - "Off-label" binder modifications can print models that match tissue X-ray attenuation coefficients. - Low print failure rate regardless of model complexity.	- Only rigid or practically rigid models possible. - Extremely fragile models; small vessels/features (<3–4 mm diameter/thickness) are unlikely to survive postprocessing.

Continued

TABLE 2.1
Relevant 3D Printing Modalities for Cardiovascular Models and Their Relative Strengths and Weaknesses.—cont'd

Technology	Model (Material Cost for Typical Model)	Model-Specific Pros	Model-Specific Cons
Cons: Siting; effort to operate; ineffective cost-to-utility ratio if dedicated to CV models (can print ~25–40% of required models)	Cardiac ($$$)	- Readily available through commercial printing services. - *Same as vascular.*	- Only useful for depicting anatomy (rigid material only).
Fused deposition modeling Printer cost: $–$$$ *Pros:* Cheap; easy to site and operate. *Cons:* Limited utility for CV models (~10–20%); highly prone to model print failure for nonprofessional (<$$$ cost) systems.	Vascular ($)/ Cardiac ($–$$)	- Low cost. - Easy to produce models with dual-extrusion printers that offer on-label soluble support material. - Ideal cost for blood pool models to display anatomy. - Readily available at low cost through commercial printing services.	- Single-color, single-material models. - Available materials resemble tissue mechanical properties less effectively than vat photopolymerization or material jetting. - Anisotropic mechanical properties more strongly dependent on print orientation than vat photopolymerization or material jetting. - Models have striated surfaces that are limit opportunity for endovascular simulation. - Endovascular models need postprocessing/infiltration with sealants for smoothness and water tightness. - Anisotropic mechanical characteristics of printed models.
	Devices and implants ($$$)	- Short- and long-term biocompatible materials. - Strong materials. - Materials can be impregnated with bioactive substances.	
Powder bed fusion Printer cost: $$$–$$$$$$ *Pros:* Synthetic polymer and metal printing for implants and devices. *Cons:* Cost; limited opportunity for anatomic models.	Devices and implants ($$$$)	- Short- and long-term biocompatible materials. - Strong materials. - Isotropic mechanical characteristics. - New technologies (multi jet fusion) can produce colored anatomic models similar to binder jetting but made of biocompatible nylon. - New technologies (multi jet fusion) can print embedded electronics for smart medical devices.	- Cost. - Printed material is porous complicating biocompatibility and sterilization.

Printer costs - $: <1000; $$: 5–10,000; $$$: 25–75,000; $$$$: 150–250,000; $$$$$: 250–750,000; $$$$$$: >750,000.
Material costs per medium-size model (e.g., abdominal aorta or pediatric myocardium) - $: <20; $$: 20–75; $$$: 75–150; $$$$: 150–500; $$$$$: 500–1000. Note: "off-label" and "on-label" refer to printer manufacturer procedures and commercially available materials, and are not related to Food and Drug Administration regulations or regulated uses.

bottom-up) or lowered into the vat holding the resin by one layer thickness, and the process repeats to cure the next layer of the object.

Equipment

Desktop systems exist that are efficient and easy to site and operate at a low, reasonable cost ($\sim$\$5000–10,000 USD and \$200/kg of material). A model of, for example, the coronary arteries can often be printed with \$10-\$50 worth of materials. An example of this technology is the Form 2 (Formlabs, Cambridge, MA). These systems have a smaller build platform (12–17 cm per axis), which complicates the printing of larger models such as an entire cardiac model or an entire aorta. With judicious selection of the anatomy necessary for a clinical model, they can however fulfill requests for a large percentage of models in a clinical practice. Industrial systems with large build volumes (up to $2\,m^3$) exist but even those with moderate-sized build platforms (e.g., $\sim$20 cm per axis) are very costly to procure (>\$400,000 USD). An example of such a system is the iPro 800 (3D Systems, Rock Hill, SC). These systems are also expensive to operate, as they are typically top-down printers, wherein the top surface of the resin is cured and the printed model recedes into the vat. Thus, the large vat holding the photopolymer must be completely filled and maintained at a constant level, rendering swapping materials between models difficult.

It is important to note that vat photopolymerization printers can only print models from a single material, as only one resin can be held in the machine's vat. Thus, it is not possible to readily for example highlight specific anatomy or pathology using color, unless the model is hand-painted after printing, or if it can be separated into different objects that can be assembled after printing (Fig. 2.3). For some industrial systems, transparent resins exist that allow highlighting anatomy by tinting the model in selected locations (e.g., DSM Somos Material Group, Elgin, IL) by overexposing the resin during printing (Fig. 2.3). Notably, apart from the (however limited) opportunity for different coloring of structures in vat photopolymerization-printed models, it is not at all possible to print models where for example soft tissues are printed in an elastic material while calcified lesions are printed in rigid material. A related technology, material jetting described later, allows multimaterial/multicolor printing while retaining the desirable material and resolution properties of vat photopolymerization.

Postprocessing

Vat photopolymerization printers are straightforward to use and to postprocess the printed models, although postprocessing is more involved compared to other modalities used for anatomic models. Postprocessing involves first a solvent or alcohol rinse (10–20 min) to remove any viscous resin remaining on the model, followed by manually breaking off and removing the support struts that are printed to support overhangs. Typically, support struts have the form of a scaffold (Fig. 2.2) and attach to the model in small point sizes of 0.6–1 mm that are easy to remove. Support is only needed at a few contact points as the object's extent in a layer can grow by a small amount (e.g., <45–65° or <0.2 mm) in the $x-y$ plane compared to the prior layer as the polymerization process creates sufficient cohesive forces to hold small cross-sectional size

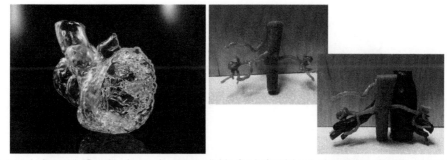

FIG. 2.3 Left panel: Certain photopolymers available for industrial vat photopolymerization printers allow highlighting anatomy in a printed model by overexposing the resin in desired locations thereby creating a tint, such as in this heart where the chordae tendinae are highlighted. Right-hand-side panel: Alternatively, for some models, multiple anatomical structures can be printed separately, such as the arteries and veins in this bilateral renal aneurysm model, and later assembled if the individual objects are designed with appropriate matching indentations and extrusions to allow spatially correct assembly. (*Left panel* Image courtesy of Materialise NV, Belgium.)

extensions in place. Light sanding, though not necessary, can be used to remove the small imperfections on the model surface at those contact points. Most materials require a final curing step (<30 min to 1 h) in an ultraviolet bath to reach their specified mechanical properties. Some materials, for example, those intended to be heat resistant or have high impact strength may also similarly require a heat treatment.

Materials

Various photopolymers are available in a range of colors and opacities, including translucent material. Similarly, different material mechanical properties are available for different resins, such as flexible or rigid (Fig. 2.4). Vat photopolymerization leads to largely isotropic characteristics in the printed material, but most materials are somewhat brittle, so some care is required in handling and using them. Elastomeric, flexible materials are readily available (Young's modulus 0.5−8 MPa) but they can only roughly replicate the clinically relevant parameters of vascular tissue such as distensibility and compliance.[24] Moreover, controlling these properties in printed models is most readily presently achieved by changing the thickness of the printed model,[10] and this approach has been preferred due to its simplicity even with multimaterial material jetting systems[25] in lieu of more involved approaches based on material mixing[26] further described with the next technology.

With current materials, it is possible to simulate the compliance of vessel wall tissue by printing a fictional vessel wall designed with a thickness of the order of

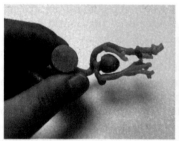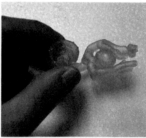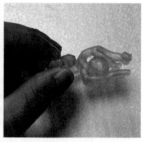

FIG. 2.4 Renal artery aneurysm models printed with different materials using stereolithography. Left panel: blood pool printed with a hard gray material. Middle- and Right-hand panels: fictional 1.5-mm-thick wall created around the blood pool is printed with a flexible clear material producing a hollow model for endovascular simulation. Right-hand panel: model is readily elastically deformed by squishing.

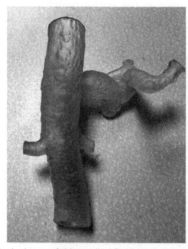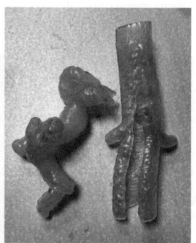

FIG. 2.5 Typical tear of thin-walled flexible photopolymer endovascular model of a hepatic artery aneurysm after light handling. Tear resistance and tensile strength are often significantly reduced due to small imperfections in the printing process, as well as due to the small thickness (~1 mm) of vascular models that is necessary to achieve physiologic tissue mechanical properties such as distensibility using current materials.

0.5−1 mm, which will yield similar properties as, for example, aortic wall tissue using currently available materials.[10,24,25,27] However, such thin-walled models are often particularly prone to tear (Fig. 2.5), and thus for many materials (primarily those available for the related material jetting printers described in the next section) the resulting models often cannot handle physiologic arterial pressures without failing (e.g., >30 mmHg). This renders the printing and use of models that closely mimic tissue properties for endovascular procedure simulation a difficult task with a low success yield. Nonetheless, vat photopolymerization is at present the best-fit modality to produce endovascular models in providing realistic guidewire and catheter manipulation capabilities.[28]

Conversely, printing the whole thickness of the, for example, myocardium or a valve leaflet is unlikely to yield properties similar to tissue, and will instead yield a comparatively stiff model, as the elastic modulus of currently available materials is typically an order of magnitude higher than that of soft tissues. Opportunities to simulate soft tissue mechanical properties are being developed primarily using the related material jetting technology, described in the next section. Despite the present limitations in available photopolymer materials, a number of studies have found that with commercially available photopolymers for both vat photopolymerization and material jetting printers, it is possible to readily fabricate models that have acceptable (if not realistic) tactile feel for surgical simulation.[29−31] One "off-label" strength of vat photopolymerization is the ability to mix small amounts of additives (<1%−5%) into the resin placed in the vat, such as for example gypsum powder, various (e.g., Kevlar and glass) fibers, or even carbon nanotubes and cellulose nanocrystals[32,33] to modify the mechanical and/or imaging (further discussed in material jetting section) properties of the printed model.

Acrylates that are the most commonly encountered materials for vat photopolymerization and material jetting systems are cytotoxic. These materials are sufficient for most anatomic surgical planning models, and if desired can often be sterilized using standard procedures, although it is important to note that models may deform and their mechanical properties altered during sterilization depending on the procedure used.[34] Less reactive methacrylates and other photoreactive monomers that have minimal in vivo biological reactivity exist, and many have undergone testing for US Pharmacopeia Convention (USP) Class VI or International Standards Organization (ISO) 10993,[35] and are commercially available as short-term biocompatible materials (e.g., Formlabs Dental SG, DSM Somos WaterShed XC 11122, and, for material jetting, Stratasys MED610). These can be used for the production of surgical guides and tools, or anatomic models that are brought into the operative field for intraoperative navigation when manufacturer's specifications for proper material postprocessing, cleaning, and sterilization are followed.

Print time and resolution

Printing time for vat photopolymerization is relatively average compared to other printing modalities, for example requiring ∼3−4 h to print a coronary artery tree. Print time is primarily driven by the time required to prepare the next layer, which involves the mechanical movement of the object along the slice dimension and allowing sufficient time for the viscous resin to flow in the void created in the vat surface so that the next layer can be printed. For this reason, although high resolutions of 50 μm are readily available in the layer dimension, one typically uses lower resolutions of, for example, 100 μm. Lower layer resolutions of, for example, 200 μm are not typically available with most resins, as light needs to penetrate the resin to the given depth to cure the layer, and opportunities to increase light intensity and illumination time to achieve larger curing depths are limited.

A recently developed advance in vat photopolymerization technology, termed continuous liquid interface production (CLIP)[36] can continuously grow the printed object by using an oxygen layer above a membrane that sits at the bottom of the vat holding the resin and that inhibits polymerization at the interface of the membrane and the printed object. This technique offers printing one order of magnitude faster than other 3D printing technologies.[2] Nonetheless, it is currently only available at a very high equipment cost (Carbon 3D Inc) that is unlikely to be viable in a clinical environment and is limited to a small rectangular build volume cross-sectional area (e.g., 8 × 14 cm) that does not lend itself to most cardiovascular models. However, commercial printing services offer this technology, which can be desirable particularly for endovascular simulation models because the model layers are printed continuously rather than iteratively (i.e., slice by slice), thereby reducing the small striations that otherwise occur due to the iterative layering process in vat photopolymerization (Fig. 2.6).

Vat photopolymerization also has a high in-plane resolution compared to other 3D printing modalities. In laser-based systems, $x-y$ resolution is determined by the laser beam spot size (diameter), which is roughly

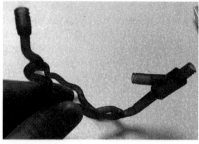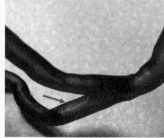

FIG. 2.6 Vat photopolymer printers yield extremely smooth models such as this coronary flow model. However, striations because of the 100-μm-thick layers that are iteratively printed are sometimes visible, even though can be barely perceptible by touch. Continuous liquid interface production (CLIP) technology can further improve high model smoothness of vat photopolymerization 3D printing.

75−150 μm at full width half maximum for commercial systems. In DLP systems, resolution is measured in dots-per-inch (dpi) based on the individually controlled dots of the light projection device, and current systems have dpi's that yield typical in-plane resolutions of 50−75 μm. It is also important to note that printer resolution (across all printing modalities) does not accurately describe the minimum size of features that can be successfully printed, as features need to be structurally stable. This is typically larger than printer resolution, of the order of 150−300 μm in vat photopolymerization systems.

Material Jetting

This process, which shares the chemical process of vat photopolymerization, is the most versatile for printing cardiovascular anatomic and simulation models. It extends 3D printing of photopolymers with multimaterial and multicolor abilities that can be used to produce models that not only readily convey anatomy and pathology, but, with new advances, also biomechanical and functional properties of the anatomy.

Process

The material jetting process is similar to vat photopolymerization in that it employs the same process of photopolymerization. The difference is that the photopolymer resin is jetted onto the build tray only in those locations occupied by the object at a given layer, much like an inkjet printer jets ink onto paper only in those paper locations occupied by text and images. The print heads scan across the build tray, jetting microdroplets of resin at the regions occupied by the object in the layer being printed, and are followed by a UV lamp that illuminates the jetted droplets to induce the photopolymerization reaction. Once a layer has thus been printed,

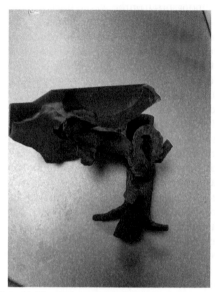

FIG. 2.7 Multimaterial model of hepatic artery aneurysm printed with material jetting printer.

the build tray recedes by one layer thickness, and the next layer is printed.

In contrast to vat photopolymerization, where support material takes the form of a scaffold (Fig. 2.2), material jetting needs to fully enclose the printed object in support material, as droplets must first rest on a surface before the material is polymerized. Thus, all material jetting printers have dedicated print heads that jet only support material, which is a gel- or wax-like material.

Equipment

Material jetting printers are among the most expensive. Single-material systems that do not offer the versatility of the technology (e.g., Objet30, Stratasys, Eden Prairie, MN) and that have a smaller build volume (14 × 19 × 29 cm) are available for reasonable cost (<$70,000); however, the strength of material jetting printing lies in multimaterial systems, which allow different jetting heads to concurrently jet different materials. Those systems are significantly more costly (>$250,000). Multimaterial examples of this technology are the Projet 5500X (3D Systems, Rock Hill, SC) and the Objet 500 Connex 3 (Stratasys, Eden Prairie, MN), while a flagship example of this technology capable of printing the full range of colors and multimaterials at each individual voxel is the Stratasys J750 (Stratasys, Eden Prairie, MN).

Materials for this technology are among the most costly amongst 3D printing technologies (>$300/kg). A typical model of a cerebral aneurysm or aortic root and valve will readily cost of the order of $100−200 in materials, in part due to the large amount of support material that must be expended in the printing process, while a larger model such as a whole heart will exceed $1000. In multimaterial printers, a single model can be printed with different portions of the model using any one of the materials loaded in the independent sets of jetting heads. For example, models can be readily printed showing different vascular territories in different colors, or with transparent organs showing internal elements such as nerves and vessels in different opaque colors (Fig. 2.7). High-end printers allow mixing of the materials loaded across the sets of jetting heads during printing, enabling tens to thousands of "digital" material combinations (e.g., colors, or mechanical properties) in a single model. The digital materials are created on the fly by controlling the multiplexing of the droplets jetted from each head when printing each "pixel" of the layer being printed. Specifically, the multiple materials are jetted in a matrix fashion to form each quantized "pixel" of the layer of the model being printed. Current development of this technology by the manufacturers has given rise to unique medical model printing techniques, for example that directly translate clinical imaging data such as CT Hounsfield units (HU) into colors and transparencies.[37] This and other more clinically relevant applications enabled by multimaterial printing are discussed in the materials section later.

Finally, although material jetting systems are easy to use and models can be used without much effort for model postprocessing, they do require significant effort to maintain, for example requiring daily print head cleaning.

Postprocessing

Material jetting model postprocessing primarily involves support material removal. The composition of the support dictates the removal process, which is typically either manual plus using a pressurized water spray in a special work station or soaking in a caustic solvent bath in an agitation station. Different from vat photopolymerization, there is no left over resin to rinse, and also, a UV postcuring step is not required, although a heat treatment is again required for heat-resistant materials.

Unfortunately, although material jetting enjoys the highest resolution among 3D printing modalities (see below), models have a matte surface finish on the sides of the models printed resting onto support material (Fig. 2.8). For most anatomic and many surgical simulation models, this does not pose a limitation. It is however undesirable in transparent models that require either sanding or application of a clear coat of resin to enhance transparency, as well as in models intended for use in endovascular procedures. A second limitation posed by material jetting postprocessing relevant to cardiovascular applications involves in general the printing of hollow vascular models. Different from vat photopolymerization, where supports can be avoided within the lumen of the printed model by judicious orienting of the model for printing (e.g., with its long axis along the z-axis of the printer), with material jetting the support material needs to fill every model cavity regardless of printing orientation. In many medical models, small cavities are extremely difficult to reach even with a pressurized water jet, and often support removal will be incomplete. More importantly, given the wax-like consistency of currently available support material with this technology, principally based on polyethylene glycol, it is extremely difficult to remove the support material from longer (>5−6 cm) vessels with relatively small calibers (<2−3 mm diameter) or tortuous vessels,[38,39] especially without damaging the model (Figs. 2.5 and 2.8).

Materials

The material properties available for material jetting fully share the previous discussion for vat photopolymerization, as both technologies use similar photopolymer chemistries. This includes rigid and flexible materials, multiple colors, and short-term biocompatible materials. Materials with low Young's modulus of the order of 0.5 MPa exist[40] that are ideal for models for cardiac surgery simulation.[41] However, the multimaterial capability of material jetting is the exceptional strength of this technology, which has led to immense

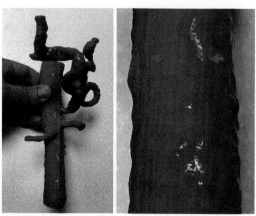 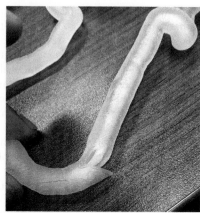

FIG. 2.8 Left panel: Model of hepatic artery aneurysm printed with material jetting after support removal exhibits uneven finish on the side of the model that had support material printed underneath it (middle panel, blue arrow), and shiny smooth finish on top side where no support was necessary (middle panel, red arrow). Right panel: model of vertebral arteries printed with a flexible semitranslucent material on a material jetting printer. The model tore during cleaning, exposing the lumen. Support material that is required in every cavity of a material jetting printer complicates printing hollow vascular models as the support, seen here as the white material in the phantom lumen, is difficult to remove.

strides in the last few years by deploying this capability for medical models. Despite these opportunities, described later, one limitation of material jetting printers compared to vat photopolymerization that counteracts some of the benefit of multimaterial printing is that materials for this type of printer are provided in sealed cartridges so that the resins cannot be doped or mixed with other substances to achieve mechanical or functional characteristics other than those intended by the manufacturer. Later, we review some of the advances based on multimaterial printing and their implications for the practicing clinician as well as some limitations.

Of particular interest in the cardiovascular 3D printing arena is the ability to generate models that mimic the mechanical, functional, and/or clinical imaging properties of vascular wall tissues. A single material for example cannot be used to reproduce the variability of elastic moduli encountered in a single tissue, which can vary by up to two orders of magnitude between for example the vessel wall and a calcified lesion. Similarly, a single material will have homogeneous signal intensity when imaged with a clinical imaging modality. Material jetting technologies address this problem via two approaches.

The first approach involves using different materials or different material mixtures to print each individual location of a 3D-printed model. The simplest example of this approach is instructing the printer to print a vessel wall with a flexible material, and the e.g., calcified

lesion or thrombus with a rigid material.[42] This approach requires that the vessel wall and lesion be individually segmented into separate objects to be printed that precisely touch at their surfaces, or with one object being partially or fully encompassed in a cavity of the other object. This is straightforward to accomplish with current medical imaging segmentation software and the approach has been successfully used to design, for example, models of the calcified aortic valve that replicate the hemodynamics of severe aortic valve stenosis,[43] or valve leaflets that when printed as an outer shell and a separate inner core using different photopolymers can achieve similar elastic modulus as porcine valve leaflets.[26]

The same approach has been used to print models that have different imaging characteristics for different anatomic structures, for example different HU or magnetic resonance imaging (MRI) signal intensities for different tissue components[11,13] that can be used to simulate image-guided therapies.[12,44] It is noted that at present photopolymer materials available yield only a small range of X-ray attenuation coefficients and MR relaxation properties that cannot replicate those of human tissues except in a relative manner.[12,13,45] Photopolymer HUs are in the 80−140 HU range,[11,13] and for at least one photopolymer known to produce an MR signal, T2 and T1 values of ∼30 and 200 ms have been reported.[11]

It is in this context that the lack of opportunity to impregnate the photopolymers with an additive, as is

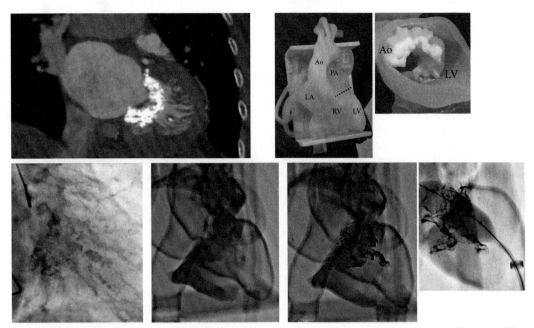

FIG. 2.9 Multimaterial model of calcified mitral valve printed with material jetting printer. Top row: CT angiogram used to produce the model (left-hand panel) and resulting 3D-printed model printed with a flexible yellow-tinted material (right-hand panel); inset shows detail of the valve printed inside the model, with the calcification printed in white rigid material. Bottom row: from left to right, fluoroscopy images acquired with C-arm during: patient catheterization procedure, 3D-printed multimaterial model, and 3D-printed model with calcification coated with tantalum powder after printing. Inset shows a 23 mm balloon-expandable SAPIEN XT valve being deployed in the mitral orifice. (Images courtesy of Ciprian Ionita, PhD, Jacobs School of Medicine & Biomedical Sciences, The State University of New York at Buffalo, adapted and reprinted with permission from Izzo R et al[46].)

possible with vat photopolymerization, is a disadvantage. Specifically for cardiovascular applications, replication of dense calcified plaque radio-attenuating properties is highly desirable for endovascular procedure simulation, as calcifications are often useful in spatial comprehension during a procedure. With current material-jetting (as well as for vat photopolymerization) models, large density variations cannot be achieved through the available materials, but can instead be achieved specifically for use with angiographic imaging by painting the e.g., calcifications with a metal, for example, tantalum powder,[46] as calcifications are typically accessible in the luminal side for painting while the projection nature of X-ray angiography does not necessitate the entire thickness of the tissue to have a higher density (Fig. 2.9).

More recent technology developed by material jetting printer manufacturers and briefly mentioned earlier enables direct translation of image signal intensities into materials to be printed via a lookup table (e.g., GrabCAD Voxel Print, Stratasys, Eden Prairie, MD). This can significantly improve the fidelity of multimaterial cardiovascular models, as, for example, it is no longer necessary to segment vessel wall and calcified lesion separately and to then assign a single material or single material mixture with which to print each tissue. One can instead segment the vessel wall plus lesion from a CT scan as a single object, and assign a continuum of materials with which to print each voxel of the model, that are in turn selected based on the HU of the corresponding voxel in the CT scan. In this manner, a mixed plaque could be printed for example so that voxels with low HU (such as the necrotic core) are printed in a very flexible, colored semitransparent material; voxels with high HU (e.g., microcalcifications) are printed in a rigid white material; and voxels with intermediate HU (e.g., wall tissue) are printed in a transparent flexible material, while each voxel with an HU between those three selections can be printed in a mixture of these base materials.

We posit that a significantly more powerful application of this new technology will be the ability to use it to translate functional or imaging properties into the materials that will be used to print each voxel of the model, so that each voxel of the printed model possesses (at least relatively) the functional or imaging properties of the tissue. For example, a model can be printed so that each voxel is printed in a material that reflects the acoustic impedance or the X-ray attenuation coefficient of the tissue in that particular voxel. Such a model can then be used for ultrasound-guided or angiographic procedure simulation. The tissue properties to translate into the printed model can be obtained from example from standard reference physiologic values (e.g., elastic modulus of aortic wall tissue vs. thrombus), or from patient-specific values, derived directly from example from imaging data such as e.g., MR elastography or distensibility measurements, obtained with an appropriate clinical imaging modality. Cardiovascular phantoms employing this 3D printing approach are already being developed and may soon become commercially available, for example for cerebral aneurysms and left atrial appendage closure simulations (Biomodex EVIAS and LAACS, respectively, Biomodex, Paris, France).

The second approach offered by multimaterial printing to enable 3D-printed models that replicate specifically tissue mechanical properties is to interweave strands printed with different materials or material mixtures in the shape of specially designed microarchitectures within the walls of the 3D-printed model. These strands can be used to control the mechanical properties of the printed model in a nonisotropic manner. For example, wavy strands of a semirigid material printed inside a vessel wall that is itself printed with a flexible material can, based on the pattern and shape of the strands, robustly replicate the nonlinear longitudinal and circumferential stress–strain relationships of vascular wall tissue.[47] Using this technique, mechanically realistic aortic root models can be produced from CT imaging acquired for transcatheter aortic valve replacement (TAVR) planning that can be used to predict post-TAVR aortic root strain and paravalvular leaks.[9]

It is reasonable to expect that as printer manufacturers become more interested in medical applications, new materials that can better-replicate tissue properties will be developed, and, in conjunction with the earlier techniques, one might expect that in the future it will be possible to print models of the cardiovascular system that can replicate both tissue anatomy and function for planning most surgical and endovascular procedures.

Print time and resolution

Material jetting is one of the slowest 3D printing modalities. A model of the aortic root apparatus might require of the order of 5−6 h to print, while a whole heart model can require 20 h or more to print in single-material mode. In multimaterial mode, where the available jetting heads must be apportioned to the multiple materials, those times are often doubled. This is also one of the highest-resolution 3D printing modalities, with typical z-axis layer resolutions of up to 1600 dpi (16 μm) and in-plane resolution of 600 dpi (40 μm). However, as mentioned earlier, sides of the model printed resting against support material have a rough surface that impacts resolution. Minimum feature sizes that can be successfully printed are roughly 100−300 μm, i.e., similar to, or potentially smaller than possible with vat photopolymerization. However, this limitation is due to very different factors, specifically, tolerances on the dimensions of the jetted droplets and droplet spread characteristics, as well as material shrinkage properties during photopolymerization. Despite the small minimum feature size possible to reproduce with this technology, thin-walled features (<1−1.5 mm thick) are unlikely to survive model post-processing with the common pressurized water jet cleaning process. Finally, this modality has the least control available for selecting layer size, as there is a limit to the amount of material that can be jetted with each droplet. Typical systems offer only 16 or 28 μm layer thicknesses, which as already mentioned lead to some of the longest print times among 3D printing modalities.

Material Extrusion

Material extrusion printers, most commonly fused deposition modeling (FDM) systems, represent the most consumer friendly and least costly 3D printing modality and as such have been widely used in medical 3D printing research. Limitations of the technology for cardiovascular models are the limited resolution and rough, striated surface finish quality, porosity and therefore lack of water tightness,[48] and anisotropic mechanical properties[21,49] of the printed models. Nonetheless, they are ideal for a number of applications in cardiovascular modeling, partly due to their low cost, and partly due to the available materials that have desirable mechanical strength and biocompatibility properties.

Process

Material extrusion printers have one or more heated extrusion heads that melt and extrude thermoplastic filaments. The filaments are wound in spools that are

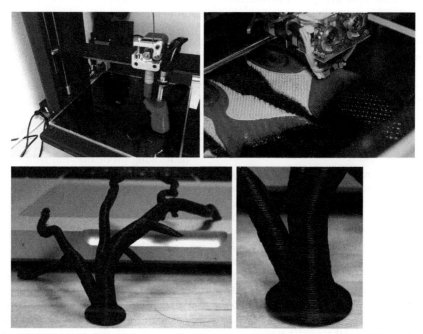

FIG. 2.10 Material extrusion printers (top row) and coronary model printed at high resolution using material extrusion (bottom row). Top right-hand panel shows a dual-extrusion system where one extrusion head is used to deposit clear support material. (Image courtesy of Materialise NV, Belgium.)

unreeled by motors thereby feeding the material to each extrusion head. Mechanical motion of the heads or printer build platform in the $x-y$ plane allows the extruded material to be selectively deposited in the shape of the layer of the object being printed (Fig. 2.10). The extruded material quickly hardens by cooling, typically aided by fans that follow the extrusion heads.

Most anatomic models are challenging to print with these printers, as printing the complex overhangs of human anatomic structures (e.g., visceral aortic branches) in thermoplastics will most likely deform as the extruded material cools if inappropriately supported. Most professional machines offer a second extrusion head that extrudes separate, for example, polyvinyl acetate or high-impact polystyrene support material that is typically soluble in a hot water or other mildly caustic solvent bath. However, soluble supports are often available for use with only a subset of model materials. Rarely, machines possess additional print heads that can be used to print a model that contains multiple colors and/or materials. However, many combinations of materials, both in terms of support plus model as well as multimaterial models are not possible as different thermoplastics have different thermal

expansion coefficients and will tend to naturally warp and separate during cooling. For this reason, most professional systems contain the build platform in a heated chamber. Because thermoplastics are susceptible to shrinkage and warping deformation during the cooling process, in machines without a heated chamber, or when models are inadequately supported by support material during the print can easily result in prints with bulk geometric inaccuracy of portions of the model.

Equipment

Material extrusion offers the most economical and easy to use 3D printing solution. Good "prosumer" systems are available for <$3500 (e.g., Ultimaker, The Netherlands), although professional systems ($\sim$$25-75,000) are preferred in a clinical setting (e.g., uPrint SE, Stratasys, Eden Prairie, MN). Materials are stronger than photopolymers, and cost less than $100/kg. Even entry-level printers have sufficiently large build platforms (>30 cm per axis) to accommodate most medical models, and professional systems offer some of the largest build volumes among 3D printing modalities, measuring in the meters. Appropriate medical applications of this technology are the printing of patient-specific guides and surgical tools due to material strength, durability, biocompatibility, and cost. Although FDM systems are the systems most commonly used and discussed in medical 3D printing applications, material extrusion encompasses the 3D deposition of many other classes of materials including silicones, hydrogels, and even biologically active materials and living cells used for bioprinting.[50] These processes, which we do not discuss here, achieve solidification via widely different physical and chemical processes.

Postprocessing

The effort required for material extrusion medical model postprocessing is primarily determined by the model intended use. Most models are ready to use after printing without requiring any treatment; the bulk of postprocessing effort involves supports removal. As mentioned earlier, this is either a solvent bath when soluble support material is available for a given printer and model material, or manual removal of support struts that resemble those described in vat photopolymerization. It is important to note that when nonsoluble supports are used, a larger contact area of each support strut to the printed model is required than with vat photopolymerization, which renders support removal difficult.

For intended model uses that require water tightness or smooth model surfaces, such as models for endovascular procedure simulation, an acidic bath treatment and/or impregnation with a sealant is necessary.[48] The popularity of material extrusion despite these disadvantages is largely due to the availability of strong, durable, and biocompatible materials.

Materials

The variety of thermoplastic materials available is an asset of the technology. Materials range from acrylonitrile butadiene styrene (ABS) and polylactic acid (PLA) to polyethylene terephthalate (PET, not to be confused with positron emission tomography) plastic, nylon, polyether ether ketone (PEEK), and elastic polyurethanes. Many materials such as PEEK, ABS, or PET (a polymer common in, for example, plastic beverage bottles) that are commercially available have been ISO 10993/USP Class VI certified biocompatible. These materials can be readily gamma or ethylene oxide sterilized.[51] Polyetherimide materials that can withstand steam autoclaving are also available (e.g., ULTEM 1010, Stratasys, Eden Prairie, MN) and may be suitable for long-term implantation. PLA and PET are also used in Food and Drug Administration (FDA)-approved devices for human implantation.

In terms of utility for specific applications relevant in cardiovascular printing, elastic polyurethanes can be used to print endovascular simulation models[52] as they have high tear resistances that can exceed those of silicone rubbers. However, the utility of the modality for these models is primarily limited by the resolution, porosity, and uneven surface finish of the resulting models (Fig. 2.10). Conversely, the strength of rigid ABS materials allows the modality to be used to print models for preshaping devices, such as microcatheters for internal carotid artery coiling procedures.[20]

In imaging properties, the radio-opacities of most thermoplastics are limited ($\sim$-60–200 HU) similar to photopolymers, although specialty filaments with much higher HU (>3000) are commercially available.[53] Furthermore, material extrusion allows lowering the HU of the printed material in the range of -600 HU via incomplete filling of the internal regions of the printed models (i.e., infill density <100%), a standard printing option in FDM systems that leaves air gaps in the internal spaces of the print in order to reduce material usage.[54] Conversely, thermoplastics can also be doped with other materials such as barium sulfate to precisely control the radio-opacities of the printed model through a large range of high HU.[55] However, this requires machinery that is not readily available to process raw thermoplastic material pellets into ready-to-use printer filaments. It is important to note that either commercial or appropriately doped materials can be used to produce a model with a single X-ray attenuation coefficient, or at most containing as many coefficients independent print heads as the printer possesses. Additionally using infill density to reduce attenuation will only be able to replicate a limited number of the continuum of X-ray attenuation coefficients encountered in an organ (limited by the intended imaging resolution), so that it is unlikely that material extrusion can be used to faithfully produce the CT imaging characteristics of human anatomy. Alternative technologies, such as binder jetting technology discussed in the next section, offer a direct approach to reproduce the minutiae of biologic tissue image characteristics.

A related, more exciting opportunity available with material extrusion involves impregnating a thermoplastic material with a bioactive substance such as antibiotics, chemotherapeutics, or antiproliferative drugs, which can then be used to print patient-specific catheters or stents.[56] If a bioresorbable material is used to print the device, it would elute new layers of the bioactive material as the device degrades, a potential advantage compared to current surface-coated devices.

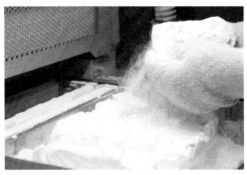
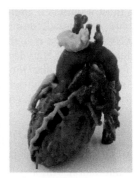

FIG. 2.11 Binder jetting model being removed from printer (left panel), and example pediatric heart model printed with binder jetting (right-hand panel). Gray support cylinders designed in the digital model in order to support the coronary arteries in the heart model are noted with red arrows. (Images courtesy of Materialise NV, Belgium.)

Print time and resolution

Print time for material extrusion tends to be average among 3D printing modalities. This is partly due to the larger typical layer thickness of prosumer FDM systems, approximately 0.2−0.5 mm. Professional printers with z-axis resolutions of 100 μm exist, but print time quickly becomes a limiting factor. The $x−y$ resolution of material extrusion printers is also much lower than other modalities, typically 0.2 mm. For most printers, it is possible to change this resolution by changing the tip of the material extruder, with extruders of 0.1−0.4 mm diameter usually available.

Binder Jetting

Binder jetting is a popular modality to reliably and cost-efficiently 3D print colorful models for visualization of anatomy that are particularly useful for surgical planning in cardiovascular applications. However, it presently only holds a niche in the field due to the limited uses of models printed with this technology, as the technology is limited to rigid models made of bonded powder materials that are neither biocompatible nor have any biomechanically realistic functional utility.

Process

Binder jetting is most similar to document inkjet printers, where a thin layer of fine powder such as gypsum acts as the paper, and a liquid binder is the jetted ink. The print heads jet binding agent only in those regions occupied by the object in the layer being printed. The build plate is then lowered by a layer thickness, a roller lays a new layer of powder, and the process is repeated to print the next layer. Just as in a color document inkjet printer, binder jetting can produce a large

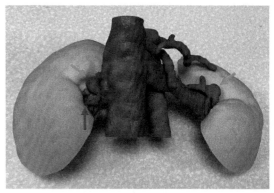

FIG. 2.12 Model of bilateral renal aneurysms (green arrows) printed with binder jetting. Due to the fragility of the bonded powder, small features can easily break from these models (red arrow), requiring much care in handling throughout the lifecycle of the model.

range of colors via mixing colored binders, or mixing colored ink onto the binder during the jetting process. An advantage of the process is that the unbonded powder continually supports the model being printed, so that intricate anatomic models can be reliably printed with little effort (Figs. 2.11 and 2.12). However, the models are extremely fragile before postprocessing so that small features such as vessels can be easily damaged (Fig. 2.12).

Equipment

Binder jetting is the most economical multicolor 3D printing modality, with professional equipment costs in the $20,000—100,000 range, and material costs of ~$150/kg. Build volumes even for entry-level systems are sufficient for most cardiovascular models (e.g., 12 × 18 × 23 cm). An example of this technology is the ProJet CJP 660Pro (3D Systems, Rock Hill, SC).

Postprocessing

Binder jetting model postprocessing involves first clearing unbonded powder from the model (Fig. 2.11), and then infiltration with a cyanoacrylate, wax, or resin to strengthen the printed model. As mentioned earlier, recovering the printed model from the powder volume requires care to ensure that it is not damaged. Support structures can be incorporated in a model so that small features such as vessels will not fracture and break during the powder removal process (Fig. 2.11).

Materials

Binder jetting models are composed of only the base powder, usually primarily consisting of gypsum, ceramic, or light organic compounds such as cornstarch and cellulose. It is not possible to print translucent or flexible models, and there are no readily available opportunities to print biocompatible models. One potentially relevant application enabled by binder jetting involves the printing of models that can fully replicate X-ray, CT, and nuclear imaging characteristics of tissues by modifying the binder with, for example, sodium iodide to achieve different X-ray attenuation coefficients that can faithfully reproduce tissue HU,[57] or radioactive tracers such as [^{18}F]FDG to reproduce activity concentration in positron emission tomography (PET).[58] With binder jetting systems that mix different-colored binders to achieve color, it is possible to translate the entire range of desired e.g., HU or activity concentrations encountered in the patient's images in a one to one fashion into printer colors and thereby reproduce the entire range of gradations of the imaging quantity (e.g., HU)[57] so that the printed model will fully replicate the patient's images when imaged with that imaging modality. This requires that one binder is doped with the additive that controls imaging characteristics in the desired imaging modality, and that a lookup table be calibrated that translates printing colors (as these are achieved by mixtures using different amounts of the doped binder) into the imaging quantity.[57]

Print time and resolution

Typical binder jet layer resolutions are 0.1—0.18 mm and printing speed that is relatively slow, at 20—40 mm per hour. In-plane (x–y) resolutions are of the order of 40—85 μm (300—600 dpi). One limitation of the modality is that the frailty of the printed material before infiltration limits the minimum feature size that can be printed compared to other 3D printing modalities, with typical minimum feature sizes of 0.5—0.8 mm.

Powder Bed Fusion

Powder bed fusion includes a number of 3D printing technologies that generally fuse material in powder form via the use of energy, typically delivered by a laser or other heat source. Commonly encountered technologies within this modality for medical applications are selective laser sintering (SLS) and direct metal laser sintering (DMLS), and the more recently developed technology, multi jet fusion (MJF), among others. To date, this technology is encountered in the clinical setting primarily in the context of the production of patient-specific surgical guides, devices, and implants, although MJF printing may lead to anatomic model applications in the future.

Process

In this process, a material in powder form is held in a build platform like in binder jetting. The powder is typically preheated to just below the material melting point. An energy source such as a laser or electron beam then traces the shape of the object in the slice being printed to selectively fuse or melt the powder. Similar to binder jetting, the build platform is lowered by one layer thickness and a roller lays a new layer of powder to prepare for printing the next layer. MJF relates to SLS similarly to how material jetting relates to vat photopolymerization. Specifically, instead of fusing the powder with a highly selectively targeted energy beam such as a laser, a liquid "fusing" agent that is able of facilitating the melting/sintering process (by capturing and distributing heat) is jetted onto the powder using inkjets. The fusing agent is jetted in the shape of the object at the layer being printed, and concurrently, a liquid "detailing" agent that is able of inhibiting the sintering process is jetted onto the powder around the contour of the regions occupied by the object. A nonselective heat source (e.g., infrared lamp) then provides the energy to sinter the powder permeated with the fusing agent.

Powder bed fusion machines produce some of the strongest models available by 3D print today. Most of the metals and synthetic polymers printed with this modality are biocompatible and can yield permanent or bioresorbable implants. Typically, models printed with SLS have a rough surface finish. However, the finely jetted detailing agent in MJF enables printing models with exceptionally smooth surfaces without postprocessing.

Equipment
With the exception of MJF that was designed to be more accessible ($50,000−200,000), industrial powder bed fusion machines are expensive, costing $250,000−800,000 for polymer SLS, and >$500,000 for metal DMLS. Most systems require extensive resources and know how to use and maintain. Lower-price point machines that are aiming to also be more user friendly are now appearing, in the price range of $100,000 for metal printing (e.g., Metal X, Markforged, Watertown, MA) and $10,000 for nylon SLS (e.g., Fuse 1, Formlabs, Somerville, MA). MJF instead provides industrial capacity but with reduced costs partly as expensive lasers are not required. An example of an MJF system is the multicolor Jet Fusion 380 (HP Inc, Palo Alto, CA), while examples of SLS systems are the P 396 (Electro Optical Systems [EOS] Gmbh, Munich, Germany) and sPro 230 (3D Systems, Rock Hill, SC), and an example of a metal DMLS system is the M 290 (EOS Gmbh, Munich, Germany). Materials are relatively costly (>$200−400/kg), and most powder bed fusion machines have large build platforms (≥20 cm in each axis) that suffice for most medical applications.

Postprocessing
Most materials do not require support structures in powder bed fusion, as the model is surrounded by unsintered powder throughout printing. This allows the modality to reliably print any structure even a thin lattice. Similar to binder jetting where some models may require embedded supports to avoid fracture (Fig. 2.11), printing in metals with powder bed fusion may require the design of embedded "supports" that will dissipate heat and reduce swelling of the object during printing. Although this modality enables printing various materials that can be used for surgical tools and guides or devices that can be implanted (see later), ensuring biocompatibility and adequate sterilization requires extensive postprocessing to remove unsintered powder remaining in small model cavities and porous surfaces.[59]

Materials
Many clinically relevant material groups that are biocompatible, sterilizable, and that can be safely implanted can be printed with SLS, including synthetic polymers such as polyamides (nylon), polyether ketone ketone (PEKK), and for DMLS, metals such as titanium and cobalt-chrome alloys. Recently, interest has concentrated on bioresorbable materials that offer exciting advances for patient-specific temporary devices[60] such as splints or stents. Whether it is possible to add bioactive substances to the raw printing material before sintering, as can be done for example in FDM,[56] has not been explored but it is unlikely due to the high temperatures involved in SLS compared to FDM.

Of note, at present, MJF is limited to nylon (Polyamide 12), although ceramics and other materials are expected to become available. MJF models, although having very low porosity compared to SLS, still require impregnation to be made watertight. However, a particularly exciting opportunity with MJF is that the liquid fusing agent can carry additional agents, for example an electrically conductive material. Such conductive traces can be used to print objects that have embedded, printed electronics within their internal structure or their surface. For example, an implantable device could be printed with embedded strain sensors to measure loads on the device in real time and communicate it to an external device.

Print time and resolution
Powder bed fusion systems are slow (typical 10−30 mm/h z-axis build speed) and layer thicknesses are typically 0.12 mm, although many systems offer selectable layer thicknesses of 0.06−0.18 mm. Laser spot sizes of 40−100 μm are commonly encountered in commercial systems. Features of size less than 300 μm can be printed with high resolution machines in part because SLS materials are stronger than for other printing modalities. Models printed with powder bed fusion tend to have a rough surface finish, and they typically possess isotropic mechanical qualities. MJF has very high in-plane resolution, with current systems offering a minimum layer thickness of 0.08 mm, and in-plane resolution of 1200 dpi (21 μm) at faster print times than typical SLS (40 mm/h). However, minimum recommended feature sizes are somewhat larger than SLS (0.5 mm). Finally, MJF model properties are highly isotropic.

Generating 3D-printable models from a patient's DICOM images

The previous section introduced the reader to the details of the various 3D printing modalities, listing their capabilities, limitations, as well as a number of current research directions that are significantly expanding their applicability in the medical field. Nonetheless, 3D printing is only one of the techniques that must be mastered to create a physical model of a patient's anatomy to enhance intervention planning, or a device to be used for treatment. 3D printers cannot interpret DICOM images. Instead, printers interpret digital 3D models. The process by which an operator creates the model to print from a patient's DICOM images is technically challenging and at present requires a number of distinct steps.

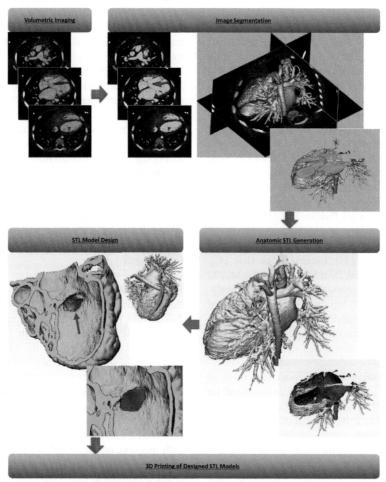

FIG. 2.13 Generating a clinically useful 3D printable model from patient imaging. First, an appropriate volumetric dataset (top left panel) is segmented to identify those voxels belonging to each tissue of interest, for example, the blood pool in a contrast enhanced CT of a double outlet right ventricle syndrome patient with a subpulmonic ventricular septal defect (VSD; top right-hand panel, red arrow). The segmented voxels are then converted into a surface model that can be manufactured by the 3D printer (e.g., STL model). Different from the segmented voxels, this model is simply an infinitesimally thin surface that encloses the space occupied by the segmented voxels (bottom right panel, inset shows the surface cut open, with red indicating the inner side of the surface). Finally, based on the STL models of the segmented anatomy, CAD software is used to design models that are more directly clinically useful, for example a hollow model of the intracardiac anatomy and a patch fitting the VSD (bottom left panel). These models are then 3D-printed for use, for example, for surgical planning.

A number of requirements are placed on the image acquisition to ensure that this multistep process has the highest chance of succeeding, for example ensuring images are volumetric without any gaps, acquired at sufficient resolution, and that steps are taken to minimize metal artifacts in CT or MR, or reconstructing CT images with an appropriate soft tissue algorithm rather than a sharp kernel.[1,5,16] Here, we assume that an appropriate 3D volumetric imaging dataset has been acquired, for example, with 3D US, MRI, CT, or rotational angiography that has been stored in DICOM format, and describe the techniques to produce a 3D-printable model from the DICOM images. This 3D model will need to be stored as an STL or an AMF file that the 3D printer can actualize. With the exception of current research and new software from printer manufacturers that aim to print objects from voxel descriptions as described earlier, to date STL or AMF models are limited to 3D surfaces that enclose a region of space. Those regions are where the printer will deposit material. With AMF files, the particular material can potentially also be specified in the file, whereas with STL files, material selection needs to be performed at printing time through the printer control software.

The process of designing clinical 3D-printed models

A number of steps are commonly followed for the production of a clinically useful 3D digital model from the patient images (Fig. 2.13). The first step is to acquire an appropriate volumetric dataset. This should be able of imaging the specific anatomy that is necessary for surgical planning with sufficient contrast to differentiate the anatomic structures of interest. The second step involves segmenting the relevant structures in the volumetric dataset, that is, demarcating their individual spatial extents in the images. The third step involves generating a surface model for each segmented structure. The fourth step is to use those models of the patient anatomy to design a clinically useful model of the anatomy, for example, a hollow model of the intracardiac volumes or of the vascular lumen, since, for example, only the blood pool will have been possible to segment from a set of clinical angiographic images. In this step, any devices that will be useful to the surgical team, for example, a correctly sized patch that will be suffice for the closure of a ventricular septal defect, can also be designed. These designed models can then be manufactured using an appropriate 3D printing modality as reviewed earlier.

Segmentation and STL Generation

Given an appropriate 3D volumetric imaging dataset, segmentation of each tissue demarcates all voxels in the dataset that belong to that tissue and excludes voxels occupied by adjacent tissues (Fig. 2.13). A number of techniques implemented in various software can achieve this step. A common initial technique is thresholding whereby for example all voxels with a value in the range of 250–700 HU in a contrast enhanced CT dataset are selected to segment the blood pool. More involved algorithms exist, for example dynamic region growing where the user selects a set of "seed" voxels in the images that lie within the tissue to be segmented. The algorithm then grows this seed to semiautomatically segment the entire extent of the target tissue. Manual editing of the segmentation is often necessary with most current software algorithms.

Depending on the planned use of the model, at present it may be necessary to separately segment each tissue relevant to the model. For example, to generate a model of a calcified aorta from a CT angiogram to be used to test a stent graft deployment, it will likely be necessary to print a hollow lumen model using a flexible material, and the calcifications in a rigid material. To design such a model, the blood pool and calcifications would first need to be separately segmented, so that two different models can be designed for the printer to print using the different materials.

Once the relevant anatomic structures have been segmented, the segmentation software must be able to produce an STL (or other file format) model representing that anatomy. STL models are surface models that enclose the segmented voxels in the images (Fig. 2.13). Software used to design 3D printable models (see next section) almost exclusively uses these surface models as inputs at present.

Although a number of software exist for segmentation of DICOM images, FDA-approved software that can output STL models should ideally be used in a clinical setting. Some of the FDA-approved software currently available for this purpose are Mimics (Materialise NV, Belgium), Vitrea (Vital Images, Minnetonka, MN), and TeraRecon (TeraRecon, Foster City, CA).

STL postprocessing for model and device design

Rarely, once STL models of the segmented anatomic structures have been produced, they can be directly 3D printed to confer a clinical benefit. Most often, the segmented anatomy must instead be used as a template from which to design a more clinically useful model that will be 3D printed (Fig. 2.13). This step uses so-called CAD software. The most common CAD operations that are usually beneficial to the referring clinician are for example trimming the segmented anatomy to reveal the underlying pathology, or creating shells around the segmented anatomy, such as for example creating a hollow vessel wall around the segmented blood pool. Augmenting the designed models with labels that can be traced to the patient and pathology, such as medical record number and laterality of the anatomy, are another common use of CAD software in the clinical setting. More complex operations that are often useful include adding geometric shapes such as cylinders to support overhanging anatomy (Fig. 2.11) or to join otherwise disjoint anatomic structures whose spatial relationship must be maintained after printing. An example is adding cylindrical connections between the arterial and venous models for example in a renal aneurysm model so that they can remain in one piece after printing.

Commercial CAD software offer a full-range of engineering capabilities that allow the user to design models that will for example conform to the contour of the anatomic STL models, for example to design a custom-fit implant that will match the patient. Many of these softwares offer significantly more advanced functionality, for example offering the ability to perform a finite element simulation of a designed device to assess its mechanical characteristics or the forces it will be subjected to when implanted. Although a number of such commercial software are available in the engineering space (e.g., SolidWorks, Dassault Systems, Waltham, MA), at present only a single such software is FDA-approved (3-matic, Materialise NV, Belgium) and although it is straightforward to use in a clinical setting, it still requires an engineering-oriented workflow. It is nonetheless expected that more clinically oriented CAD software with a workflow amenable to the busy clinical setting will become increasingly available in the future.

As is clear from the earlier description, the earlier steps involve both interpretation of the anatomy based on the image data, as well as the design of models (e.g., custom devices) that accurately represent or conform to that interpretation. The subjective nature of this process necessitates that a clinical 3D printing service have appropriate quality assurance systems in place to ensure that this is indeed the case. Such systems are in any case necessary to continually ensure the proper function of the software and hardware used to produce clinical 3D models.

Establishing the quality of medical 3D-printed models

In a clinical practice, imaging is ideally performed using equipment and procedures accredited by the American College of Radiology (ACR). This includes specific equipment quality control (QC) procedures, defined as "distinct technical procedures that ensure the production of a satisfactory product," that is, high-quality diagnostic images, as well as quality assurance (QA) procedures, such as assessment of the agreement between interpreters and comparison to surgical or pathological findings whenever possible.[61,62] Going forward, clinical applications of 3D printing, even if these are limited to anatomic models used to facilitate procedure planning should be considered to be of "diagnostic use" (i.e., affecting diagnosis, patient management, or patient treatment), and will likely be considered class II devices by the FDA.[63] Thus, appropriate QC and QA procedures should be incorporated in a clinical 3D printing service. The ACR model provides an established blueprint to this end, and 3D printing techniques are being developed that mirror the procedures in that model.

Equipment QC

As discussed in each printing modality, 3D printer resolution, that is, the smallest scale that a 3D printer can reproduce, exceeds that of most medical imaging modalities (typically ~0.5-1 mm). 3D printers also yield models with high reproducibility.[15] Thus, for a well-maintained 3D printer, technical QC procedures similar to the ACR model, based on 3D printing calibration phantoms have been described in the medical literature[5,16] and should suffice for in-hospital 3D printing services. Phantoms should be printed at regular intervals, possibly along with every model for high-risk scenarios such as when printing surgical guides. Physical measurements of the printed phantom can be compared with the design dimensions of the digital model or alternatively, phantoms containing features that can be fit-tested against a "negative" template can also be designed. The printed phantom's extruding features and depressions can be quickly fit-tested against a template that contains matching negative mirror features.[16] However, the template should not be 3D printed, as the fit test would for example pass if the 3D printer has a fixed geometric inaccuracy such as an incorrect size scaling.

It is noted that 3D printing dimensional accuracy may differ depending on print orientation even in a well-maintained printer, for example due to the thermal, chemical, or other process used to bond layers, or the amount of support struts designed to support overhangs. Thus, phantoms should (a) be printed with slicing along two orthogonal orientations, with both orientations required to pass the measurement or fit test, and (b) phantoms should be designed to be application- and printing modality-specific, for example with vessel-like overhangs to support the accuracy of vascular models, or with cylindrical holes to support the accuracy of drilling guides. Second, successful phantom testing with one material does not translate to another material. For example, flexible photopolymers exhibit different shrinkage characteristics during printing than rigid ones.[64] Thus, phantoms should be material-specific for each given clinical application for which quality control is being performed.[65]

Interpretive QA

Interpretive QA is significantly more difficult for cardiovascular 3D printing. Printed models of soft tissues cannot be readily compared against pathologic specimens or against intraoperative measurements, as tissue shape is not fixed.[15] Printed model measurements can nonetheless be compared against measurements performed on the source images from which the model was generated.[66–68] Measurements reported by the interpreting radiologist should ideally be confirmed in the printed model, particularly since the operator of the 3D printing software at present inevitably interprets the image data independently of the radiologist's interpretation. Image-based measurements are also most pertinent for cardiovascular applications, as they are used to guide treatment plans or select device sizes, while current results indicate that models can vary significantly from expert interpretation. For example, the diameter of the aortic annulus can differ by as much as 4 mm from the interpretation of the source CT angiography images,[66] while intracardiac defect models designed from 3D transthoracic echocardiography have been reported to differ by as much as 2–3 mm from source image measurements, with, for example, a 1.6 mm short axis diameter perivalvular leak depicted as 3.4-mm-wide in the printed model.[69] Anatomic details that are relevant to a procedure should be measured and compared to the reported findings as part of an in-hospital 3D printing service's QA program. Nonetheless, discrepancies between model measurements and expert interpretation can be considered in the context of the intra- and interobserver variability of image-based measurements for the given imaging study.[70]

An equivalent of secondary review of a study to assess the agreement of the original report and the subsequent review dictated in ACR QA procedures[61] is more difficult to translate to 3D printing. Mathematical techniques can be used that compare the "distance" between digital models. These techniques detect the minimum distance from an arbitrary point located on the surface of one model to the other models' surface. Current CAD software canautomatically compute these distances for a number of representative points (typically the nodes of the triangles composing the STL model), providing a distribution of differences that quantitatively conveys the spatial agreement between two models.[11,15,16] This can be used to compare a model derived from a second segmentation (secondary review) to the initial model derived from an imaging study. Different mathematical techniques, based on set theory and considering a 3D model as a subset of 3D space, can be used to define more familiar measures of agreement and disagreement between models, as well as true and false positive and false negative volumes and resultant measures such as sensitivity, specificity, and accuracy whenever a gold standard (e.g., pathology or reference model derived from the images by experts) is available.[15,71] An advantage of this approach is that disagreement between models can be more readily related to specific actions that can improve 3D-printed model quality, such as for example increasing signal-to-noise ratio of the imaging protocol, or altering CAD software procedures.[71]

SUMMARY

Cardiovascular 3D printing today accounts for the second largest application of the technology in the hospital setting. Anatomic models are being printed in daily practice to communicate with patients and assist the informed consent procedure, devise and assess surgical plans, and simulate procedures. In-hospital production of surgical guides, tools, and devices is also quickly emerging. The diversity of 3D printing modalities and the continual technological advances places us well on our way to produce anatomic models that will possess the mechanical and imaging characteristics of cardiovascular tissue, and devices that will enhance surgical accuracy or that will release bioactive substances as they are absorbed after implantation. The techniques that form the basis of these current and future applications were thoroughly described in this chapter.

To use a 3D printer for the production of patient models, the relevant anatomy in the patient images must first be extracted into a digital format that can be understood by the 3D printers. This is achieved by segmenting the anatomy from the images and converting each segmented anatomical structure into a digital model. Those models can then be used to design models of the patient anatomy that for example better expose pathology and thus more readily convey the clinical picture, or devices that can be used for treatment. This process unfortunately still remains highly technical in nature. However, current software and approaches reviewed here enable the advanced user to design clinical models that fully take advantage of current 3D printing technologies.

Finally, quality control procedures are necessary to ensure delivery of high-quality, safe 3D-printed clinical models for appropriate indications. Appropriate procedures based on the ACR model for imaging equipment, and current research to quality-check every aspect of the process were also reviewed and should provide an adequate basis for the clinician to implement safe 3D printing in their practice.

REFERENCES

1. Mitsouras D, Liacouras P, Imanzadeh A, et al. Medical 3D printing for the radiologist. *Radiographics.* 2015;35(7): 1965−1988.
2. Giannopoulos AA, Steigner ML, George E, et al. Cardiothoracic applications of 3-dimensional printing. *J Thorac Imaging.* 2016;31(5):253−272.
3. Chepelev L, Hodgdon T, Gupta A, et al. Medical 3D printing for vascular interventions and surgical oncology: a primer for the 2016 radiological society of North America (RSNA) hands-on course in 3D printing. *3D Print Med.* 2015;2(1):5.
4. Giannopoulos AA, Chepelev L, Sheikh A, et al. 3D printed ventricular septal defect patch: a primer for the 2015 Radiological Society of North America (RSNA) hands-on course in 3D printing. *3D Print Med.* 2015;1(1):3.
5. Matsumoto JS, Morris JM, Foley TA, et al. Three-dimensional physical modeling: applications and experience at mayo clinic. *Radiographics.* 2015;35(7):1989−2006.
6. George E, Barile M, Tang A, et al. Utility and reproducibility of 3-dimensional printed models in pre-operative planning of complex thoracic tumors. *J Surg Oncol.* 2017; 116(3):407−415.
7. Gillaspie EA, Matsumoto JS, Morris NE, et al. From 3-dimensional printing to 5-dimensional printing: enhancing thoracic surgical planning and resection of complex tumors. *Ann Thorac Surg.* 2016;101(5):1958−1962.
8. Gosnell J, Pietila T, Samuel BP, Kurup HK, Haw MP, Vettukattil JJ. Integration of computed tomography and three-dimensional echocardiography for hybrid three-dimensional printing in congenital heart disease. *J Digit Imaging.* 2016;29(6):665−669.
9. Qian Z, Wang K, Liu S, et al. Quantitative prediction of paravalvular leak in transcatheter aortic valve replacement based on tissue-mimicking 3D printing. *JACC Cardiovasc Imaging.* 2017;10(7):719−731.
10. Biglino G, Verschueren P, Zegels R, Taylor AM, Schievano S. Rapid prototyping compliant arterial phantoms for in-vitro studies and device testing. *J Cardiovasc Magn Reson.* 2013;15:2.
11. Mitsouras D, Lee TC, Liacouras P, et al. Three-dimensional printing of MRI-visible phantoms and MR image-guided therapy simulation. *Magn Reson Med.* 2017;77(2): 613−622.
12. George E, Liacouras P, Lee TC, Mitsouras D. 3D-Printed patient-specific models for CT- and MRI-guided procedure planning. *AJNR Am J Neuroradiol.* 2017;38(7):E46−E47.
13. Leng S, Chen B, Vrieze T, et al. Construction of realistic phantoms from patient images and a commercial three-dimensional printer. *J Med Imaging.* 2016;3(3):033501.
14. Filippou V, Tsoumpas C. Recent advances on the development of phantoms using 3D printing for imaging with CT, MRI, PET, SPECT, and ultrasound. *Med Phys Epub ahead of print.* 2018. https://doi.org/10.1002/mp.13058.
15. George E, Liacouras P, Rybicki FJ, Mitsouras D. Measuring and establishing the accuracy and reproducibility of 3D printed medical models. *Radiographics.* 2017;37(5): 1424−1450.
16. Leng S, McGee K, Morris J, et al. Anatomic modeling using 3D printing: quality assurance and optimization. *3D Print Med.* 2017;3(1):6.
17. Barker TM, Earwaker WJ, Lisle DA. Accuracy of stereolithographic models of human anatomy. *Australas Radiol.* 1994; 38(2):106−111.
18. Chepelev L, Giannopoulos A, Tang A, Mitsouras D, Rybicki FJ. Medical 3D printing: methods to standardize terminology and report trends. *3D Print Med.* 2017;3(1):4.
19. Hoashi T, Ichikawa H, Nakata T, et al. Utility of a super-flexible three-dimensional printed heart model in congenital heart surgery. *Interact Cardiovasc Thorac Surg.* 2018; 27(5):749−755. https://doi.org/10.1093/icvts/ivy160.
20. Namba K, Higaki A, Kaneko N, Mashiko T, Nemoto S, Watanabe E. Microcatheter shaping for intracranial aneurysm coiling using the 3-dimensional printing rapid prototyping technology: preliminary result in the first 10 consecutive cases. *World Neurosurg.* 2015;84(1):178−186.
21. Somireddy M, Czekanski A. Mechanical characterization of additively manufactured parts by FE modeling of mesostructure. *Manuf Mater Process.* 2017;1:18.
22. Bass L, Meisel NA, Williams CB. Exploring variability of orientation and aging effects in material properties of multi-material jetting parts. *Rapid Prototyp J.* 2016;22(5): 826−834.
23. American Society for Testing and Materials (ASTM). F2792-12a standard terminology for additive manufacturing technologies. In: *Electronics; Declarable Substances in Materials; 3D Imaging Systems.* Volume 10.04. West Conshohocken, PA: ASTM; 2014.
24. Baeck B, Lopes P, Verschueren P. State of the art in 3D printing of compliant cardiovascular models: HeartPrint. 3rd Joint Workshop on New Technologies for Computer/Robot Assisted Surgery; 2013; Verona, Italy. (3rd Joint Workshop on New Technologies for Computer/Robot Assisted Surgery).

25. Sommer K, Izzo RL, Shepard L, et al. Design optimization for accurate flow simulations in 3D printed vascular phantoms derived from computed tomography angiography. *Proc SPIE-Int Soc Opt Eng.* 2017:10138.

26. Vukicevic M, Puperi DS, Jane Grande-Allen K, Little SH. 3D printed modeling of the mitral valve for catheter-based structural interventions. *Ann Biomed Eng.* 2017;45(2): 508−519.

27. Cloonan AJ, Shahmirzadi D, Li RX, Doyle BJ, Konofagou EE, McGloughlin TM. 3D-Printed tissue-mimicking phantoms for medical imaging and computational validation applications. *3D Print Addit Manuf.* 2014;1(1):14−23.

28. Mafeld S, Nesbitt C, McCaslin J, et al. Three-dimensional (3D) printed endovascular simulation models: a feasibility study. *Ann Transl Med.* 2017;5(3):42.

29. Yoo SJ, Spray T, Austin 3rd EH, Yun TJ, van Arsdell GS. Hands-on surgical training of congenital heart surgery using 3-dimensional print models. *J Thorac Cardiovasc Surg.* 2017;153(6):1530−1540.

30. Shiraishi I, Yamagishi M, Hamaoka K, Fukuzawa M, Yagihara T. Simulative operation on congenital heart disease using rubber-like urethane stereolithographic biomodels based on 3D datasets of multislice computed tomography. *Eur J Cardiothorac Surg.* 2010;37(2): 302−306.

31. Costello JP, Olivieri LJ, Su L, et al. Incorporating three-dimensional printing into a simulation-based congenital heart disease and critical care training curriculum for resident physicians. *Congenit Heart Dis.* 2015;10(2):185−190.

32. Hofstätter T, Pedersen DB, Tosello G, Hansen HN. State-of-the-art of fiber-reinforced polymers in additive manufacturing technologies. *J Reinf Plast Compos.* 2017; 36(15):1061−1073.

33. Kumar S, Hofmann M, Steinmann B, Foster EJ, Weder C. Reinforcement of stereolithographic resins for rapid prototyping with cellulose nanocrystals. *ACS Appl Mater Interfaces.* 2012;4(10):5399−5407.

34. Shaheen E, Alhelwani A, Van De Casteele E, Politis C, Jacobs R. Evaluation of dimensional changes of 3D printed models after sterilization: a pilot study. *Open Dent J.* 2018; 12:72−79.

35. U.S. Food and Drug Administration, Use of International Standard ISO-10993. *Biological Evaluation of Medical Devices Part 1: Evaluation and Testing.* 2013. Replaces #G87-1 #8294) (blue book memo.

36. Januszewicz R, Tumbleston JR, Quintanilla AL, Mecham SJ, DeSimone JM. Layerless fabrication with continuous liquid interface production. *Proc Natl Acad Sci U S A.* 2016;113(42):11703−11708.

37. Hosny A, Keating SJ, Dilley JD, et al. From improved diagnostics to presurgical planning: high-resolution functionally graded multimaterial 3D printing of biomedical tomographic datasets. *3D Print Addit Manuf.* 2018;5(2): 103−113.

38. Shepard L, Sommer K, Izzo R, et al. Initial simulated FFR investigation using flow measurements in patient-specific 3D printed coronary phantoms. *Proc SPIE-Int Soc Opt Eng.* 2017:10138.

39. O'Hara RP, Chand A, Vidiyala S, et al. Advanced 3D mesh manipulation in stereolithographic files and post-print processing for the manufacturing of patient-specific vascular flow phantoms. *Proc SPIE-Int Soc Opt Eng.* 2016:9789.

40. Slesarenko V, Rudykh S. Towards mechanical characterization of soft digital materials for multimaterial 3D-printing. *Int J Eng Sci.* 2017;123:62−72.

41. Yoo SJ, Thabit O, Kim EK, et al. 3D printing in medicine of congenital heart diseases. *3D Print Med.* 2015;2(1):3.

42. Maragiannis D, Jackson MS, Igo SR, Chang SM, Zoghbi WA, Little SH. Functional 3D printed patient-specific modeling of severe aortic stenosis. *J Am Coll Cardiol.* 2014;64(10):1066−1068.

43. Maragiannis D, Jackson MS, Igo SR, et al. Replicating patient-specific severe aortic valve stenosis with functional 3D modeling. *Circ Cardiovasc Imaging.* 2015;8(10): e003626.

44. Guenette JP, Himes N, Giannopoulos AA, Kelil T, Mitsouras D, Lee TC. Computer-based vertebral tumor cryoablation planning and procedure simulation involving two cases using MRI-visible 3D printing and advanced visualization. *AJR Am J Roentgenol.* 2016;207(5): 1128−1131.

45. Kim MJ, Lee SR, Lee MY, et al. Characterization of 3D printing techniques: toward patient specific quality assurance spine-shaped phantom for stereotactic body radiation therapy. *PLoS One.* 2017;12(5):e0176227.

46. Izzo RL, O'Hara RP, Iyer V, et al. 3D printed cardiac phantom for procedural planning of a transcatheter native mitral valve replacement. *Proc SPIE-Int Soc Opt Eng.* 2016:9789.

47. Wang K, Zhao Y, Chang YH, et al. Controlling the mechanical behavior of dual-material 3D printed meta-materials for patient-specific tissue-mimicking phantoms. *Mater Des.* 2016;90:704−712.

48. Frolich AM, Spallek J, Brehmer L, et al. 3D printing of intracranial aneurysms using fused deposition modeling offers highly accurate replications. *AJNR Am J Neuroradiol.* 2016; 37(1):120−124.

49. Cai L, Byrd P, Zhang H, Schlarman K, Zhang Y, Golub M, Zhang J. Effect of Printing Orientation on Strength of 3D Printed ABS Plastics. In: The Minerals, Metals & Materials Society, ed. *TMS 2016 145th Annual Meeting & Exhibition.* Cham: Springer; 2016:199−204 (The Minerals, Metals & Materials Society (Eds.) TMS 2016 145th Annual Meeting & Exhibition).

50. Panwar A, Tan LP. Current status of bioinks for micro-extrusion-based 3D bioprinting. *Molecules.* 2016;21(6): E685.

51. Perez M, Block M, Espalin D, Winker R, Hoppe T, Medina F, Wicker RB. Sterilization of FDM-Manufacured Parts. 29th Annual International Solid Freeform Fabrication Symposium - an Additive Manufacturing Conference; 2012 August 13−15; Austin, TX. (29th Annual International Solid Freeform Fabrication Symposium - an Additive Manufacturing Conference).

52. Chung M, Radacsi N, Robert C, et al. On the optimization of low-cost FDM 3D printers for accurate replication of

patient-specific abdominal aortic aneurysm geometry. *3D Print Med.* 2018;4(1):2.

53. Lam K. MO-F-CAMPUS-I-03: CT and MR characteristics of some specialty 3D printing filaments. *J Med Phys.* 2015; 42(6):3579.

54. Okkalidis N, Chatzigeorgiou C, Okkalides D. Assessment of 11 available materials with custom three- dimensional-printing patterns for the simulation of muscle, fat, and lung Hounsfield units in patient-specific phantoms. *J Eng Sci Med Diagn Ther.* 2018;1, 011003-011001.

55. Hamedani BA, Melvin A, Vaheesan K, Gadani S, Pereira K, Hall AF. Three-dimensional printing CT-derived objects with controllable radiopacity. *J Appl Clin Med Phys.* 2018; 19(2):317–328.

56. Weisman JA, Ballard DH, Jammalamadaka U, et al. 3D printed antibiotic and chemotherapeutic eluting catheters for potential use in interventional radiology: in vitro proof of concept study. *Acad Radiol.* 2019;26(2):270–274. https://doi.org/10.1016/j.acra.2018.03.022.270-274.

57. Yoo TS, Hamilton T, Hurt DE, Caban J, Liao D, Chen DT. *Toward quantitative X-ray CT phantoms of metastatic tumors using rapid prototyping technology.* 2011:1770–1773, 2011 IEEE International Symposium on Biomedical Imaging: From Nano to Macro. Chicago, IL.

58. Miller MA, Hutchins GD. *Development of anatomically realistic PET and PET/CT phantoms with rapid prototyping technology.* 2007:4252–4257, 2007 IEEE Nuclear Science Symposium Conference Record. Honolulu, HI.

59. Di Prima M, Coburn J, Hwang D, Kelly J, Khairuzzaman A, Ricles L. Additively manufactured medical products - the FDA perspective. *3D Print Med.* 2016;2.

60. Zopf DA, Hollister SJ, Nelson ME, Ohye RG, Green GE. Bioresorbable airway splint created with a three-dimensional printer. *N Engl J Med.* 2013;368(21): 2043–2045.

61. ACR American College of Radiology. *Computed Tomography Quality Control Manual.* 2012.

62. ACR American College of Radiology. *Magnetic Resonance Imaging Quality Control Manual.* 2015.

63. Kiarashi N. *FDA Current Practices and Regulations*; 2017. https://http://www.fda.gov/downloads/MedicalDevices/ NewsEvents/WorkshopsConferences/UCM575723.pdf. FDA/CDRH–RSNA SIG Joint Meeting on 3D Printed Patient-Specific Anatomic Models.

64. Pang T, Guertin MD, Nguyen HD. *Accuracy of stereolithography parts: mechanism and modes of distortion for a "letter H" diagnostic part.* Solid Freeform Fabrication Proceedings. 1995:170.

65. Wake N, Rude T, Kang SK, et al. 3D printed renal cancer models derived from MRI data: application in pre-surgical planning. *Abdom Radiol (NY).* 2017;42(5):1501–1509. https://doi.org/10.1007/s00261-016-1022-2.

66. Ripley B, Kelil T, Cheezum MK, et al. 3D printing based on cardiac CT assists anatomic visualization before transcatheter aortic valve replacement. *J Cardiovasc Comput Tomogr.* 2016;10(1):28–36.

67. Hakansson A, Rantatalo M, Hansen T, Wanhainen A. Patient specific biomodel of the whole aorta – the importance of calcified plaque removal. *VASA Zeitschrift fur Gefasskrankheiten.* 2011;40(6):453–459.

68. Koleilat I, Jaeggli M, Ewing JA, Androes M, Simionescu DT, Eidt J. Interobserver variability in physician-modified endograft planning by comparison with a three-dimensional printed aortic model. *J Vasc Surg.* 2015. https://doi.org/10.1016/j.jvs.2015.09.044. epub ahead of print.

69. Olivieri LJ, Krieger A, Loke YH, Nath DS, Kim PC, Sable CA. Three-dimensional printing of intracardiac defects from three-dimensional echocardiographic images: feasibility and relative accuracy. *J Am Soc Echocardiogr.* 2015;28(4):392–397.

70. Cai T, Ripley B, Cheezum M, et al. Accuracy of 3D printed models of the aortic valve complex for transcatheter aortic valve replacement (TAVR) planning: comparison to computed tomographic angiography (CTA). *Circulation.* 2015 (Chicago, IL).

71. Cai T, Rybicki FJ, Giannopoulos AA, et al. The residual STL volume as a metric to evaluate accuracy and reproducibility of anatomic models for 3D printing: application in the validation of 3D-printable models of maxillofacial bone from reduced radiation dose CT images. *3D Print Med.* 2015;1(1):2.

CHAPTER 3

From Multiplanar Imaging to Physical 3D Models: 3D Printing as an Adjunct to Congenital Heart Surgery

SHI-JOON YOO, MD • CHRISTOPHER Z. LAM, MD • NABIL HUSSEIN, MBCHB (HONS) • GLEN VAN ARSDELL, MD

3D printing is highly valuable in preoperative assessment for congenital heart disease.[1–6] As an adjunct to routine imaging, it provides physical replicas of the heart and major vessels to the operators' hands in advance. Although echocardiograms usually provide excellent anatomical and physiological information, surgical decision-making often relies on mental reconstructions of the 3D anatomy, with confirmation of the plan only possible intraoperatively during physical exploration of the abnormal heart. Owing to significant improvements in image quality in regards to spatial and temporal resolution, CT and MR angiograms have increasingly been used for morphological assessment of cardiac anatomy in the last decade.[7] Both CT and MR are superior to echocardiography in visualization of cardiovascular anatomy, except only for the anatomy and function of the cardiac valves. When appropriately performed, both CT and MR angiograms provide excellent image data for 3D reconstruction with multiplanar reconstruction and volume rendering. With further 3D modeling, the patient's heart and major vessels are displayed on a computer screen or in space for virtual demonstration and, when required, 3D printed. Virtual demonstration and 3D printing significantly reduces the difficulties faced when attempting to describe the complex anatomy of the congenital heart disease and minimizes the chances of misinterpretation and miscommunication.

This chapter introduces the applicable imaging techniques, basics of postprocessing and 3D printing, and current applications and limitations, including future possibilities in the utilization of 3D printing in congenital heart surgery.

IMAGING

The applicable imaging modalities used for 3D printing are computed tomography (CT), magnetic resonance (MR), ultrasound, and 3D rotational angiography. It is ideal to acquire the images with electrocardiographic (ECG)-gating and breath-holding or respiratory navigation. It is preferable to target ECG-gating to end-diastole instead of the end-systole to simulate the relaxed status of the heart at surgery. The parameters of 3D imaging should be prescribed for the highest spatial and temporal resolutions possible without significant compromise of the signal-to-noise ratio.

ECG-gated CT angiography is the most commonly used imaging modality for 3D modeling. It is important to time the scanning so that all cardiac chambers and major vessels are opacified as homogeneously as possible (Fig. 3.1). A generous amount of contrast medium (>2 cc/kg) is injected for a prolonged period (15–20 s). It is important to avoid streak artifacts from undiluted contrast medium in the superior or inferior vena cave and the tributaries. This can be achieved by injecting normal saline or 5%–10% diluted contrast medium following injection of the undiluted contrast medium.[8] Although it is not ideal, non-ECG-gated CT can still be used for 3D printing, albeit with abbreviated detail.

Contrast-enhanced MR angiography is also an excellent imaging modality for 3D modeling and printing. Although the achievable spatial resolution is not as good as that of CT, an ECG-gated respiration-navigated MR angiography using inversion recovery fast low angle shot (IR-FLASH) technique provides excellent image quality. Opacification of the cardiac chambers and vessels are usually far more

3-Dimensional Modeling in Cardiovascular Disease. https://doi.org/10.1016/B978-0-323-65391-6.00003-X

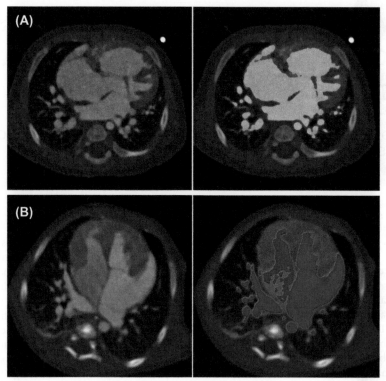

FIG. 3.1 Computed tomographic angiograms showing the effects of homogeneous **(A)** versus inhomogeneous **(B)** opacification of the cardiovascular systems at threshold-based segmentation. Note that a part of the right atrium (arrow) in B is not highlighted at segmentation as the signal intensity is not within the thresholding window.

homogeneous in MR angiograms than in CT angiograms (Fig. 3.2).[9,10] With this technique, delivery of an accurate amount of contrast medium is paramount. As the total amount of contrast medium used is usually far less than the dead space volume in the delivery system, the tube should be primed with saline accurately so that the exact amount of contrast medium is loaded at the end of the tube. Accepting that there is limited accuracy due to cardiac motion artifact, conventional non-ECG-gated MR angiograms can be used. Noncontrast MR angiography using 3D steady-state free precession sequences are usually not applicable in most patients with congenital heart disease because of dephasing artifact from turbulent flow across stenotic valves or vessels, septal defects, or regurgitant valves.

Ultrasound is extremely useful for 3D demonstration of the cardiac valves. However, ultrasound is of limited use in 3D printing because of ubiquitous artifact from strong interfaces such as the surface of the bones and air, and nonuniformity of the axial and lateral resolutions. However, use of 3D ultrasound data for printing of limited parts of the heart such as valves has been attempted.[11–15] The raw Digital Imaging and Communications in Medicine (DICOM) data obtained from nonlinear transducers are composed of anisotropic voxels with the size varying with distance from the transducer.[14] For 3D modeling and printing, the raw DICOM data should be converted to Cartesian DICOM format with isotropic voxels.

Finally, rotational CT angiograms obtained from modern X-ray angiographic equipment can also be used for 3D printing.[16]

As each imaging modality has its inherent strengths and weaknesses, the data from more than two imaging modalities can be integrated to produce a more comprehensive dataset for visualization of all cardiovascular structures.[17]

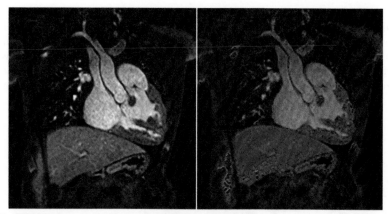

FIG. 3.2 Magnetic resonance angiograms showing homogeneous opacification of cardiovascular system allowing easy segmentation despite its lower spatial resolution as compared to computed tomographic angiograms.

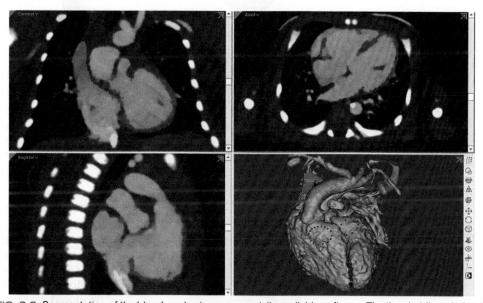

FIG. 3.3 Segmentation of the blood pool using commercially available software. The thresholding window is chosen relative to the signal intensities within the contrast-enhanced blood pool. Inhomogeneous signal intensity requires additional manual segmentation using local thresholding, drawing, and erasing. The sites of the mitral and tricuspid valvar attachment are marked with dots on the multiplanar reconstruction images. By connecting these dots with additional fine adjustment, the valve annuli can accurately be defined.

POSTPROCESSING

Postprocessing consists of segmentation and computer-aided design (CAD) process. For 3D modeling and printing, raw Cartesian DICOM datasets are required. Segmentation relies primarily on thresholding and region growing. In both CT and MR angiograms, high signal intensity from the contrast medium allows easy thresholding for segmentation of cardiac chamber cavities and blood vessel lumens (Fig. 3.3). However, thresholding does not work well for the outer boundaries of the heart and vessels because of low-level signal intensity differences between the wall of the heart and adjacent structures. Alternatively, a shell with a uniform thickness is added to the surface of the segmented blood pool (Figs. 3.4 and 3.5). The inner surface of the shell thus produced is a precise representation of the endocardial surface of the heart and vessels, whereas the outer surface is fictionalized. As most intracardiac procedures are performed from the endocardial side of the heart, the endocardial representation is mostly sufficient for assessment of the surgical anatomy and for surgical practice in most congenital heart diseases.

Signal-intensity-based thresholding usually requires additional work with erasing, drawing, and regional thresholding tools. Once the segmentation process is complete, the data are further processed with CAD tools

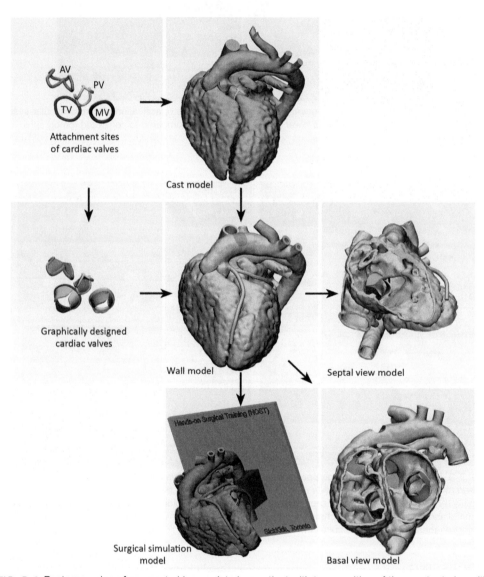

FIG. 3.4 Postprocessing of segmented image data in a patient with transposition of the great arteries with ventricular septal defect. Upper middle panel shows a cast model with superimposed cardiac valve annuli. A wall model in the center middle panel is produced by adding a thin wall outside the cast model. The sepal and basal view anatomy can be exposed by removing the free wall of the heart or the apex of the ventricles (right middle and lower panels). The surgical simulation model is produced by mounting the model on a plate with support columns, while the surgical area is kept intact (center lower panel). Graphically designed cardiac valve leaflets and coronary arteries can be added. Corresponding 3D print models are shown in Fig. 3.5.

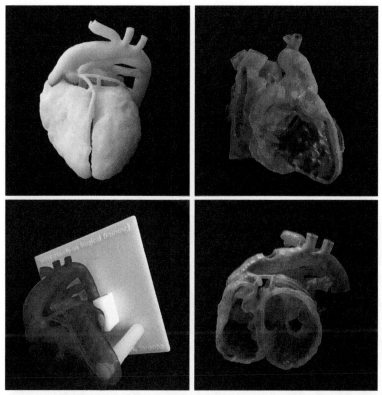

FIG. 3.5 Models printed from the dataset shown in Fig. 3.4. Cast model in left upper panel, septal view model in right upper panel, basal view model in right lower panel, and surgical simulation model in left low panel.

that include volume rendering, generation of curves and planes, hollowing, wrapping, and trimming. Volume rendering is a basic component of most 3D imaging programs. The volume rendered images are reviewed during the segmentation process to check the appropriateness of the initial processing and to guide further refinements. If the results seen on volume rendered images are satisfactory, the file is saved in a file format that can be used for further CAD and 3D printing. Stereolithography or Standard Tessellation Language (STL) is the most commonly used file format. Using the volume rendered image, unnecessary parts are trimmed. 3D modeling of the cardiac valves is the most challenging aspect. Although the cardiac valves may appear well reconstructed on a computer screen, they are far from satisfactory when they are 3D printed. In contrast to this, the sites of attachment of the cardiac valve are identifiable and can be marked on the model (Figs. 3.3 and 3.4). The atrioventricular valve attachments are usually identifiable in cross-sectional images (Fig. 3.3). Using multiple imaging planes, 6–10 attachment points are marked and connected with a curved

line. The semilunar valvar attachment is easier to mark on the 3D volume rendered image. The curves thus created are then given a 1–2 mm thickness so as that they are identifiable in the 3D images and printed models (Fig. 3.4). The cardiac valve leaflets can be graphically designed and added to the model (Figs. 3.4 and 3.5). Although the images and models thus created are not based on true image data, they may serve as an approximate representation of the cardiac valves. If the attachment points of chordae tendinae to the valve leaflets and papillary muscles are identifiable in the reference images, including echocardiograms, simulated chords can be added (Fig. 3.6).

For preoperative assessment and planning of congenital heart surgery, we produce a cast model of the whole heart and major vessels, an endocardial surface anatomy model for the atrial and ventricular septal anatomy, and an endocardial surface anatomy for the anatomy of the base of the ventricles (Fig. 3.5). For surgical simulation, the endocardial surface anatomy model is mounted on a platform base so that the model can be plastered to a table (Figs. 3.4 and 3.5).[18]

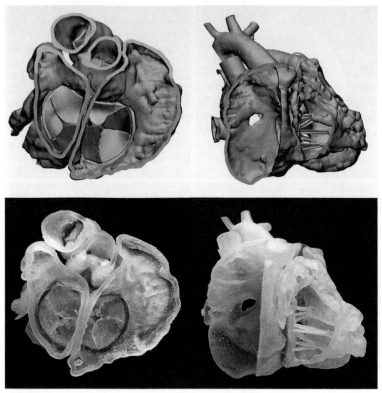

FIG. 3.6 Complete form of atrioventricular septal defect with graphically designed cardiac valves and tension apparatuses.

3D PRINTING

Most commercially available 3D printers are capable of a printing with a resolution that is higher than that achievable by clinical CT scanners. Therefore, printer resolution is usually not a limiting factor for 3D printing applications using medical image data. Printers that can produce models of variable softness and flexibility are ideal for application for surgical planning and simulation of congenital heart diseases. Currently, the printers using polyjet technology offer photopolymer resin materials that can be mixed in various ratios to represent the different physical properties of the components of the heart and vessels.[5] Silicone is an attractive material for representation of various components of human soft tissues. However, high-quality printers using silicone have not yet arrived in the market.

Using currently available 3D printers, it typically takes 6–10 h to print a set of heart models for an infant case of congenital heart disease. After the models are printed, the supporting material around the surface of the model is removed using a high-pressure waterjet or chemical solvent, or both. Depending on the materials used and complexity of the structure, it may take only a few minutes or up to multiple hours to remove the support material. Careful cleaning is very important as fine structures can easily be broken or washed out during this removal process. Therefore, given the delicateness of fine complex structures, the detail quality of the final product is not necessarily equal to the greatest resolution capable of the printer.

Some printers build models with multiple colors, while others provide limited color options. The surface anatomy is usually better appreciated in models with slightly dark color than white or lightly colored ones. Lightly colored models can easily be colored using commercially available dyes for clothes or food.

Heart models can also be manufactured using 3D printed molds.[19,20] The major advantage of a molding technique is the ability to use highly flexible materials such as silicone and urethane. However, it requires additional steps for production, and a degree of inaccuracy is unavoidable.

UTILIZATION OF 3D MODELING AND PRINTING IN SURGICAL MANAGEMENT OF CONGENITAL HEART DISEASES

Surgical decision-making in management of congenital heart diseases consists of two hierarchic levels. The first-level decision is mostly a binary decision regarding biventricular versus univentricular repair. Although univentricular repair is an innovative palliative procedure with excellent predictable surgical results, the Fontan circulation requires high systemic venous pressures and is uniformly associated with low cardiac output, resulting in impaired forms and function of all body organs.[21] However, there are situations when the intraoperative and postoperative risks of a complex biventricular repair outweigh the long-term disadvantages of a univentricular repair.[22] Furthermore, intraoperative conversion of a biventricular to a univentricular repair is associated with high operative risk. Therefore, the decision for a biventricular versus univentricular is crucially important. The second-level decision is to personalize the surgical procedure based on the precise understanding of the surgical anatomy and the potential risks along with short- and long-term outcomes of the intended surgery.

Among many pathological entities, double outlet right ventricle is the most frequently encountered indication for 3D printing (Fig. 3.7).[1,23] Double outlet right ventricle is not a specific pathological entity but a collection of various pathologies showing one specific form of ventriculoarterial connection: that is, the origin of both the aorta and pulmonary arterial trunk from the right ventricle. Hearts described as double outlet right ventricle thus encompass a heterogeneous group of malformations. Consequently, there is a long list of the essential features to take into consideration in the preoperative assessment of double outlet right ventricle.[24] The primary goal of the surgical repair is to establish unobstructed inlets and outlets of the ventricles, competent cardiac valves, adequate ventricular volumes, and good coronary arterial perfusion. The major determinant in achieving biventricular repair is the feasibility of intraventricular baffling of the ventricular septal defect (VSD) to the aortic valve. The right ventricle should have enough space to accommodate an unobstructed baffle without compromising the form and function of the tricuspid valve and the future right ventricular outflow tract. In addition, there needs to be adequate volume of the functional right and left ventricles after completion of the surgery. When the VSD is not able to be baffled to the aortic valve, the feasibility of baffling to the pulmonary valve along with an arterial switch operation should be considered.

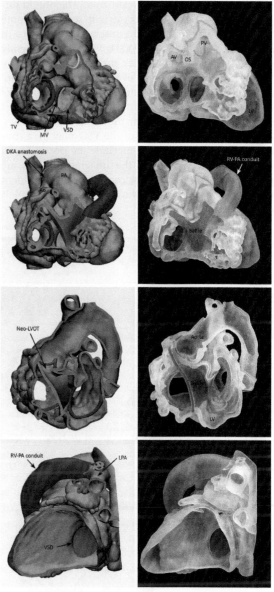

FIG. 3.7 Graphics and corresponding photos of 3D print models of a clinical case with double outlet right ventricle with a remote ventricular septal defect who previously underwent bidirectional cavopulmonary and Damus–Kaye–Stansel (DKS) aortopulmonary anastomoses. After reconstruction of the cardiovascular structures (first pair of panels), an intracardiac baffle and right ventricle-pulmonary artery (RV-PA) conduit were graphically designed and printed with the heart to assess the feasibility of biventricular repair. *Ao*, ascending aorta; *MV*, mitral valve annulus; *LPA*, left pulmonary artery; *LV*, left ventricle; *LVOT*, left ventricular outflow tract; *OS*, outlet septum; *PA*, pulmonary arterial trunk; *TV*, tricuspid valve annulus; *VSD*, ventricular septal defect.

3D modeling and printing is particularly helpful in surgical decision-making of the cases with so-called remote VSD. There is currently no consensus on criteria to define the remoteness of a VSD. VSDs are frequently defined as remote when they predominantly involve the inlet or trabecular part of the ventricular septum. Alternatively, remoteness can be defined as when the distance between the margin of the VSD and nearest semilunar valve is greater than the aortic valve diameter. Although the "remoteness" of the VSD may be a concerning finding, it does not preclude the possibility of biventricular repair. When the imaging findings are not sufficient for a definitive conclusion, it is prudent to reassess the imaging findings with 3D print models directly in hand.

The second most common indication for 3D modeling and printing is for complex forms of transposition of the great arteries. Typical examples of transpositions do not usually require 3D print models. However, there are number of unusual forms of transposition. As in patients with double outlet right ventricle, the major indication for 3D modeling is to assess the feasibility of maintaining an unobstructed left ventricular outflow tract leading to the aorta, with or without arterial switch or aortic translocation. One rare example is the so-called "posterior" transposition in which the aortic root and valve are located posteriorly in relation to the pulmonary arterial trunk and valve (Fig. 3.8).[25] The heart with posterior transposition shows an unusual external appearance for the diagnosis

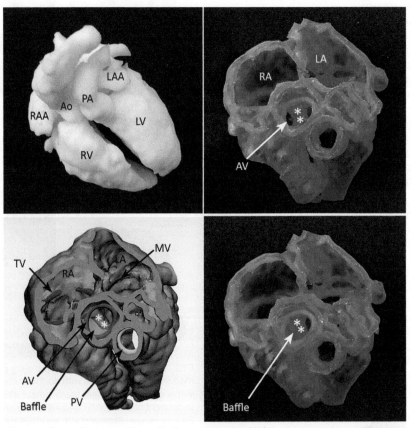

FIG. 3.8 Unusual form of transposition with the aortic valve (AV) in the posterior position overriding the ventricular septum (asterisks). The case model and basal view model seen from the top show the rightward and posterior location of the aortic valve in relation to the pulmonary valve. As the small ventricular septal defect was not able to be enlarged due to the conduction tissue located along the posteroinferior margin of the ventricular septal defect, the ventricular septal defect was baffled to the aortic valve and the ascending aorta and pulmonary arterial trunk were anastomosed (so-called Yasui operation). The intracardiac procedure was simulated by placing a graphically designed baffle before the surgery (lower panels). *LA*, left atrium; *LAA*, left atrial appendage; *MV*, mitral valve annulus; *PA*, pulmonary arterial trunk; *PV*, pulmonary valve annulus; *RA*, right atrium; *RAA*, right atrial appendage; *TV*, tricuspid valve annulus.

of transposition, as the arterial trunks appear normally related. The intracardiac anatomy is different from the usual anatomy of transposition with the aorta arising from the right ventricle with a short or absent muscular infundibulum and the pulmonary trunk arising from the left ventricle with a long muscular infundibulum. The unusual external appearance and intracardiac anatomy for the given diagnosis of transposition may require a longer time for assessment during surgical exploration or may potentially lead to misinterpretation of the surgical anatomy and incorrect decision-making if not informed beforehand.

The third most common indication for 3D printing as an adjunct to surgical planning is in the setting of situs abnormalities such as isolated dextrocardia, situs inversus, and heterotaxy. These types of abnormally positioned hearts are usually associated with complex forms of congenital heart disease showing nonuniform characteristics. The descriptive terms used in situs abnormalities are frequently confusing and often not uniformly or clearly defined, leading to unnecessarily long discussions or misunderstanding among the responsible medical teams. In addition, heterotaxy is typically associated with abnormal systemic and pulmonary venous connections that need to be clearly understood preoperatively regardless of whether biventricular or univentricular repair is planned (Fig. 3.9). 3D modeling is crucially important when biventricular repair is considered in heterotaxy or other forms of cardiac malposition.

There are rare situations in which the cardiac chambers and major vessels are abnormally related for the given situs and segmental connections. They include twisted or criss-cross heart, superoinferior ventricles, and topsy-turvy heart. These rare conditions are definite indications for 3D modeling and printing. As the morphology, spatial relationship among cardiac chambers and arterial trunks, and the connections at the atrioventricular and ventriculoarterial junctions are so complicated, it is extremely difficult to understand solely from imaging findings and requires extensive description to explain the findings to others.

MORPHOLOGY TEACHING OF CONGENITAL HEART DISEASES USING 3D MODELING AND PRINTING

Both imaging and surgical treatment of patients require precise understanding of the morphological features of various congenital heart diseases. Pathological specimens have been the major resource for traditional morphology teaching of imagers and surgeons. However, the availability of specimens are limited to a few major centers throughout the world. Although existing specimens are damaged by repeated use for teaching and research, new specimens are barely available owing to improvements in surgical and medical treatment of congenital heart diseases. Furthermore, the pathological specimens do not represent the usual pathological spectrum as they include hearts only from deceased patients or removed at the time of cardiac transplantation. As 3D print models are from living patients, the collection of available cases is rapidly increasing and any number of replicas can be printed and distributed without restriction. Attendees of morphology teaching courses that use both specimens and 3D print models find that 3D print models and pathological specimens are equally important and complimentary (Fig. 3.10).

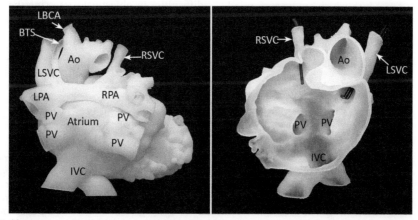

FIG. 3.9 Heterotaxy with atrial right isomerism and atrioventricular septal defect. 3D print models were used to plan intraatrial routing of the systemic and pulmonary venous returns. *Ao,* aorta; *BTS,* Blalock-Taussig shunt; *IVC,* inferior vena cava; *LBCA,* left brachiocephalic artery; *LPA,* left pulmonary artery; *LSVC,* left superior vena cava; *PV,* pulmonary vein; *RPA,* right pulmonary artery; *RSVC,* right superior vena cava.

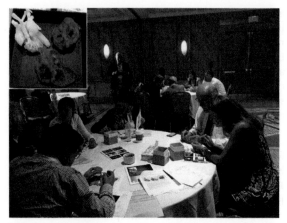

FIG. 3.10 Morphology teaching using 3D print models. The inset in the left upper corner of the figure shows a typical set of models for morphology teaching that includes a cast model (in white), and basal and septal view models (in red).

HANDS-ON SURGICAL TRAINING OF CONGENITAL HEART SURGERY WITH 3D PRINT MODELS

Congenital heart surgery training relies on exposure to surgical procedures in the operating room under the close tutelage of experienced supervisors. However, such preceptor-apprenticeship on the operating table is reliant on opportunistic encounters because of the relative rarity of individual lesions. More importantly, training in the operating room inevitably carries a risk to the patient's health. Therefore, surgical simulation has increasingly been demanded in training programs. However, the surgical simulation programs for congenital heart surgery have been extremely scarce and are limited to a few procedures such as the arterial switch operation and Ross procedure, which can be performed on the explanted animal hearts.

3D print models made of flexible rubber-like material are excellent for surgical training.[18] Although the physical properties of the currently available print materials are significantly different from those of human myocardial and endocardial tissue, 3D print models are regarded as acceptable for surgical simulation. For surgical simulation, original models are modified to represent cardiovascular structures as close to surgical reality as possible by adding graphically designed cardiac valves, chordae tendinae, and coronary arteries.

The preliminary data from the most recent hands-on surgical training course in the authors' institution showed remarkable improvement of the end-point results of arterial switch operation and reduced procedural time measured at the end of the course as compared to initial attempts for most attendees (Fig. 3.11). Repeated practice on 3D print models will be extremely helpful in achieving surgeons' common goal of masterful performance of the procedure in the least amount of time. Overall, this has the potential to reduce patient morbidity and mortality globally in congenital heart surgery.

CURRENT LIMITATIONS AND FUTURE DIRECTIONS

3D modeling and printing has brought a new paradigm for preoperative assessment, surgical practice, and simulation in congenital heart surgery. However, the utilization of 3D modeling and printing does not seem as high as was expected, considering its obvious benefits. Current major limitations include the labor-intensive nature of postprocessing and 3D printing, the high costs of postprocessing software programs, 3D printing equipment and print materials, and the difficulties in objectively assessing the accuracy of the process and the impact of its utilization on patient

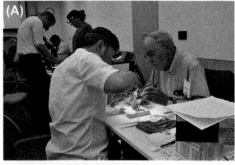
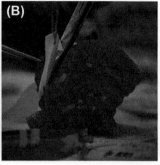

FIG. 3.11 Hands-on surgical training (HOST) course for congenital heart surgery. **(A)** An attendee is guided and assisted by Dr. William Williams, a retired pediatric cardiac surgeon for a simulation procedure. **(B)** Surgical simulation on a model of truncus arteriosus.

management. These limitations will gradually be overcome by continuous improvement of technology, introduction of new print materials, expanded utilization with decreased costs, and recognition of 3D printing as a necessary standard medical service that will qualify for reimbursement by insurance companies or government.

Software programs will continue to improve in function and speed. The knowledge-based programs will eventually allow detailed and enhanced representation of the fine structures such as cardiac valves, chords, and papillary muscles and coronary arteries and veins that are difficult to clearly define using individual patient's image data alone. Using image fusion technology, the strengths of multiple imaging modalities can be integrated to generate a comprehensive model. Improved CAD tools will enable fabrication of patient-specific surgical baffles, patches, and prostheses in advance of surgery.

With growing utilization of 3D printing in medicine, print materials with physical properties that are similar to those of human tissue will emerge. Myocardial fiber orientation might be able to be reflected in 3D print models by integrating data from diffusion tensor imaging obtained with magnetic resonance.[26] Endocardial and epicardial layers will one day be able to be represented by adding thin coats of different print materials on the surfaces of the myocardium.

3D printing of living tissues and organs, known as 3D bioprinting, has emerged as a promising technology that holds a great potential for personalized medicine such as partial or total replacement of the diseased heart that is not amenable to the existing medical or surgical management.[27] Furthermore, 3D bioprinting may allow fabrication of congenital heart models for surgical simulation and outcome assessment.

REFERENCES

1. Yoo SJ, Thabit O, Kim EK, et al. 3D printing in medicine of congenital heart diseases. *3D Print Med.* 2015;2(1):3. https://doi.org/10.1186/s41205-016-0004-x.
2. Anwar S, Singh GK, Varughese J, et al. 3D printing in complex congenital heart disease: across a spectrum of age, pathology, and imaging techniques. *JACC Cardiovasc Imaging.* 2017;10(8):953–956. https://doi.org/10.1016/j.jcmg.2016.03.013.
3. Anwar S, Singh GK, Miller J, et al. 3D printing is a transformative technology in congenital heart disease. *JACC Basic Transl Sci.* 2018;3(2):294–312. https://doi.org/10.1016/j.jacbts.2017.10.003.
4. Valverde I, Gomez-Ciriza G, Hussain T, et al. Three-dimensional printed models for surgical planning of complex congenital heart defects: an international multicentre study. *Eur J Cardiothorac Surg.* 2017;52(6):1139–1148. https://doi.org/10.1093/ejcts/ezx208.
5. Meier LM, Meineri M, Qua Hiansen J, Horlick EM. Structural and congenital heart disease interventions: the role of three-dimensional printing. *Neth Heart J.* 2017;25(2):65–75. https://doi.org/10.1007/s12471-016-0942-3.
6. Lau IWW, Liu D, Xu L, Fan Z, Sun Z. Clinical value of patient-specific three-dimensional printing of congenital heart disease: quantitative and qualitative assessments. *PLoS One.* 2018;13(3):e0194333. https://doi.org/10.1371/journal.pone.0194333.
7. Han BK, Rigsby CK, Hlavacek A, et al. Computed tomography imaging in patients with congenital heart disease Part I: rationale and utility. An expert consensus document of the society of cardiovascular computed tomography (SCCT): endorsed by the society of pediatric radiology (SPR) and the North American society of cardiac imaging (NASCI). *J Cardiovasc Comput Tomogr.* 2015;9(6):475–492. https://doi.org/10.1016/j.jcct.2015.07.004.
8. Goo HW. Cardiac MDCT CT in children: CT technology overview and interpretation. *Radiol Clin.* 2011;49(5):997–1010. https://doi.org/10.1016/j.rcl.2011.06.001.
9. Tandon A, James L, Henningsson M, et al. A clinical combined gadobutrol bolus and slow infusion protocol enabling angiography, inversion recovery whole heart, and late gadolinium enhancement imaging in a single study. *J Cardiovasc Magn Reson.* 2016;18(1):66.
10. Lam CZ, Pagano J, Gill N, Vidarsson L, de la Mora R, Seed M, Grosse-Wortmann L, Yoo SJ. Dual phase infusion with bolus tracking: technical innovation for cardiac and respiratory navigated magnetic resonance angiography using extracellular contrast. *Pediatr Radiol.* 2019;49(3):399–406. https://doi.org/10.1007/s00247-018-4293-7.
11. Olivieri LJ, Krieger A, Loke YH, Nath DS, Kim PC, Sable CA. Three-dimensional printing of intracardiac defects from three-dimensional echocardiographic images: feasibility and relative accuracy. *J Am Soc Echocardiogr.* 2015;28(4):392–397. https://doi.org/10.1016/j.echo.2014.12.016.
12. Farooqi KM, Sengupta PP. Echocardiography and three-dimensional printing: sound ideas to touch a heart. *J Am Soc Echocardiogr.* 2015;28(4):398–403. https://doi.org/10.1016/j.echo.2015.02.005.
13. Mashari A, Montealegre-Gallegos M, Knio Z, et al. Making three-dimensional echocardiography more tangible: a workflow for three-dimensional printing with echocardiographic data. *Echo Res Pract.* 2016;3(4):R57–R64. https://doi.org/10.1530/ERP-16-0036.
14. Muraru D, Veronesi F, Maddalozzo A, et al. 3D printing of normal and pathologic tricuspid valves from transthoracic 3D echocardiography datasets. *Eur Heart J Cardiovasc Imaging.* 2017;18(7):802–808. https://doi.org/10.1093/ehjci/jew215.
15. Zhu Y, Liu J, Wang L, et al. Preliminary study of the application of transthoracic echocardiography-guided three-dimensional printing for the assessment of structural heart disease. *Echocardiography.* 2017;34(12):1903–1908. https://doi.org/10.1111/echo.13715.

16. Parimi M, Buelter J, Thanugundla V, et al. Feasibility and validity of printing 3D heart models from rotational angiography. *Pediatr Cardiol.* 2018;39(4):653—658. https://doi.org/10.1007/s00246-017-1799-y.

17. Gosnell J, Pietila T, Samuel BP, Kurup HK, Haw MP, Vettukattil JJ. Integration of computed tomography and three-dimensional echocardiography for hybrid three-dimensional printing in congenital heart disease. *J Digit Imaging.* 2016;29(6):665—669.

18. Yoo SJ, Spray T, Austin 3rd EH, Yun TJ, van Arsdell GS. Hands-on surgical training of congenital heart surgery using 3-dimensional print models. *J Thorac Cardiovasc Surg.* 2017;153(6):1530—1540. https://doi.org/10.1016/j.jtcvs.2016.12.054.

19. Shiraishi I, Yamagishi M, Hamaoka K, Fukuzawa M, Yagihara T. Simulative operation on congenital heart disease using rubber-like urethane stereolithographic biomodels based on 3D datasets of multislice computed tomography. *Eur J Cardiothorac Surg.* 2010;37(2):302—306. https://doi.org/10.1016/j.ejcts.2009.07.046.

20. Hoashi T, Ichikawa H, Nakata T, et al. Utility of a super-flexible three-dimensional printed heart model in congenital heart surgery. *Interact Cardiovasc Thorac Surg.* 2018. https://doi.org/10.1093/icvts/ivy160.

21. Rychik J. The relentless effects of the fontan paradox. *Semin Thorac Cardiovasc Surg Pediatr Card Surg Annu.* 2016;19(1):37—43. https://doi.org/10.1053/j.pcsu.2015.11.006.

22. Delius RE. 2-V or not 2-V: that is the question…plus some musings on thinking out of the box. *J Thorac Cardiovasc Surg.* 2017;154(2):583—584. https://doi.org/10.1016/j.jtcvs.2017.03.010.

23. Yoo SJ, van Arsdell GS. 3D printing in surgical management of double outlet right ventricle. *Front Pediatr.* 2018;5:289. https://doi.org/10.3389/fped.2017.00289. eCollection 2017.

24. Yim D, Dragulescu A, Ide H, et al. Essential modifiers of double outlet right ventricle: revisit with endocardial surface images and 3-dimensional print models. *Circ Cardiovasc Imaging.* 2018;11(3):e006891. https://doi.org/10.1161/CIRCIMAGING.117.006891.

25. Van Praagh R, Perez-Trevino C, López-Cuellar M, et al. Transposition of the great arteries with posterior aorta, anterior pulmonary artery, subpulmonary conus and fibrous continuity between aortic and atrioventricular valves. *Am J Cardiol.* 1971;28(6):621—631.

26. Mekkaoui C, Jackowski MP, Kostis WJ, et al. Myocardial scar delineation using diffusion tensor magnetic resonance tractography. *J Am Heart Assoc.* 2018;7(3):e007834. https://doi.org/10.1161/JAHA.117.007834. pii.

27. Ong CS, Nam L, Ong K, et al. 3D and 4D bioprinting of the myocardium: current approaches, challenges, and future prospects. *BioMed Res Int.* 2018;2018:6497242. https://doi.org/10.1155/2018/6497242. eCollection 2018.

CHAPTER 4

3D Modeling as an Adjunct to Complex Congenital Catheter Interventions

COLIN J. MC MAHON, MD, FRCPI, FAAP, FACC • DARREN BERMAN, MD •
FRANCESCA PLUCINOTTA, MD • DAMIEN KENNY, MD, FACC

KEY POINTS

- Imaging formats that may act as a template for generation of 3D models to help guide complex congenital catheter-based interventions are freely available.
- Evolving to generation of 3D printed models to preperform these interventions has to date been limited to case reports or associated with preparing for newer techniques and has not reached mainstream as yet.
- It is unclear if newer computer-generated 3D models with techniques such as finite element analysis will supersede the need for printed models.
- The ultimate goal may be personalized interventions and 3D modeling is essential to achieving this goal. However, much work is needed to move beyond sole focus on anatomical details and to understand interaction with tissue interfaces and flow dynamics.

INTRODUCTION

Cardiac catheterization since its inception has required some form of imaging to guide catheter manipulation and provide imaging of the heart and surrounding vessels. Werner Forssmann's "self-catheterization" was only possible with the use of X-ray to guide a urinary catheter into his right heart. Since that time, imaging systems have evolved to include biplane image intensifiers through to digital flat panel detectors, with focus on radiation reduction and image optimization. However, the limitations of identifying and treating pathology within a 3D structure with 2-D images have remained. More advanced forms of cross-sectional imaging have contributed to understanding complex anatomy; however, a disconnect between preprocedural and intraprocedural imaging has persisted. The advent of 3D rotational angiography has made possible the generation of intraprocedural CT like volume-rendered images to guide catheter interventions. Evolution to generation of 3D printed models from diagnostic 3D rotational angiograms, MRIs, or preprocedural CT angiograms have contributed to physician and patient confidence in developing new catheter-based techniques for complex congenital heart lesions. The technology will continue to evolve, with computerized 3D modeling providing opportunities to simulate not only the anatomical but also the physiological impact of a particular intervention. Whether more futuristic forms of 3D modeling such as virtual reality and holography will move into the mainstream to provide intraprocedural guidance for complex interventions remains to be seen. This chapter will discuss these topics and provide examples of the current state as well as future potentials of 3D modeling in complex congenital cardiac catheter interventions.

3D Modeling in Congenital Heart Disease

Congenital heart disease is a perfect fit for 3D modeling as congenital cardiac interventional cardiologists deal with a wide variety of complex abnormal cardiac anatomies requiring high-stake interventions. The initial application of 3D modeling has been predominantly to assist preoperative surgical planning in complex anatomies. Its use in determining potential for septation in double outlet right ventricle with remote or challenging ventricular septal defect (VSD) arrangement and to aid in creation of a pathway for conduit placement in total cavopulmonary connection are two classic

3-Dimensional Modeling in Cardiovascular Disease. https://doi.org/10.1016/B978-0-323-65391-6.00004-1

examples of 3D printing assisting the cardiac surgeon in caring for children with congenital heart disease.[1,2] It is still unclear, however, if these models alter surgical approach and improve outcomes. A recent international multicenter study designed to evaluate the impact of 3D printed models on surgical planning in complex congenital heart disease demonstrated that although 3D models are accurate replicas of the cardiovascular anatomy and improve the understanding of complex CHD, the models did not change the surgical decision in most cases.[3] The challenges in designing a study to objectively demonstrate benefit of 3D models in surgical outcomes have been outlined[4] and must be considered as this technology gains acceptance in guiding complex catheterization. 3D models have also been used as teaching tools for medical students,[5] surgical trainees,[6] and as an adjunct for patients and parents with congenital heart disease.[7] These issues are discussed in much greater detail in subsequent chapters (Chapters 10 and 11).

3D Modeling in Congenital Catheterization

3D modeling as an adjunct to complex congenital catheterization was stimulated by the development of transcatheter pulmonary valve replacement. Desire for greater understanding of the unique anatomical challenges of the dysfunction right ventricular outflow tract required additional forms of advanced cross-sectional imaging, which subsequently provided the raw data for segmented models (Chapter 5). This facilitated valve stent implantation within a 3D printed model and helped predict patients who were unsuitable for transcatheter pulmonary valve replacement.[8] As transcatheter pulmonary valve replacement has evolved with introduction of multiple newer valve systems to cover the variety of anatomies encountered,[9–12] 3D modeling has remained an important part of the landscape. Introduction of new valve platforms has often been assisted by development of 3D models to predict performance of new technologies in patient-specific models augmenting appropriate patient selection.[12,13] Advances have also been made with modeling the dynamic nature of the contractile right ventricular outflow tract, with the use of systolic and diastolic *virtual models* generated to assess valve stent performance at various phases throughout the cardiac cycle.[14] These computer-generated virtual models reduce the need for printing multiple 3D physical models and may overcome the limitations of nonphysiological interaction of stented valve with synthetic 3D printed materials. Current virtual models, however, have underestimated device volumes relative to actual device implant volumes and

further refinement of these models is necessary before they supersede physical models.[14]

As has been stated in previous chapters, the accuracy of 3D models is dependent on the quality of the source imaging. To date CT has been regarded as the optimal source imaging platform as it has excellent temporal and spatial resolution. However, more recently with the introduction of 3D rotational angiography in many catheterization laboratories, this appears to be quite useful for generating 3D printed models[15] as well as provide intraprocedural "real-time" virtual 3D procedural guidance. Flat plane detectors allow tomographic slices to be routinely reconstructed with superior spatial resolution exceeding that of multidetector CT.[15] Indeed, some groups have used angiographic CT, generating cross-sectional CT images from a rotational angiography run using a C-arm-mounted flat-panel detector. The volume set can be processed to generate a 3D angiographic image with CT quality soft tissue imaging that can augment subtle anatomical details and also be used as a 3D overlay on the to guide interventions.[16]

Complex Congenital Interventions

If the last two decades provide any insight into the next generation, a major focus in congenital cardiology will be to deliver less invasive therapy to higher risk patients.[17] Development of more suitable devices and delivery platforms for smaller patients will help counter this risk; however, in marginal cases, optimal outcomes will only be achieved with comprehensive understanding of the anatomy. Understanding how hard the limits of safety can be pushed will be greatly assisted with the use of accurate 3D modeling providing preprocedural simulation. Indeed this approach has already been described in a number of complex interventions such as transverse aortic arch stenting,[18] transcatheter atrial septal defect (ASD) closure in a patient with a deficient posteroinferior rim,[19] and more recently in the context of covered stent implantation to treat patients with a sinus venous ASD.[20] In each instance preprocedural simulation provided confidence to the operator that the approach was feasible and in each example, the actual clinical intervention was successful.

Transcatheter VSD closure is evolving. 3D models have been used to guide postmyocardial infarction VSD closure with good result.[21] In complex VSDs in smaller congenital patients, 3D modeling can also be used to assess optimal approach and deployed device configuration. Recently we encountered an infant with clinical signs of congestive cardiac failure secondary to a large apical muscular VSD. While there may be

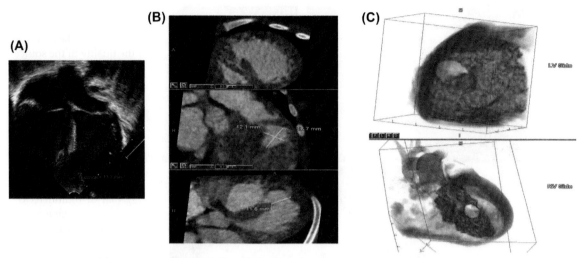

FIG. 4.1 **(A)** Transesophageal echocardiography apical 4-chamber view of the large apical muscular ventricular septal defect (VSD) measuring 13.7 mm. **(B)** Series of CT cuts highlighting the VSD from varying views. **(C)** STL files generated from CT source data.

advantages to a periventricular approach for such defects,[22] in some cases the right ventricular disc may not conform appropriately due to limited space. In the case described, a cardiac CT was performed and an STL file was created to print a 3D model of the heart (Fig. 4.1). The model provided excellent anatomical information regarding the defect and it was clear that the optimal approach to access the defect was from the right atrium as opposed to a direct right periventricular approach (Fig. 4.2). Based on these observations, a hybrid periatrial approach was planned using a 16 mm Amplatzer muscular VSD occluder which had occluded the defect appropriately during the preprocedural simulation (Fig. 4.3). A limited median sternotomy was performed and following placement of a purse-string suture in the right atrium, a 6Fr sheath was placed in the right atrium. The VSD was crossed from the right ventricle and the 16 mm VSD occluder was deployed in a good position with full occlusion of the defect (Fig. 4.4). The procedure time was 45 min.

Preprocedure Patient and Parental Communication and Informed Consent

One further value proposition of bespoke 3D printed models in congenital interventional cardiology includes the capacity to use these models to explain to patients, where old enough, and their parents the strategic plan for a given catheter procedure and intervention. This may give patients and their families further insight into the procedure particularly in situations which are

challenging, e.g., ASD with marginal rims or a malaligned VSD. Biglino et al. reported on the beneficial use of a 3D printed model prior to surgical intervention to communicate with multiple stakeholders, including the surgeon, cardiologist, and family in a complex case of truncus arteriosus.[23] However, others have reported that although there are measured improvements in parental engagement, this is countered by longer clinic times and no measurable improvement in parental understanding of their child's congenital heart lesion.[7] However, we believe that with wider acceptance it is likely that such models may prove helpful in communicating with the catheterization laboratory team the strategic plan for the catheter intervention. The model could be incorporated into the precatheterization pause before the case begins so everyone is aligned in understanding the aim of a particular catheterization procedure (Fig. 4.5).

The Future of 3D Modeling and Congenital Interventions
Computer generated 3D modeling and finite element analysis

Once a 3D model has been reconstructed, there are two possible outputs: the 3D model can be printed or used for a virtual simulation of the outcomes of the percutaneous procedure. Finite element (FE) models may be generated to simulate the structural dynamics of clinically relevant scenarios, including native heart valve biomechanics as well as the effects of surgical or

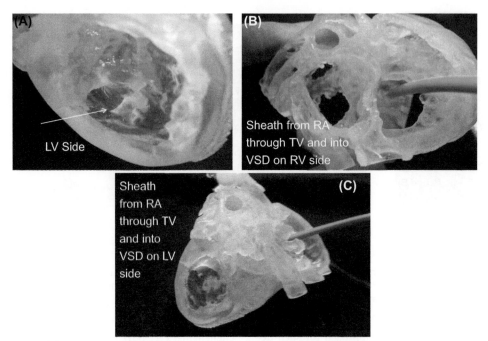

FIG. 4.2 **(A)** 3D printed model demonstrating the ventricular septal defect (VSD) from the left ventricular view. **(B)** 3D printed model simulation with long sheath passed from the right atrium across the VSD. **(C)** 3D printed model simulation demonstrating the delivery sheath form the left ventricular aspect after it has crossed the VSD.

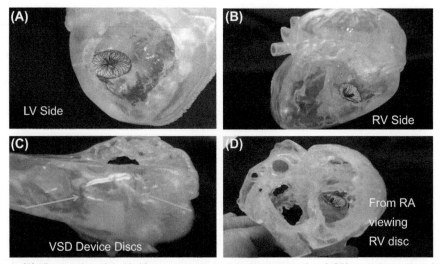

FIG. 4.3 **(A)** 3D printed model with 16 mm muscular ventricular septal defect (VSD) occluder in place from the left ventricular view. **(B)** 3D printed model with 16 mm muscular VSD occluder in place from the right atrial (RV) view. **(C)** 3D printed model with 16 mm muscular VSD occluder in place from the RV free wall. **(D)** 3D printed model with 16 mm muscular VSD occluder in place viewed from the RA.

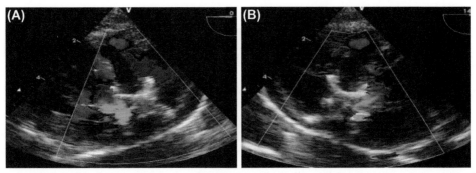

FIG. 4.4 **(A and B)** Transesophageal echocardiography color flow transgastric view of the device across the defect with no residual leak.

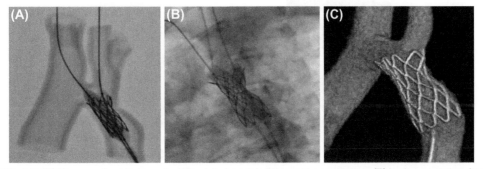

FIG. 4.5 **(A)** Preprocedural tests on the 3D printed model of the aortic coarctation. **(B)** In vivo procedure from the catheterization laboratory. **(C)** Result of aortic coarctation stenting from CT rotational angiography reconstruction.

percutaneous treatments.[24,25] To build up an FE analysis, the reconstructed 3D virtual model is meshed into nodes and elements, and material properties are endowed to each element. By further applying the boundary conditions and mechanical loadings on the corresponding nodes or elements, FE computation of the mechanical stress and strain is possible, thus enabling the prediction of the cardiac structures dynamics. FE modeling has been used to analyze stent fracture phenomena in patients undergoing percutaneous pulmonary valve implantation.[26,27] Advancements in these analyses have recently demonstrated not only the behavior of the stent once implanted but also the patient-specific response to the stenting procedure in terms of potential complications and their clinical implications.[28] In particular, a patient-specific FE framework has been built for patients undergoing attempted percutaneous pulmonary valve implantation due to calcific conduit failure in the right ventricle outflow tract (Fig. 4.6). Balloon angioplasty can be simulated to test the procedure feasibility;

subsequently, prestenting of the outflow tract is performed expanding the stent through a balloon-in-balloon delivery system. In the enrolled patients, simulated results were consistent with intraprocedural in vivo fluoroscopy, and in one patient the FE framework was able to predict the most worrisome complication of coronary compression, which indeed was registered during the balloon testing in vivo.[28]

Bespoke Device Creation

Although the morphology and shape of atrial and VSDs vary from patient to patient, the design of devices is standardized rather than unique to a patient's specific defect size and shape. Some defects may in fact be spherical rather than circular in shape. Additionally, in the instance of ASDs, there may be a deficient rim which is not taken into account by standard device design.[19] Potential future developments could include the generation of an STL file and 3D print of the patient's specific atrial or VSD. Preliminary reports have already been published which support this approach.[29] A bespoke

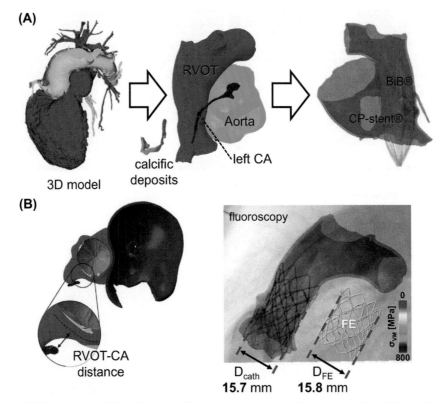

FIG. 4.6 **(A)** Finite element (FE) patient-specific framework to simulate the stenting of a calcific right ventricle outflow tract. **(B)** FE results predicted in a patient successfully submitted to the percutaneous stenting procedure. σ_I, maximum principal stress.

defect occlude could be printed in the catheterization laboratory overnight in preparation for implantation into the patient the following day. Such bespoke devices would truly represent an era of personalized patient-centered medicine.

Stent Printing

Similarly, at the current time stents are standardized in their shape and indeed somewhat limited in the materials used in their manufacture. Many lesions, e.g., pulmonary artery stenosis or coarctation of the aorta for which stents are implanted, are not straight cylindrical structures. Additionally, many vessels which are stented have important side branches, e.g., right upper pulmonary arterial branch or the head and neck vessels arising from the transverse aorta, which are not taken into account during stent design. Potentially in the future bespoke stents could be engineered specific to patients with a lumen within the stent to accommodate the origin of the right upper lobe branch in the right

pulmonary artery or the strap vessels of the aortic arch in transverse arch stenting. Use of resorbable materials (polylactic acid) and other resorbable materials may fashion stents which can be implanted in small children and resorb within 6 months allowing further stent implant when the child is a bigger size. In vivo preclinical testing of 3D-printed polymeric stents has been reported demonstrating favorable mechanical and degradation properties.[29a,b] Specific challenges such as guaranteeing sufficient radial strength particularly in congenital heart lesions remains problematic but should be circumvented with the development of new materials employed in stent design.

Device Creation in Under-resourced Countries

Traditionally devices have been engineered by specific vendors under tight regulatory conditions. Such devices may prove highly expensive and outside the reach of a developing country's budget. In the future it may be possible to significantly underwrite the cost of devices by printing devices locally under guidance of local healthcare authorities. This could prove a new paradigm in making catheterization procedures available to children from resource-depleted countries, including those in the developing world.

Regulation

Current regulatory authorities include the FDA and the European regulatory authority. In order to broaden the capacity to implant 3D printed bespoke devices, much work will need to be completed to ensure safe production, testing, and monitoring of the use of these devices. Collaboration between medical professionals, engineers, and regulatory bodies will be required to bring this vision to realization. Needless to say the juxtaposition of opening therapies for children throughout the world may conflict with loss for revenue for device companies given the costs involved in standard device design.

CONCLUSION

The full potential for 3D modeling in complex congenital interventions is as yet unrealized. Printed models provide the opportunity to simulate the proposed intervention and provide greater confidence of success, with less learning during the case and potentially shorter procedural times. As computerized modeling develops, we may be able to develop a greater understanding of the potential physiological effects of our interventions optimizing flow patterns and minimizing inflammation. Ultimately bespoke 3D printed devices, designed for a patient-specific defect, provide the opportunity for truly personalized medicine; however, navigating the necessary regulatory concerns that such technology will generate will be a challenge. Despite such challenges the potential positive disruptive effect of 3D printing in patients undergoing cardiac catheterization remains exciting.

DISCLOSURE STATEMENT

None.

REFERENCES

1. Farooqi KM, Nielsen JC, Uppu SC, et al. Use of 3-dimensional printing to demonstrate complex intracardiac relationships in double-outlet right ventricle for surgical planning. *Circ Cardiovasc Imaging.* 2015;8(5):e003043.
2. McGovern E, Kelleher E, Snow A, et al. Clinical application of three-dimensional printing to the management of complex univentricular hearts with abnormal systemic or pulmonary venous drainage. *Cardiol Young.* 2017;27(7): 1248−1256.
3. Valverde I, Gomez-Ciriza G, Hussain T, et al. Three-dimensional printed models for surgical planning of complex congenital heart defects: an international multicentre study. *Eur J Cardiothorac Surg.* 2017;52:1139−1148.
4. Batteux C, Haidar MA, Bonnet D. 3D-printed models for surgical planning in complex congenital heart diseases: a systematic review. *Front Pediatr.* 2019;7:23.
5. Costello JP, Olivieri LJ, Krieger A, et al. Utilizing three-dimensional printing technology to assess the feasibility of high-fidelity synthetic ventricular septal defect models for simulation in medical education. *World J Pediatr Congenit Heart Surg.* 2014;5:421−426.
6. Yoo SJ, Spray T, Austin 3rd EH, Yun TJ, van Arsdell GS. Hands-on surgical training of congenital heart surgery using 3-dimensional print models. *J Thorac Cardiovasc Surg.* 2017;153:1530−1540.
7. Biglino G, Capelli C, Wray J, et al. 3D-manufactured patient specific models of congenital heart defects for communication in clinical practice: feasibility and acceptability. *BMJ Open.* 2015, 5e007165.
8. Schievano S, Migliavacca F, Coats L, et al. Percutaneous pulmonary valve implantation based on rapid prototyping of right ventricular outflow tract and pulmonary trunk from MR data. *Radiology.* 2007;242:490−497.
9. Cao QL, Kenny D, Zhou D, et al. Early clinical experience with a novel self-expanding percutaneous stent-valve in the native right ventricular outflow tract. *Cathet Cardiovasc Interv.* 2014;84:1131−1137.
10. Bergersen L, Benson LN, Gillespie MJ, et al. Harmony feasibility trial: acute and short-term outcomes with a self-expanding transcatheter pulmonary valve. *JACC Cardiovasc Interv.* 2017;10:1763−1773.
11. Kim GB, Kwon BS, Lim HG. First in human experience of a new self-expandable percutaneous pulmonary valve implantation using knitted nitinol-wire and tri-leaflet porcine pericardial valve in the native right ventricular outflow tract. *Cathet Cardiovasc Interv.* 2017;89:906−909.
12. Zahn EM, Chang JC, Armer D, Garg R. First human implant of the Alterra Adaptive Present™: a new self-expanding device designed to remodel the right ventricular outflow tract. *Cathet Cardiovasc Interv.* 2018; 91:1125−1129.
13. Gillespie MJ, Benson LN, Bergersen L, et al. Patient selection process for the harmony Transcatheter pulmonary valve early feasibility study. *Am J Cardiol.* 2017;120: 1387−1392.
14. Jolley MA, Lasso A, Nam HH, et al. Toward predictive modeling of catheter-based pulmonary valve replacement into native right ventricular outflow tracts. *Cathet Cardiovasc Interv.* 2019;93:E143−E152.
15. Parimi M, Buelter J, Thanugundla V, et al. Feasibility and validity of printing 3D heart models from rotational angiography. *Pediatr Cardiol.* 2018;39:653−658.
16. Glatz AC, Zhu X, Gillespie MJ, Hanna BD, Rome JJ. Use of angiographic CT imaging in the cardiac catheterization laboratory for congenital heart disease. *JACC Cardiovasc Imaging.* 2010;3:1149−1157.

17. Kenny D, Hijazi ZM. Going beyond the high-risk patient: the new boundaries for transcatheter device focused therapy. *Expert Rev Med Devices*. 2018;15:645–652.

18. Valverde I, Gomez G, Coserria JF, et al. 3D printed models for planning endovascular stenting in transverse aortic arch hypoplasia. *Cathet Cardiovasc Interv*. 2015;85:1006–1012.

19. Chaowu Y, Hua L, Xin S. Three-Dimensional printing as an aid in transcatheter closure of secundum atrial septal defect with rim deficiency: in vitro trial occlusion based on a personalized heart model. *Circulation*. 2016;133:e608–e610.

20. Velasco Forte MN, Byrne N, Valverde I, et al. Interventional correction of sinus venosus atrial septal defect and partial anomalous pulmonary venous drainage: procedural planning using 3D printed models. *JACC Cardiovasc Imaging*. 2018;11(2 Pt 1):275–278.

21. Lazkani M, Bashir F, Brady K, Pophal S, Morris M, Pershad A. Postinfarct VSD management using 3D computer printing assisted percutaneous closure. *Indian Heart J*. 2015;67:581–585.

22. Gray R, Menon S, Johnson J, et al. Acute and mid-term results following perventricular device closure of muscular ventricular septal defects: a multicenter PICES investigation. *Cathet Cardiovasc Interv*. 2017;90:281–289.

23. Biglino G, Moharem-Elgamal S, Lee M, Tulloh R, Caputo M. The perception of a three-dimensional model from the perspective of different stakeholders: a complex case of truncus arteriosus. *Front Pediatr*. 2017;5:209.

24. Sturla F, Vismara R, Jaworek M, et al. In vitro and in silico approaches to quantify the effects of the Mitraclips system on mitral valve function. *J Biomech*. 2017;50:83–92.

25. Sturla F, Ronzoni M, Vitali M, et al. Impact of different aortic valve calcification patterns on the outcome of transcatheter aortic valve implantation: a finite element study. *J Biomech*. 2016;49:2520–2530.

26. Cosentino D, Quail MA, Pennati G, et al. Geometrical and stress analysis of factors associated with stent fracture after Melody percutaneous pulmonary valve implantation. *Circ Cardiovasc Interv*. 2014;7:510–517.

27. Schievano S, Taylor AM, Capelli C, et al. Patient specific finite element analysis results in more accurate prediction of stent fractures: application to percutaneous pulmonary valve implantation. *J Biomech*. 2010;43:687–693.

28. Caimi A, Sturla F, Pluchinotta FR, et al. Prediction of stenting related adverse events through patient-specific finite element modelling. *J Biomech*. 2018;79:135–146.

29. a Sun Y, Zhang X, Li W, Di Y, Xing Q, Cao Q. 3D printing and biocompatibility study of a new biodegradable occluder for cardiac defect. *J Cardiol*. 2019.b Zhang Y, Zhao J, Yang G, et al. Mechanical properties and degradation of drug eluted bioresorbable vascular scaffolds prepared by three-dimensional printing technology. *J Biomater Sci Polym Ed*. 2019:1–14.

CHAPTER 5

Instructional Case Examples Utilizing Three-Dimensional Modeling in Congenital Heart Disease

SANJAY SINHA, MD

KEY POINTS

1. 3-Dimensional (3D) reconstruction is becoming a mainstay for preprocedural planning.
2. The 3D modeling can be accomplished using any Cartesian dataset (MRI, CT, 3D Echocardiography) as well as with reconstruction using rotational angiography in the catheterization lab.
3. For complex procedures, incorporation of 3D reconstruction, 3D printing, and bench testing using a 1:1 3D model is a useful tool.
4. Further studies are needed to assess the efficacy of the 3D modeling and printing on clinical practice and outcomes.

INTRODUCTION

The use of two-dimensional (2D) and then three-dimensional (3D) cross-sectional imaging has developed significantly in the last 10 years, and even more so in the last 5 years.[1−3] Most picture archiving and communication systems software packages utilized by hospitals throughout the world offer the ability to reconstruct cross-sectional CT, and MRI data into a 3D dataset. Moreover, these modalities can now be transformed into a physical 3D printed model with which to better understand patient's anatomy. The following represent selected cases that highlight the utility of each 3D modeling modality.

Dynamic 3D Modeling with Cardiac MRI in Infants

In addition to requiring ionizing radiation (albeit, ever increasingly lower dosages), one of the most significant limitations of CT angiographic technology is the need for a low heart rate to fully visualize small structures.[4] Patients with complex congenital heart disease are at increased risks when subjected to multiple CT scan/catheterizations over a lifetime due to a cumulative risk that can accrue an exposure of 20 mS V by adolescence.[5,6] Advances in MRI technology along with the development of longer half-life contrast media such as ferumoxytol (Feraheme, AMAG Pharmaceuticals, Waltham, MA) can provide high-quality information in a neonate in whom normal heart rates are >100 bpm without the need for ionizing radiation.[7,8] Feraheme provides a prolonged blood pool phase and with concurrent use of four-dimensional, multiphase, steady-state imaging with contrast enhancement (MUSIC), the study can achieve a temporal resolution of 65−95 ms, as well as an extremely high spatial resolution of 0.6−0.9 mm isotropic.[9,10] This results in better definition of tiny structures in an infant such as coronary arterial anatomy, hypoplastic structures vessels, and vessels with minimal flow.[11]

CASE 1

A term infant was born with a prenatal diagnosis of complex single ventricle consisting of double outlet right ventricle, left ventricular hypoplasia, pulmonary atresia, severe mitral valve hypoplasia, 3:2 heart block, and likely heterotaxy polysplenia syndrome. After birth, a neonatal echocardiogram was unable to definitively determine the atrial and ventricular morphology, as well as the complete segmental anatomy. Moreover, there was an inability to assess the status of the ductus arteriosus secondary to the complex arterial outlet anatomy. Before planning appropriate treatment, questions regarding the viability of ductal stenting and pacemaker placement needed to be answered. It was felt that a CT scan with this infant's heart-rate variability and elevated heart rate (despite the conduction delay was still 80–100 bpm) would be suboptimal. Thus, a Feraheme cardiac MRI with MUSIC cardiovascular imaging was conducted on a Siemens TIM Trio 3.0T MR scanner, utilizing general anesthesia with controlled ventilation. For optimal vascular visualization, vascular enhancement was achieved via administration of ferumoxytol 4 mg/kg, high resolution 4D MUSIC sequence and HASTE sequences of the cardiovascular structures were obtained, in addition to 4D-flow imaging, during uninterrupted positive pressure ventilation. Postprocessing included reconstruction of multiplanar images, Maximum Intensity projection (MIP) images and creation of 3D volume rendered images utilizing dedicated software (Osirix, **company name and location** and Vitrea, **company name and location**) as well as flow analysis (Arterys platform, **company name and location**). Utilizing the pooled Feraheme contrast, the entirety of the anatomy could be clearly demonstrated in both still and dynamic images (Fig. 5.1). The use of 3D imaging clearly defined this infant's complex anatomy that comprised I,L,L segmental anatomy, ventricular inversion, tricuspid valve hypoplasia, near pulmonary atresia, a large window-type ductus arteriosus, and left ventricular (LV) noncompaction. Furthermore, the level of anatomic detail produced by this study provided the entire heart team with a common understanding of this infant's quite complex anatomy making treatment decisions relatively straightforward that included surgical placement of a dual chamber biventricular pacemaker and placement of a 3.5 mm central shunt.

3D Rotational Angiography

At times, anatomical questions and concerns arise during evaluation of a patient who is already in the catheterization lab. The ability to perform a 3D anatomic evaluation in this setting, in addition to traditional biplane angiography, can be done using three-dimensional rotational angiography (3DRA). The hardware and software required to accomplish this is available on most standard cardiac catheterization lab imaging suites.[12] Typically an angiographic catheter is

positioned before or "upstream" from the area of interest. A timed injection of usually 50%–70% contrast is set up using the anteroposterior (AP) camera alone. The 3D acquisition protocol requires an automated 180–190° rotational cine acquisition, coupled with a synchronized contrast injection performed over a 5–6 s period. Typically, respirations are held and rapid ventricular pacing may be utilized to maximize opacification of the desired structures during rotational acquisition. The acquired dataset is typically available for postprocessing in <1 min on a dedicated workstation within the catheterization suite. Postprocessed images

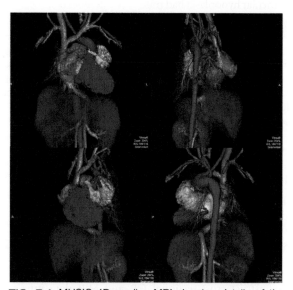

FIG. 5.1 MUSIC 4D cardiac MRI showing details of the complex anatomy (Video). There is a single dilated monoatrium that received both systemic and pulmonary venous return without an appreciable interatrial septum. There is ventricular inversion with a dilated, noncompacted right-sided morphologic left ventricle and a hypoplastic left-sided morphologic right ventricle. There was, in fact, a hypoplastic left-sided tricuspid valve, a severely hypoplastic trileaflet pulmonic valve with the pulmonary arterial supply augmented by a large ductus arteriosus inserting at the level of the bifurcation of the left and right pulmonary arteries. The aortic arch yields three branch vessels, with the right subclavian artery being without a visible connection to the aortic arch, but is patent distally, and is likely supplied by collateral flow, possibly from the right vertebral, Multiple small spleens in the right-upper quadrant, centralized transverse liver and right-sided stomach. There were duplicated abdominal IVCs that join just posterior to the liver. A right hepatic vein drains directly into the monoatrium in parallel to the hepatic IVC that receives venous return from the remaining hepatic veins.

have many of the qualities of other cardiac 3D static multiplanar images such as MRI or CT. 3DRA allows for better understanding of complex cardiac anatomy both before as well as after performance of a given transcatheter intervention. In addition, utilization of 3DRA imaging may allow for completion of catheter-based congenital interventions in a faster and safer timeframe with less radiation exposure[13-15].

CASE 2

A 14-year-old female with a diagnosis of pulmonary valve atresia and an intact ventricular septum and right ventricular hypoplasia had previously underwent a surgical pulmonary valvotomy and right ventricular outflow tract (RVOT) patch as well as modified Blalock-Taussig shunt in the new born period. At 1-year old, she underwent coil embolization of the shunt. At 13 years old she demonstrated progressively worsening pulmonary valve insufficiency, and was put forward for a transcatheter Melody valve (Medtronic, Minneapolis MN) placement. During that catheterization, the RVOT was deemed too large to undergo safe implantation of a Melody valve (which has an outer diameter of 24 mm) and she was deferred for a later attempt at Sapien valve implantation into her RVOT (which has an outer diameter as high as 31 mm). Her echocardiogram before the procedure demonstrated severe pulmonary insufficiency, no RVOT obstruction, dilation of the main and branch pulmonary arteries, and right atrial and RV dilation. She underwent a diagnostic catheterization and static balloon sizing of the RVOT using a 30 mm PTS-X balloon catheter (NuMED Inc., Hopkinton, NY, USA). Coronary compression testing was negative. The RVOT measured 27 mm using this technique, and a 29-mm Sapien XT valve was implanted in the pulmonic position. The valve was stable, and repeat angiography of the pulmonary artery (PA) showed a satisfactory result. An aortic angiogram demonstrated no aortic insufficiency with brisk filling of the coronary arteries; however, there was some concern that the Sapien valve could be impinging upon the ascending aortic lumen. Standard biplane angiography showed only a mild deformation of the ascending aorta. Given the clinical suspicion of aortic compression, a decision was made to proceed with 3DRA of aorta. This imaging modality quite clearly demonstrated severe compression of the ascending aorta from the distal struts of the Sapien valve frame (Fig. 5.2). Although the patient was asymptomatic, based on these images and a concern for possible future aortic erosion

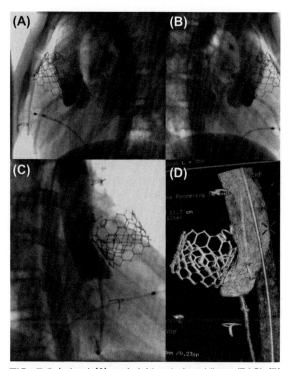

FIG. 5.2 Lateral **(A)** and right anterior oblique (RAO) **(B)** projection of the Sapien XT valve in the pulmonary position after deployment with simultaneous angiography in the ascending aorta with no evidence of significant aortic distortion. **(C)** Still image of a 3D reconstructed aortogram clearly showing a significant indentation of the superior portion of the valve frame into the ascending aorta.

secondary to the location of the Sapien valve, the patient was sent to surgery for device removal and surgical pulmonary valve replacement.

3D Overlay

The risk of contrast-induced nephropathy secondary to the use of iodinated contrast in the cath lab is an added risk to these procedures.[6,16] Moreover, there are often times when anatomic structures that are not radiopaque but influence the positioning of a device, valve, or balloon, for example, cannot be seen in real time during the deployment. The recent ability to overlay previously acquired advanced cross-sectional images over simple two-dimensional real-time fluoroscopic images has a number of distinct advantages that translate to the performance of several complex transcatheter interventions in a safe and clearer way.

CASE 3

A 50-year-old male with a history of repaired tetralogy of Fallot (TOF) presented at cardiac catheterization for placement of a transcatheter Melody valve. His initial management consisted of a Pott's shunt at age 4 and subsequent intracardiac repair at age 16 with ventricular septal defect (VSD) closure and transannular patch repair of his RVOT. In 1998, he underwent take down of a residual Pott's shunt, correction of a residual VSD, Maze procedure, and placement of a 29-mm Carpentier-Edwards in the pulmonary position (Edwards Lifesciences, Irvine CA). His most recent echocardiogram showed moderate pulmonary valve stenosis, pulmonary valve regurgitation, and a persistent small VSD patch leak. Previously, he was diagnosed with a large left pulmonary artery embolism and was maintained on warfarin. He was also known to have severe baseline renal insufficiency. In this complex patient with significant comorbidities, the decision was made to utilize 3D overlay imaging, primarily to decrease the quantity of contrast required in the hopes of preserving his renal function. Thus, before cardiac catheterization, an ECG-gated cardiac CT scan was performed on a Siemens sensation 16 multidetector scanner with non-contrast images, followed by a single vascular sequence. Multiplanar reformations were obtained, and these 3D acquisitions were loaded on to the catheterization laboratory imaging system using AW Volume Share software (GE Healthcare Systems, Chicago, IL). The images were aligned or registered to the patient's bony structures as well as this bioprosthetic valve. By registering the previously acquired 3D CT cross-sectional images, the 3D on the catheterization monitors appropriately and accurately move as the gantry angulation is adjusted throughout the case. Use of 3D overlay technology allowed for precise Melody valve implantation while limiting the amount of contrast this patient revived (Fig. 5.3). This may be even helpful when attempting transcatheter valve deployment in more complex RVOT such as those patients who present without a defined landing zone (Fig. 5.4).

3D Modeling and Rapid Prototyping

As noted in preceding chapters, the creation and availability of patient-specific 3D models are increasingly accessible with the advent of commercially available rapid prototyping printers.[17] The ability to take cross-sectional imaging of anatomical structures and convert them from a Cartesian model (datasets with an x, y, and z plane) to a physical model, has allowed for the interface of medical imaging and 3D printing to be a notable disruptive technology in the field of congenital heart disease.[17,18] Current high-fidelity 3D printers, allow the models to come within 0.07 mm of the true anatomy.[19] Moreover, new polymers or "inks" are constantly being developed and tested such that practitioners can select specific thickness and compliance qualities in their models to best approximate, for

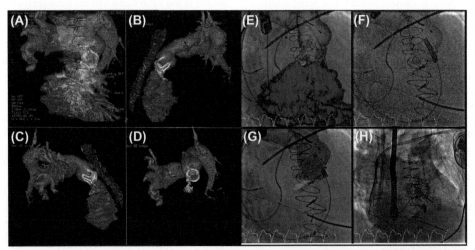

FIG. 5.3 Overlay of previously acquired CT images on the live fluoroscopy of a patient undergoing a Melody valve placement. The CT 3D reconstruction shows the AP **(A)**, lateral **(B)**, RAO **(C)** views with the sternal wires in preparation for anatomical registration. The RV is removed for a clear guide during valve placement **(D)**. Sternal wires as well as the bioprosthetic valve (BPV) act to register the CT images to the live screen and can be edited to include the RV **(E)**, reveal only the BPV and PA's **(F)**. The previously placed surgical bioprosthetic valve was able to be colorized blue **(G)** to ensure perfect alignment of the valve during deployment **(H)**.

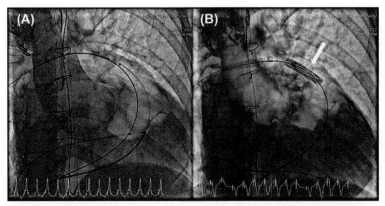

FIG. 5.4 Overlay is even more essential when there is a paucity of anatomical landmarks in the chest to guide the intervention such as this patient with a native pulmonary artery as a landing zone, dilated ascending aorta, and a dynamic narrowing (systolic image **A**). The valve is aligned **(B)** using overlay and markers indicating the branch point of the pulmonary arteries (asterisk) and the anatomical narrowing confirmed during previous injection (arrow).

example, human arterial tissues properties (Young's modulus between 0.2 and 9 MPa; pliability between 1.2×10^{-3} and 6.6×10^{-3} mmHg) with high fidelity.[20]

CASE 4

A 65-year-old 62 kg gentleman with a past medical history of Tetralogy of Fallot presented after a 20-year gap in care to reestablish care. He had a complete intracardiac repair at 5 years old that involved VSD patch closure and treatment of RVOT obstruction using a transannular patch technique. He presented with symptomatic exercise intolerance and was assessed as New York Heart Association Class II. His most recent echocardiogram showed severe pulmonary regurgitation, moderate right ventricular dilation, no pulmonary valvular stenosis, and mild tricuspid valve regurgitation. A cardiac MRI showed a right ventricular end-diastolic volume indexed (RVEDVi) of 155 mL/m^2, right ventricular end-systolic volume indexed of 55 mL/m^2, a pulmonary regurgitant fraction of 50%, with a large dynamic RVOT measuring in some dimensions in systole in excess of 30 mm. The patient was felt to be a poor candidate for commercially available balloon expandable transcatheter valves and refused surgery. He was therefore entered into the US Multicentered Harmony Valve (Medtronic, Minneapolis, MN) Pivotal Clinical trial.

The Harmony valve is a self-expanding transcatheter valve developed to treat patients with a dysfunctional RVOT that is too large for conventional transcatheter

balloon expandable valve therapy. The screening process used to access anatomic suitability for this valve integrates multiple 3D-dimensional modeling modalities. After being enrolled, this patient underwent an ECG-gated cardiac CT scan (0.3 mm slice thickness) with phase acquisition targeted in peak systole and diastole (30% and 70% of the R−R interval by ECG). Using commercially available software, the RV, RVOT, and proximal branch pulmonary arteries were reconstructed in both a systolic and diastolic model. The perimeters and circumferences of the RVOT in these models at multiple levels were determined and used to assess the degree of tissue interaction, or interference, the valve would have when fully expanded within this patient's specific unique anatomy (Fig. 5.5). The blood pool of these two models was then segmented and converted to a standard triangle language (STL) file using Mimics software (Materialize, NV Belgium) and together with a scanned virtual model of the Harmony valve stent frame, practitioners were able to visualize a virtual implant (Fig. 5.6C and D). The systolic and diastolic models were then 3D printed using a hard cast stereolithographic (SLA) material at which point a Harmony valve could be implanted into each model to assess how it would interact with the RVOT anatomy in both systole and diastole (Fig. 5.6E). Based upon this advanced 3D-imaging assessment, the patient underwent successful transcatheter placement of a Harmony valve with complete resolution of his pulmonary valvular regurgitation (Fig. 5.6F).

The meticulous 3D modeling screening process for this valve allows for the practitioner to have a complete

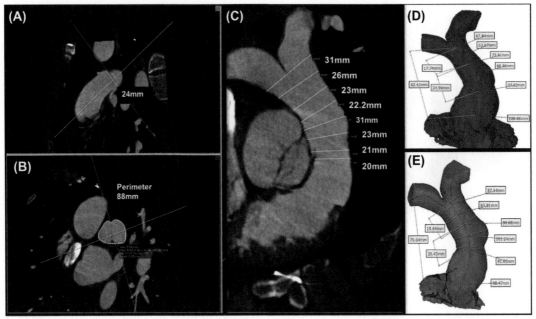

FIG. 5.5 Multiplanar reconstruction (MPR) in the sagittal **(A)**, axial **(B)**, and modified RVOT view **(C)** illustrating the multiple measurements taken along the RVOT. A virtual model in diastole **(D)** and systole **(E)** is then created with perimeter measurements made along the landing zone.

understanding of the patient's RVOT anatomy, with tactile insight into the behavior of the valve following deployment. By the time patient is on the table and ready for the implant, the practitioner has practiced multiple times on the model, and the addition of muscle memory and hands on manipulation within the printed physical model provide the operator with a more complete understanding of the device—"tissue" interaction and added comfort with the procedure. We believe that this will play an ever-increasingly important role, as device technology continues to advance and devices become increasingly complex.

CASE 5

A 17-year-old female with a history of fibromuscular dysplasia (FMD) presented initially with headaches and presyncope. A subsequent workup including brain MRI demonstrated absence of the left internal carotid artery, and Ct angiography of the chest revealed a right aortic arch with an aberrant left subclavian artery. The aortic arch and proximal descending aorta were diffusely abnormal with multiple small aneurysms and membranes consistent with FMD.

It was thought that these aneurysms posed a lifetime risk of progressive enlargement and possible rupture,

prompting a decision to pursue transcatheter exclusion of these aneurysms. Given the complexity and uniqueness of the underlying anatomy, a 3D reconstruction was created based upon CT data. The CT data were segmented to an STL file, and printed as a 3D model using hard plastic SLA material (Materialize, NV Belgium) (Fig. 5.7). A simulated procedure was performed placing three telescoping covered Cheatham Platinum stents (NuMED Inc., Hopkinton, NY, USA) across the area using a "retrograde approach." Use of the physical model in this case allowed for the operators to approximate the number of stents required as well as to precisely gauge their positioning to avoid impingement upon the aberrant subclavian or spinal arteries while completely excluding the effected aorta (Fig. 5.8). The patient subsequently underwent this procedure in the exact fashion as tested in the model and had successful complete exclusion of the multilobulated aneurysmal complex without evidence of residual flow into aneurysm (Fig. 5.8).

CASE 6

A 1-year-old boy with a prenatal diagnosis of dextrocardia, double outlet right ventricle with dextro-malposed vessels, as well as a mildly unbalanced atria-ventricular

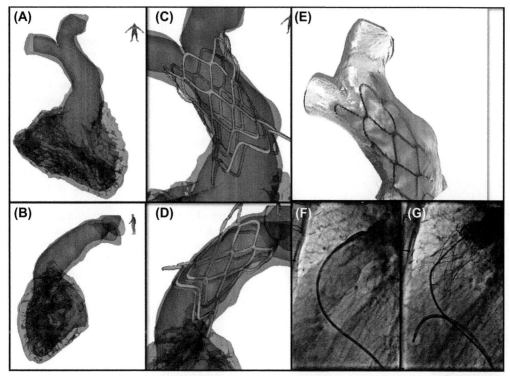

FIG. 5.6 Simultaneous systolic and diastolic model in an RVOT angulation **(A)** and lateral projection **(B)**. The virtual stent frame of the Harmony valve is then placed in the ideal landing zone to visualize the positioning **(C, D)**, and then a physical stent frame is deployed in the an SLE model in both diastole (not shown) and systole **(E)**. The valve was then placed percutaneously in the patient with a large native RVOT **(F)** in perfect position with no regurgitation **(G)**.

canal defect and moderate pulmonary valve stenosis was presented for a potential biventricular repair. The patient's echocardiogram demonstrated much of the anatomy well; however, based solely upon this imaging alone, the distance from the left ventricle to the aortic valve and the three-dimensional nature of the VSD, two elements critical to successful surgical repair, were unclear. A cardiac MRI was performed as described previously, from which a dataset was segmented and a model was created (Mimics software, Materialize, NV Belgium). The model was transected along the axial plane with isolation and colorization of the AV valve, and aortic valve to gain a clearer understanding of the interface between the VSD/LV/Aortic valve (Fig. 5.9). Using this technology, it became clear that any VSD patch would have to traverse a significant distance within the heart and result in important encroachment upon both the right atrioventricular valve as well as the right ventricle. With this enhanced knowledge, this patient was referred for a single ventricle palliation. The

ability to create transection planes along any access using these advanced imaging and processing techniques assists the heart team in making more accurate complex decision-making in settings such as these which are not uncommon in congenital heart disease.

CASE 7

A 62-year-old male presented with a history of an unrepaired partial anomalous pulmonary venous return and a sinus venosus atrial septal defect (ASD). The patient underwent an ECG-gated CT scan that confirmed the diagnosis of a persistent sinus venosus ASD with anomalous pulmonary venous return of the right-upper and right-middle veins draining directly into superior vena cava (SVC); however, the patient was unwilling to undergo surgical repair. A 3D SLA model was printed with a 2.5-mm thickness and soft compliant material to emulate the venous structures. Utilizing this physical model, the feasibility of transcatheter exclusion of the pulmonary veins from the systemic venous return as well as closure of the ASD using a large covered stent could be demonstrated (Fig. 5.10).

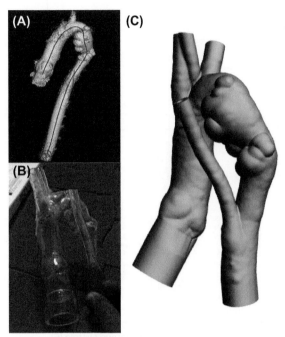

FIG. 5.7 3D reconstruction from a CTA showing the dilated aneurysms and anatomy of the thoracic aorta in this patient with FMG **(A)**. This CT data are then used to reconstruct the virtual model **(C)** and print a hard plastic SLA model **(B)**. The aneurysms, as well as the proximity to the aberrant subclavian vessel, are clearly seen.

This particular model was printed such that the ostium of the anomalous pulmonary veins as well as the borders of the sinus venosus defect was colorized. After some practice, a large covered Cheatham Platinum (CP) stent (NuMED Inc., Hopkinton, NY, USA) was able to be deployed into the precise location within the SVC resulting in baffling of SVC flow into the right atrium while simultaneously excluding the anomalous pulmonary venous flow across the sinus venous ASD into the left atrium.

The patient subsequently underwent uncomplicated placement of the covered stent CP stent utilizing an anchoring open cell stent in the manner described earlier resulting in (Fig. 5.11) elimination of the left to right shunt and successful baffling of the SVC flow to the RA without and obstruction of the anomalous veins as they entered into the left atrium. 3D models and bench testing such as this was essential in preprocedural planning, particularly when there is a possibility of occluding adjacent structures, causing obstruction with covered stents, or when attempting to understand the size of a communication/defect being closed (Fig. 5.12).

CONCLUSION

It is clear that 3D modeling techniques are being used in an increasingly wide variety of ways to improve the understanding of complex congenital and postsurgical anatomy as well as for improved surgical and interventional procedural decision-making and planning. As noted in previous chapters, virtual modeling and rapid prototyping technology were developed outside of the

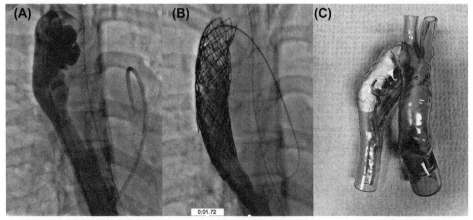

FIG. 5.8 Aortic angiogram at the level of the aneurysms in a patient with FMD **(A)**, and after exclusion using covered stents **(B)**. The deployment was conducted in the exact same fashion as performed on the SLA model **(C)**.

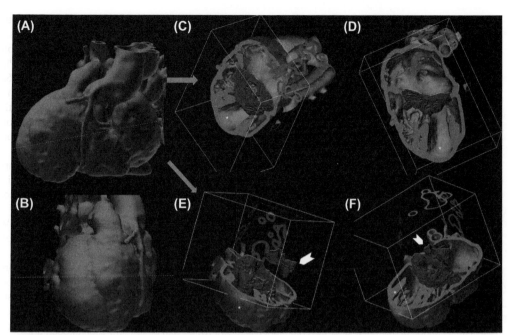

FIG. 5.9 3D model of a patient with complex DORV anatomy **(A, B)** with a slice along the axial plan (dotted line). The superior portion **(C, D)** shows the relative size of the RV to the LV (asterisk) and the AV valve (blue). The inferior portion **(E, F)** is segmented to show the distance between the LV and the aortic valve (arrowhead).

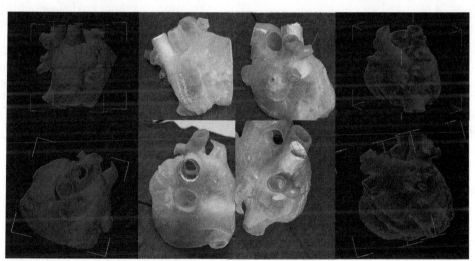

FIG. 5.10 Multiple views of the 3D virtual model and the soft polymer SLA model showing a patient with PAPVR (pink coloration) with a 10 Zig covered CP stent placed in the SVC, excluding the pulmonary veins to the LA.

medical field and only relatively recently adopted into practice within congenital heart disease.[21] The power of these modalities has been realized and companies entirely dedicated to medical modeling have begun to burgeon in this potential market, and the potential of

3D modeling and printing rests in the fact that the technology is rapidly evolving. Companies have begun to incorporate virtual or augmented reality technology, tactile simulators to replicate a virtual operating room for surgeons, and even cellular bioprinting.[22-25] This

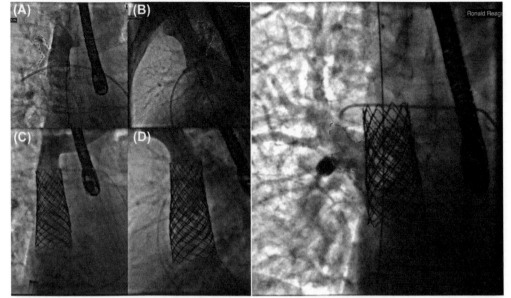

FIG. 5.11 Angiogram in the SVC showing some reflux of contrast into the anomalous pulmonary veins **(A, B)**. There is no evidence of this reflux after covered stent placement **(C, D)** with patent flow seen through the anomalous veins in levophase to the LA.

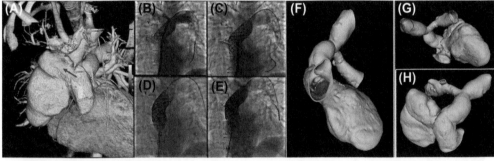

FIG. 5.12 Covered stent placement in the RVOT of a patient with a large pseudoaneurysm of the MPA. Although a 3D reconstruction was done after the case **(A)**, 3D modeling was not used and several stents had to be placed **(B–D)** before sealing the leak (red arrow). 3D modeling of the RVOT revealed the exact size and shape of the mouth of the aneurysm (red, **E–F**).

results in higher fidelity modeling with 3D prints approaching exact tissue characteristics, the ability to print living tissue, and to model procedures in an exact fashion before performing them on patient.

DISCLOSURE STATEMENT

None.

REFERENCES

1. Heintzen P, Adam WE. History of cardiovascular imaging procedures (as developed and/or applied in German cardiology). *Z Kardiol.* 2002;91(Suppl 4):64–73.
2. De roos A, Higgins CB. Cardiac radiology: centenary review. *Radiology.* 2014;273(2 Suppl):S142–S159.
3. Burchill LJ, Huang J, Tretter JT, et al. Noninvasive imaging in adult congenital heart disease. *Circ Res.* 2017;120(6): 995–1014.
4. Kanie Y, Sato S, Tada A, Kanazawa S. Image quality of coronary arteries on non-electrocardiography-gated high-pitch dual-source computed tomography in children with congenital heart disease. *Pediatr Cardiol.* 2017; 38(7):1393–1399.
5. Han BK, Lindberg J, Grant K, Schwartz RS, Lesser JR. Accuracy and safety of high pitch computed tomography imaging in young children with complex congenital heart disease. *Am J Cardiol.* 2011;107(10):1541–1546.
6. Andreassi MG. Radiation risk from pediatric cardiac catheterization: friendly fire on children with congenital heart disease. *Circulation.* 2009;120(19):1847–1849.
7. Lai LM, Cheng JY, Alley MT, Zhang T, Lustig M, Vasanawala SS. Feasibility of ferumoxytol-enhanced neonatal and young infant cardiac MRI without general anesthesia. *J Magn Reson Imaging.* 2017;45(5):1407–1418.
8. Rangamani S, Varghese J, Li L, et al. Safety of cardiac magnetic resonance and contrast angiography for neonates and small infants: a 10-year single-institution experience. *Pediatr Radiol.* 2012;42:1339–1346.
9. Zhou Z, Han F, Yoshida T, Nguyen KL, Finn JP, Hu P. Improved 4D cardiac functional assessment for pediatric patients using motion-weighted image reconstruction. *Magma.* 2018;31(6):747–756.
10. Zhou Z, Han F, Rapacchi S, et al. Accelerated ferumoxytol-enhanced 4D multiphase, steady-state imaging with contrast enhancement (MUSIC) cardiovascular MRI: validation in pediatric congenital heart disease. *NMR Biomed.* 2017;30(1).
11. Han F, Zhou Z, Han E, et al. Self-gated 4D multiphase, steady-state imaging with contrast enhancement (MUSIC) using rotating cartesian K-space (ROCK): validation in children with congenital heart disease. *Magn Reson Med.* 2017;78(2):472–483.
12. Van der stelt F, Siegerink SN, Krings GJ, Molenschot MMC, Breur JMPJ. Three-dimensional rotational angiography in pediatric patients with congenital heart disease: a literature review. *Pediatr Cardiol.* 2019;40(2):257–264.
13. Glockler M, Halbfabeta J, Koch A, Achenbach S, Dittrich S. Multimodality 3D-roadmap for cardiovascular interventions in congenital heart disease—a single-center, retrospective analysis of 78 cases. *Cathet Cardiovasc Interv.* 2013;82:436–442. https://doi.org/10.1002/ccd.24646.
14. Goreczny S, Morgan GJ, Dryzek P, Mo Initial experience with live three-dimens lay for ductal stenting in hypoplastic lef *EuroIntervention.* 2016;12:1527–1533. F 4244/EIJ-D-15-00101.
15. Nguyen HH, Balzer DT, Murphy Shahanavaz S. Radiation exposure by rotational angiography (3DRA) during t ody pulmonary valve procedures (TMF cardiac catheterization laboratory. *Pedi* 37:1429–1435.
16. Prasad A. Acute kidney injury following tration in pediatric congenital heart dis to move beyond the serum creatinine. *Interv.* 2014;84(4):620–621.
17. Shin J, Truong QA. Manufacturing b cardiovascular intervention: 3D printi tice today. *Curr Treat Options Cardi* 20(12):95.
18. Anwar S, Singh GK, Miller J, et al. 3D pr mative technology in congenital heart c *Transl Sci.* 2018;3(2):294–312.
19. Farooqi KM, ed. *Rapid Prototyping in Car* Switzerland: Springer International Pul
20. Sinha S, Aboulhosn J, Levi DS. Transc valve replacement in congenital heart *diol Clin.* 2019;8(1):59–71.
21. Garner K, Singla DK. 3D modeling: a fu lar medicine. *Can J Physiol Pharmacol.* 20
22. De paolis LT, De luca V. Augmented depth perception cues to improve th mance in minimally invasive surgery. *M* 2018;57(5):995–1013.
23. Grant EK, Olivieri LJ. The role of 3-D he ning and executing interventional pro *diol.* 2017;33(9):1074–1081.
24. Tandon A, Burkhardt BEU, Batsis M, e defects: anatomic variants and transca bility using virtual reality planning. *JAC* *ing.* 2018;12(5):921–924.
25. Ong CS, Krishnan A, Huang CY, et al. R in congenital heart disease. *Congenit He* 357–361.

CHAPTER 6

Is There Role for 3D Modeling in Planning Acquired Heart Disease Surgery?

ANDREAS A. GIANNOPOULOS, MD, PHD • RONNY R. BUECHEL, MD • AHMED OUDA, MD • DIMITRIS MITSOURAS, PHD

Cardiovascular surgery has closely followed the cardiac intervention field, transforming substantially over the last two decades.[1] Minimally invasive surgical procedures are increasingly replacing more traditional surgical approaches across nearly the entire spectrum of acquired heart disease.[2] Although technically more challenging, such novel surgical approaches offer reduced morbidity, faster recovery, shorter hospital stay, and decreased costs.[3] Transcatheter management of valve diseases, for example transcatheter aortic valve replacement (TAVR), MitraClip for mitral valve replacement, and percutaneous approaches for occlusion of septal (atrial and ventricular) defects and the left atrial appendage are quickly replacing open-heart surgeries in a significant proportion of appropriately selected patients. Similarly, minimally invasive coronary artery bypass surgery and hybrid coronary revascularization approaches have also been introduced. A common theme across these interventions is that they necessitate collaborative work with interventional cardiologists in hybrid operating suites or even utilization of surgical robots (such as the DaVinci Robotic Surgical System).[4]

This paradigm shift in cardiac surgery has blurred the lines between interventional cardiologists and cardiac surgeons. Today, Heart Teams incorporating surgeons, cardiologists, and cardiovascular imagers represent a critical part of the management of cardiac surgery patients. The contribution of imagers is substantial given the importance of pre- and perioperative imaging. In this landscape, cardiovascular three-dimensional (3D) printing, or more accurately, rapid prototyping, has recently been brought to clinical practice as an adjunct to standard imaging, enhancing the horizons of preoperative planning in acquired heart disease surgery. Interestingly, as noted previously, some 3D printing technologies that are actively used in this setting today have existed for more than 30 years. Nonetheless, utilization of this technology in cardiovascular medicine can still be considered to be at its infancy, and many exciting opportunities exist that have not yet been exploited.

Most clinical cardiovascular 3D printing to date has been in the field of congenital heart diseases (CHDs), for both pediatric as well as adult patients. This is presented in detail in other chapters in this book. In the surgical treatment of acquired heart disease, it is only recently that 3D printing has started moving from niche applications to more standardized implementation. In particular, diagnosis, planning, and simulation of surgical operations and interventions in acquired heart disease patients have been shown to benefit from the advanced imaging insight and tactile feedback that can be provided by printed models. These models improve understanding of patient-specific anatomical relationships and allow for highly individualized surgical management to be planned well in advance of the patient entering the operating room.

The imaging utilized in 3D printing for cardiac surgical planning is high-resolution cross-sectional imaging, primarily computed tomography (CT), and magnetic resonance imaging (MRI). Increasingly, modeling with the use of echocardiography is also being reported for appropriate indications. When considering construction of a 3D-printed model for an individual patient with acquired heart disease, careful planning of both imaging modality type as well as the parameters used for raw image data acquisition can significantly help increase the accuracy and ease of generating and interpreting the printed model. For example, CT allows for superior visualization of extracardiac structures, MRI provides for a more detailed evaluation of myocardial architecture, while echocardiography (transthoracic or transesophageal) enhances the creation of models that will clearly convey the valvular structures and their functional relationships. Thus, a model requested for planning a complex transcatheter mitral valve replacement might benefit from fusing a CT from which a highly accurate model of the entire ventricular cavity can be created, in conjunction with a transesophageal echocardiogram (TEE) study from which a precise model of the valve can be created, and fusing the corresponding models to produce a combined model.[5]

This chapter describes the current clinical application and the role of cardiovascular 3D printing in the planning of cardiac surgery for treatment of acquired heart disease and the future directions of the field. Their wide spectrum and the need for optimization of interventions to treat acquired heart disease render 3D printing a potential game-changer for patient-specific preoperational/interventional assessment.

VALVES

Rapid prototyping of valvular pathologies has become particularly attractive in recent years with applications evolving mainly around aortic and mitral valve disorders. The atrioventricular valves have complex anatomic relationships pertinent to surgical/interventional management including the mitral annular area, the aortic—mitral angle, the anterior mitral leaflet length, the left ventricular outflow track (LVOT) area, and the location and extent of subvalvular and annular calcifications. 3D visualization software, currently in clinical use, can clearly delineate and evaluate the atrioventricular valves, but they do not readily provide insight on how a device will deform or alter the native anatomy. 3D printing allows for the creation of anatomically accurate, deformable, patient-specific 3D models that maintain all the attributes of a detailed digital model, but additionally provide the opportunity for a bench-top evaluation of the deformation of the critical anatomic relations influenced by the implanted device, such as for example the extent of anterior leaflet displacement into the LVOT.

Physical models are of added value for planning and simulating cardiac valve interventions, spanning from open valve replacement or repair surgery to minimal invasive percutaneous valve procedures such as TAVR and transcatheter mitral valve repair (TMVR).[6,7] Planning of surgical repair or replacement of cardiac valves is challenging as surgeons examine the anatomical structures in a noncontractile unfilled heart, and intraoperative decision-making is common practice. Printed

models that accurately represent patient-specific valvular anatomy from any field of view that an operator selects offer a nearly in vivo, intraoperative assessment of the anatomy in a preprocedural setting, providing an operating surgeon or interventional cardiologist a huge advantage in decision-making.

Aortic Valve

TAVR is already a safe alternative to surgical repair of aortic stenosis in high-risk populations[8,9] and is constantly evolving in technique, equipment, and target population.[10] That being said, there remain important aspects of the procedure that are open to improvement, such as patient selection and prosthesis sizing and refinement.[11] Relatively simple anatomical 3D-printed models can assist in preinterventional identification of potential complications in complex cases,[7] while full-heart models can provide training opportunities, such as transapical replacement approaches.[12] Valve-in-valve procedures, though particularly challenging, will potentially be more common in the near future. For those procedures, simulation and planning utilizing 3D printing can thus provide significant advantages in identifying risks and selecting optimal prostheses parameters.[13]

In a retrospective study of TAVR patients, simulations of balloon valvuloplasty in 3D-printed models of the aortic root including calcifications were assessed for identifying risk factors that could predict postprocedural necessity for permanent pacemaker implantation.[14] Beyond anatomically accurate representations of the pathology, 3D models printed in flexible material can now replicate functional properties of severe degenerative aortic valve stenosis,[15] and these can be used to improve patient-specific TAVR planning.[16] Notably, printing of functionally accurate models for valve pathologies that yield less fixed cusp anatomy, such as valve regurgitation, remains challenging as most available materials exhibit different stress—strain relationships compared to human tissue. However, as discussed in previous chapters, research currently underway may soon render it possible to replicate the mechanical characteristics of valve leaflets. Furthermore, 3D printouts can aid in aortic valve replacement surgery that require resternotomy.[17] In those cases, models can limit the risk of accidental graft dissection from a previous coronary artery bypass grafting or accidental incision of the aorta.

Improvements in both prosthetic valve technology and increasing interventional experience have reduced the frequency of severe paravalvular leaks following surgical repair and percutaneous replacement of aortic valves.[18] Nonetheless, mild and moderate leaks remain common and the latter can impact functional benefit and late survival.[11] Percutaneous approaches are particularly attractive for management of paravalvular leaks[19] and 3D printing can assist either by preinterventional prediction of leak or by optimizing management approaches once a leak has been identified. Models have been reported to be advantageous in both instances. Flexible 3D-printed models of the aortic root complex derived from routine planning CT were able to retrospectively predict post-TAVR paravalvular aortic regurgitation.[20,21]

Mitral Valve

Similar to aortic valve and aortic annulus models, successful efforts have been made toward 3D printing mitral valve models for intervention planning.[22–24] Although, the mitral valve was among the first heart structures to be 3D printed,[25] given the anatomical complexity of the valve and the apparatus, the advancement in the field has been slower.[22–24,26,27] Both 3D TEE and CT imaging data have been used to replicate the morphology of the papillary muscles and LV, with CT being superior for the replication of chordae tendineae and pathologic calcification, and echocardiography for the mitral leaflets. In a study by Mahmood et al.[23] the mitral valve annulus was printed and postoperative alterations in shape and diameter of annulus were evaluated. Those were shown to represent with high fidelity the anticipated actual geometries as well as the features of the annuloplasty devices used. Static printed phantoms of normal and diseased valves including those with ischemic and mitral regurgitation and myxomatous degeneration[24] can help objectifying annuloplasty ring selection and aid decision-making during mitral valve repair surgery.[28]

Minimally invasive percutaneous techniques represent an alternative for the treatment of functional mitral regurgitation in non-low-risk patients.[11] Heart teams have reported use of 3D-printed models to optimize the implantation of the Mitralign percutaneous mitral valve annuloplasty system (Mitralign Inc., Tewksbury, MA).[26] Sizing of catheters, the curvature of the left ventricle (LV), the location of the papillary muscles, and the degree of dilation at the base of the heart were available before the intervention by using the 3D-printed model. Similarly, a 3D physical model of the mitral valve leaflets and subvalvular calcium depositions was utilized for testing a simultaneous transseptal placement of a MitraClip (Abbott Laboratories, Abbott Park, Illinois) and an occluder device to a posterior valve leaflet perforation.[29] Accurate sizing of the mitral annulus and avoidance of LVOT obstruction

are incremental for uneventful TMVR.[30] Printed heart models provide the opportunity for patient-specific device bench testing and can help in estimating the risk of left ventricle outflow tract obstruction, and may potentially reduce procedural times.[31,32] Similar to the aortic valve, percutaneous closure of the periprosthetic mitral valve defects can be simulated in physical models to determine the optimal interventional approach and proper sizing of occluder devices.[33]

Pulmonary and Tricuspid Valves

The management of the "forgotten" semilunar valves has recently gained interest in the surgical/interventional field[34] secondary to the advancements in the aortic and mitral valve management, accounting for their complex anatomical relationships and the lack of dedicated valves and catheters. Sizing and accurate deployment for these valves is paramount, emphasizing the role of preoperative imaging. Pulmonary stenosis or regurgitation are managed with surgical valve replacement or less invasively with percutaneous valve implantation. The latter is however not suitable for most patients and management selection is primarily dictated by the size of the outflow tract in relation to the valve implant. 3D printing and modeling can provide patient-specific anatomical details of the implantation site and the dimensions of the right ventricle outflow tract (RVOT) that offer incremental benefit to planning the management approach, and, through intervention simulation, device selection.[35,36] Physical models of the RVOT were found to be advantageous when compared to assessment of surgical correction or percutaneous implantation of pulmonary valve solely using MRI.[37,38] Printouts of the RVOT have been demonstrated for assisting pulmonary valve implantation and certain patients could potentially benefit for planning with the use of similar 3D printed models.[39,40]

3D transthoracic echocardiography data have been recently used to model and fabricate physical models of normal and pathologic human tricuspid valves with highly preserved reliability.[41] Personalized interventional treatment for tricuspid valve regurgitation with the design of a braided stent has been facilitated by employing 3D modeling in an animal study.[42] For a patient with secondary tricuspid regurgitation who was not a suitable candidate for isolated tricuspid valve surgery and heart transplantation, physical models of the right atrium-inferior vena cava junction enabled preinterventional caval valve implantation sizing and likely helped in achieving an uncomplicated implantation.[43]

LEFT ATRIAL APPENDAGE

Nonpharmacological strategies that locally prevent thrombus formation in the left atrial appendage (LAA) in patients with nonvalvular atrial fibrillation include surgical excision or exclusion and percutaneous occlusion of the LAA.[44] Surgical excision or exclusion of the LAA is also recommended in atrial fibrillation patients that undergo mitral valve, coronary artery bypass, or aortic valve replacement surgery.[45,46] Several devices are available for percutaneous closure and have been approved for use.[47,48] Planning usually combines periinterventional TEE with fluoroscopy guidance or with preinterventional CT. Although the overall benefit of LAA occlusion has been demonstrated, procedural success and safety is critically dependent on comprehension of the patient's LAA anatomy, and on adequate preprocedure planning. The variable anatomy of the appendage poses a challenge for ideal occluder device sizing, and the intervention is not always free from complications.

Different types and sizes of devices have been tested in physical 3D-printed models allowing for sizing and more accurate positioning.[49,50] Small clinical studies have shown the feasibility of the approach, the ability of models to aid in sizing of LAA occluder device and the advantage in device selection and prediction of device compression.[51–53] A large ongoing prospective study (Clinical Trials ID NCT03330210) aims to demonstrate a reduction of operating time and number of prosthesis used per procedure when prior simulation testing and sizing is made on a 3D-printed model.[54] Models printed with materials that resemble the physical tissue properties could potentially further optimize procedural planning combined with standard imaging in challenging cases.

Beyond planning and simulation of occlusion, 3D printing technology has also recently been used to develop 3D-printed personalized implants for LAA occlusion (Fig. 6.1).[55] Specifically, 3D-printed molds of patient's LAAs were filled with a composite elastomeric material to generate soft, inflatable devices that would thus adopt the morphology of the LAA after cardiac implantation and inflation.[56] The authors initially validated the occlusion performance of patient-specific implants using an in vitro system replicating the communication between the left atrial and LAA chambers under pulsatile fluid flow. Next, a personalized device was surgically delivered and inflated in a canine model and the correct orientation of the implant in the LAA was confirmed postmortem. Such patient-specific occluders could offer a nonpharmacological alternative to current surgical/interventional occlusion

methods in cases wherein anatomic relationships are challenging to manage with available devices.

AORTA AND GREAT ARTERIES

Surgical management of vascular pathologies incorporating 3D printing has been shown to potentially aid diagnosis and management in challenging cases and to allow for testing device deployment as demonstrated in the last chapter. Reports to date have focused mainly on aorta pathology[57,58] whereby hollow elastic models are easily printed to represent the vessel wall using current 3D printing techniques. These models readily allow for tactile perception of the arterial wall dimensions and course and for preoperational simulation.

One of the first clinical studies in humans of an intervention enabled by the use of cardiovascular 3D printing was in fact reported in this field, involving the use of 3D models of the aorta to shape aortic root supports for Marfan syndrome patients.[57,59,60] Printed models of each patient's aorta from the annulus to the proximal aortic arch were used to knit a fitting bespoke porous fabric mesh sleeve support.[59] This personalized external support that fits accurately to the patient's aorta was then surgically implanted.[61]

A 3D-printed replica of the ascending aorta and the aortic arch was found to be useful in planning and simulating interventional occlusion of an aortic arch pseudoaneurysm.[62] Using routine-preoperatively CT images to fabricate an accurate replica of the patient's vascular anatomy, precise positioning of a transcatheter-delivered occlude device was achieved. Rapid prototyping using a patient's CT aortogram as source image data was also helpful in the differential diagnosis of a paramediastinal mass.[33] A 3D physical model that delineated the location of the aortic pseudoaneurysm was incremental in selecting the appropriate treatment approach and more specifically the dimensions of the endoprothesis implanted. Rigid and flexible models can aid in assessing optimal stent position and dimensions in endovascular interventions in cases of transverse aortic arch hypoplasia[63] and in pre- and postoperative evaluation of frozen elephant trunk procedures in patients with complex aortic anatomy.[64] Selection and sizing of excluder devices in cases of anastomotic leaks after replacement of the ascending aorta and the aortic arch using accurate vascular phantoms can potentially minimize perioperative morbidity and mortality.[62] A 3D-printed model has also been reported in a case of aortic dissection depicting the location of the aneurysm in the aortic arch, the dissection, as well as the intimal flap separating the true lumen

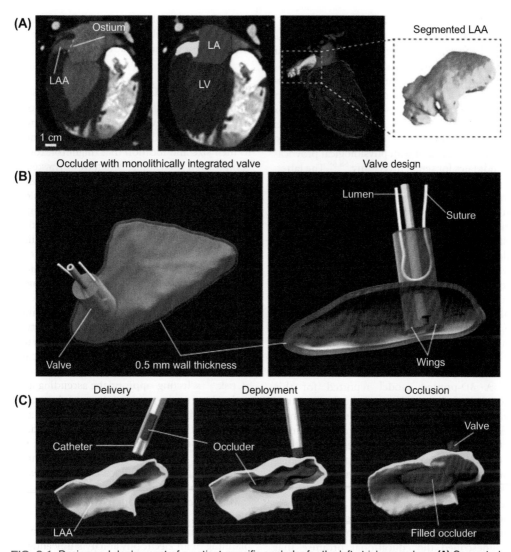

FIG. 6.1 Design and deployment of a patient-specific occluder for the left atrial appendage. **(A)** Computed-tomography segmentation of the left atrial appendage (LAA). LA, left atrium; LV, left ventricle. **(B)** A patient-specific soft occluder with an integrated valve (used for filling, anchoring, and retrieval of the occluder during deployment into the LAA). **(C)** Implantation of the occluder in the patient's LAA: the occluder is deployed into the distal tip of the LAA and filled through the valve with a biocompatible epoxy, until it fully occludes the LAA. (Figure reproduced from Ref. 56 with permission from Macmillan Publishers Ltd.)

from false lumen.[65] Nevertheless, such applications will be probably be limited to the nonacute setting as 3D printing at present requires a number of hours to produce a model of the aorta, although newer technologies (see Chapter 2) may reduce this to less than an hour.

In rare pathologies, such as the Kommerell diverticulum, an aneurysmal dilation at the origin of an aberrantly arising subclavian artery, 3D models can provide direct visibility of the aberrant aorta, the aortic branches, and the diverticulum. In one reported case,

accurate measurements of the diameter of the descending aorta distal to the Kommerell's diverticulum at different levels aided in the appropriate selection and sizing of the frozen elephant trunk.[66] Furthermore, the rigid physical model was used as a guideline in anatomy of the arch branches and Kommerell's diverticulum during exposure in a timely fashion. Finally, the 3D model indicated the optimal section that should be surgically removed as part of the preoperative planning.

HYPERTROPHIC OBSTRUCTIVE CARDIOMYOPATHY

Obstructive hypertrophic cardiomyopathy, the most common monogenic cardiovascular disorder, is heterogeneous in presentation and natural history. It is characterized by a hypertrophied, nondilated left ventricle in the absence of another cardiac, systemic, metabolic, or syndromic disease.[67] Severely symptomatic patients with impaired quality of life due to long-standing LVOT obstruction at rest or with physiological provocation are candidates for septal myectomy.[68,69] The latter, performed to abolish the gradient and mitral regurgitation, involves muscular resection from the basal ventricular septum, frequently accompanied by remodeling of the mitral valve, reconstruction of submitral intraventricular structures, or both.[70] Although the operation is considered one of the safest open-heart procedures with very low mortality in experienced centers, in cases with unique and/or challenging left ventricular outflow tract anatomy advanced imaging may be required.

In this context, 3D-printed models of the left ventricle, aortic valve and ascending aorta, and coronary arteries in cases of myocardial bridging, can provide incremental preoperative guidance and opportunities for preoperative operational simulation.[71,72] A 3D-printed model reported for this application included the LV myocardium, the intraventricular muscle band, the accessory papillary muscle, and the mitral annulus, using multicolor printing to delineate different structures, and printed in flexible, rubber-like material that enabled preoperative simulation of the surgical myectomy.[73] Small clinical studies have reported analogous benefit as well as resection volumes that were in agreement between models and patients.[74,75] Most similar studies of 3D-printed models for low-volume operations have also described the educational promise that printed models hold for training that is not otherwise possible,[74] as well as an improvement in physician–patient communication.[75]

CARDIAC TUMORS

Primary or metastatic cardiac tumors are rare, but when malignant, they have poor prognosis.[76] Benign tumors can be found incidentally or produce symptoms due to their size and location that might for example cause compression of cardiac structures. These commonly require surgical resection, for which diagnostic workup includes multimodality imaging with CT, MRI, positron emission tomography, and echocardiography.[77,78] Visualizing the tumor size and location relative to pertinent cardiac structures is critical for a complication-free operation. Recognition of anatomical alterations following resection is critical for procedural planning. 3D printing may provide a benefit in defining the tumor borders during surgical planning. Models can provide advanced understanding of the relationship between the tumor and the surrounding structures and can facilitate the therapeutic decision-making process.

3D-printed models of primary cardiac neoplasms have been utilized to identify the tumor and structures at risk,[79] selecting appropriate surgical approaches,[80] and selecting the most appropriate therapeutic option.[81,82] (Fig. 6.2). 3D-printing was shown to be of additive value in an infant with a large cardiac fibroma that was causing obstruction of the right ventricular outflow by guiding the extent of tumor resection while avoiding injury of the left descending coronary artery.[83] Similarly, in an adolescent patient with a large residual cardiac rhabdomyoma that was causing mild LVOT obstruction and refractory ventricular tachycardia, a model of the tumor and the heart facilitated proper planning of an electrophysiology study and ablation.[83]

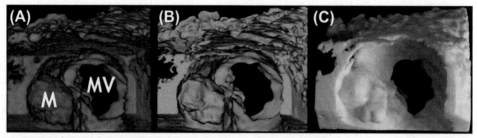

FIG. 6.2 Left atrial myxoma attached to the interatrial septum: en face view from the left atrium. **(A)** 3D echocardiographic image processed in CardioView (TomTec GmbH, Munich, Germany); **(B)** virtual model; **(C)** real 3D printout using Stereolithography. *M*, myxoma; *MV*, mitral valve. (Reproduced from Ref. 78 with permission from Oxford University Press.)

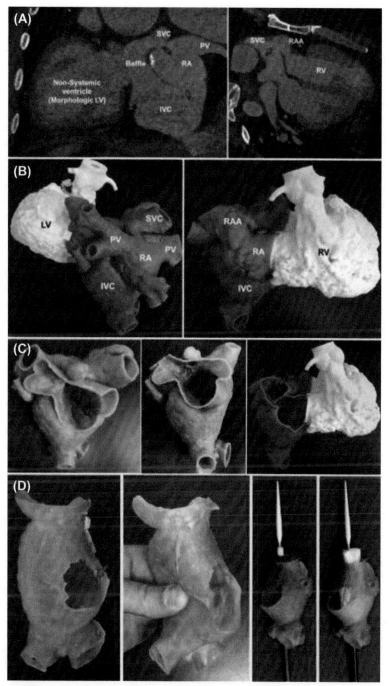

FIG. 6.3 Models for planning and simulation of stent deployment for Mustard baffle revision in a 45-year-old man with a history of complete transposition of great vessels. **(A)** Delayed venous phase CT demonstrating a large defect between the IVC and the pulmonary venous pathways at the rightward aspect of the baffle, a smaller defect between the SVC and the pulmonary venous pathways, and an intermediate-sized defect between the baffle and the right atrial appendage (red arrows). **(B)** 3D-printed model of the baffle designed as a fictitious wall around the blood pool (printed in gray) and including the ventricles (printed in white) for spatial

CARDIAC ANEURYSMS

Atrial and ventricular aneurysms, usually postmyocardial infarction pseudoaneurysms, are rather rare, space-occupying entities within the cardiac muscle that can however lead to detrimental complications.[84–86] Current diagnostic workup employs echocardiography and CT[84] while management approaches include anticoagulation[87] and, when indicated, either transcatheter occlusion procedures[88] or surgical correction.[89] 3D models derived from cardiac CT images have been used to determine the best treatment approach for atrial or ventricular aneurysms.

In a case of a fenestrated atrial septal defect accompanied by a large atrial septal aneurysm and using the patient's CT as source image data, Kim et al.[33] created a physical model that clearly depicted both the atrial septal aneurysm and the anatomic relationship to the septal fenestrations. Simulation of the percutaneous procedure allowed for proper selection of occluder device, diagnostic catheter shapes, and navigation strategy, thereby permitting closure without obstructing the tricuspid valve inflow and the mitral valve annulus.[90] Similarly, 3D printing of left ventricular aneurysms has been reported to aid the tactile appreciation of the kinetic rest volume of the left ventricle.[79] Surgeons were able to identify structures at risk, assess the ideal resection lines of the aneurysmectomy, and determine the residual shape after the reconstructive procedure using the 3D-printed model.

OTHER CARDIAC SURGICAL APPLICATIONS

Ventricular and atrial septal defects (VSD, ASD, respectively) are among the most common CHD where 3D printing has been employed, primarily in large or in unusual types of septal defects. These are presented in other chapters throughout this textbook. In addition to congenital VSD, patients with postinfarct VSDs, a rare but fatal complication of myocardial infarction, undergo usually high-mortality surgical repair.[91] Percutaneous closure devices in selected patients may permit less invasive management.[92] Nonetheless, postinfarct VSD occluder devices have high rates of failure, and thus bench testing in a 3D-printed model can potentially enable more accurate selection and successful in vivo deployment. Such an example has been reported in a case of a postinfarct VSD 1 week after coronary stenting for myocardial infarction, whereby a model assisted in selecting the appropriate size of the VSD occluder.[93]

Due to management and surgical advances, adults with repaired CHD now represent a growing population. During their extended life span, these patients frequently develop heart failure.[94] Left ventricular assist devices that could serve as bridge to transplant might be problematic to implant in these patients, due to the complexity of the anatomic relationships because of prior interventions. Preoperative planning using 3D-printed models can potentially confer a large benefit for planning of cannula and device placement in challenging patients who are candidates for such therapies.[95] Similarly, adults post-Mustard operation can present with structural issues related to the intraatrial baffles including baffle leak or baffle obstruction, and physical models have been utilized for planning and simulation of stent deployment for Mustard baffle revision.[96,97] (Fig. 6.3)

CONCLUSION AND FUTURE OUTLOOK

Cardiac surgery is evolving and personalized surgical planning for acquired heart disease with preoperative imaging will play a pivotal role to the advances in the field. 3D printing is a natural, direct evolution of cardiovascular imaging, and as such it can be expected to enable and help to further advance the field. To date, Heart Teams have reported a benefit from 3D printing in almost the entirety of both common and rare operations. The benefit of the technology is that it translates the already indispensable 3D visualization of anatomical structures possible from modern imaging into tangible, physical models that are easier for the operators to comprehend and that provide unique "hands-on" opportunities to plan and simulate an intervention.

Nevertheless, with few exceptions, reports to date have included only small numbers of patients, and only subjectively support enhanced diagnostic accuracy, procedural success, and reduction in complications. Despite the lack of objective data and randomized clinical trials, 3D printing is nonetheless being implemented into routine clinical practice because of the benefit that interventionalists and surgeons believe

orientation in this difficult case. **(C)** Removable ventricles and cutout window of the wall of the pulmonary venous pathway/right atrium demonstrate the superior small and inferior large baffle defect (red arrows) and cutout window of the right atrial wall demonstrates the third baffle defect communicating with the right atrial appendage. **(D)** A segment of the baffle was also printed in flexible material and used to simulate stent graft deployment to ensure an adequate proximal sealing zone. *IVC*, indicates inferior vena cava; *LV*, left ventricle; *PV*, pulmonary vein; *RA*, right atrium; *RAA*, right atrial appendage; *RV*, right ventricle; *SVC*, superior vena cava. (Reproduced from Ref. 75 with permission by Wolters Kluwer Health, Inc.)

they gain from it. It is thus expected that larger studies that will evaluate standardized metrics and hard outcomes, such as perioperative complications, hospitalization length, and long-term surgical outcomes, will swiftly follow. This will in turn lead to the development of clinical appropriateness guidelines, and optimization and standardization of image acquisition protocols.[90]

Current areas of active research revolve primarily around the improvement of material properties with respect to mimicking the cardiac structure(s), and the development of patient-specific implantable prostheses. Large efforts are also underway toward biofabrication of cardiac valves, as the technology provides a unique opportunity to generate anatomically accurate valvular conduits that can potentially mimic the native living tissue, with all its mechanical heterogeneity.[98–101] The field of cardiovascular 3D printing represents one of the most actively progressing areas in the field of medical 3D printing. At present, elucidating the proper indications for 3D printing in cardiac surgery planning is imperative, as not all operations require planning with a physical model and not all models will confer a benefit compared to standard imaging for preoperative planning.

REFERENCES

1. Bertrand X. The future of cardiac surgery: find opportunity in change!. *Eur J Cardiothorac Surg.* 2013;43(1): 253–254.
2. Easterwood RM, Bostock IC, Nammalwar S, McCullough JN, Iribarne A. The evolution of minimally invasive cardiac surgery: from minimal access to transcatheter approaches. *Future Cardiol.* 2018;14(1):75–87.
3. Shemin RJ. The future of cardiovascular surgery. *Circulation.* 2016;133(25):2712–2715.
4. Ishikawa N, Watanabe G. Robot-assisted cardiac surgery. *Ann Thorac Cardiovasc Surg.* 2015;21(4):322–328.
5. Gosnell J, Pietila T, Samuel BP, Kurup HKN, Haw MP, Vettukattil JJ. Integration of computed tomography and three-dimensional echocardiography for hybrid three-dimensional printing in congenital heart disease. *J Digit Imaging.* 2016;29(6):665–669.
6. Schmauss D, Schmitz C, Bigdeli AK, Weber S, Gerber N, Beiras-Fernandez A, et al. Three-dimensional printing of models for preoperative planning and simulation of transcatheter valve replacement. *Ann Thorac Surg.* 2012; 93(2):e31–e33.
7. Gallo M, D'Onofrio A, Tarantini G, Nocerino E, Remondino F, Gerosa G. 3D-printing model for complex aortic transcatheter valve treatment. *Int J Cardiol.* 2016; 210:139–140.
8. Nishimura RA, Otto CM, Bonow RO, et al. 2014 AHA/ACC guideline for the management of patients with valvular heart disease report of the American college of cardiology/American heart association task force on practice guidelines. *J Am Coll Cardiol.* 2014;63(22): e57–e185.
9. Moat NE. Will TAVR become the predominant method for treating severe aortic stenosis? *N Engl J Med.* 2016; 374(17):1682–1683.
10. Webb JG, Lauck S. Transcatheter aortic valve replacement in transition*. *JACC Cardiovasc Interv.* 2016;9(11): 1159–1160.
11. Figulla HR, Webb JG, Lauten A, Feldman T. The transcatheter valve technology pipeline for treatment of adult valvular heart disease. *Eur Heart J.* 2016;37(28): 2226–2239.
12. Abdel-Sayed P, Kalejs M, von Segesser LK. A new training set-up for trans-apical aortic valve replacement. *Interact Cardiovasc Thorac Surg.* 2009;8(6):599–601.
13. Fujita B, Kutting M, Scholtz S, et al. Development of an algorithm to plan and simulate a new interventional procedure. *Interact Cardiovasc Thorac Surg.* 2015;21(1): 87–95.
14. Fujita B, Kutting M, Seiffert M, et al. Calcium distribution patterns of the aortic valve as a risk factor for the need of permanent pacemaker implantation after transcatheter aortic valve implantation. *Eu Heart J Cardiovasc Imaging.* 2016;17(12):1385–1393.
15. Maragiannis D, Jackson MS, Igo SR, Chang SM, Zoghbi WA, Little SH. Functional 3D printed patient-specific modeling of severe aortic stenosis. *J Am Coll Cardiol.* 2014;64(10):1066–1068.
16. Maragiannis D, Jackson MS, Igo SR, et al. Replicating patient-specific severe aortic valve stenosis with functional 3D modeling. *Circ Cardiovasc Imaging.* 2015; 8(10).
17. Schmauss D, Haeberle S, Hagl C, Sodian R. Three-dimensional printing in cardiac surgery and interventional cardiology: a single-centre experience. *Eur J Cardiothorac Surg.* 2015;47(6):1044–1052.
18. Leon MB, Smith CR, Mack M, et al. Transcatheter aortic-valve implantation for aortic stenosis in patients who cannot undergo surgery. *N Engl J Med.* 2010;363(17): 1597–1607.
19. Sorajja P, Cabalka AK, Hagler DJ, Rihal CS. Long-term follow-up of percutaneous repair of paravalvular prosthetic regurgitation. *J Am Coll Cardiol.* 2011;58(21): 2218–2224.
20. Ripley B, Kelil T, Cheezum MK, et al. 3D printing based on cardiac CT assists anatomic visualization prior to transcatheter aortic valve replacement. *J Cardiovasc Comput Tomogr.* 2015;10(1):28–36.
21. Qian Z, Wang K, Liu S, et al. Quantitative prediction of paravalvular leak in transcatheter aortic valve replacement based on tissue-mimicking 3D printing. *JACC Cardiovasc Imaging.* 2017;10(7):719–731.
22. Kapur KK, Garg N. Echocardiography derived three-dimensional printing of normal and abnormal mitral annuli. *Ann Card Anaesth.* 2014;17(4):283–284.

23. Mahmood F, Owais K, Taylor C, et al. Three-dimensional printing of mitral valve using echocardiographic data. *JACC Cardiovasc Imaging.* 2015;8(2):227−229.

24. Witschey WR, Pouch AM, McGarvey JR, et al. Three-dimensional ultrasound-derived physical mitral valve modeling. *Ann Thorac Surg.* 2014;98(2):691−694.

25. Binder TM, Moertl D, Mundigler G, et al. Stereolithographic biomodeling to create tangible hard copies of cardiac structures from echocardiographic data: in vitro and in vivo validation. *J Am Coll Cardiol.* 2000;35(1):230−237.

26. Dankowski R, Baszko A, Sutherland M, et al. 3D heart model printing for preparation of percutaneous structural interventions: description of the technology and case report. *Kardiol Pol.* 2014;72(6):546−551.

27. Mahmood F, Owais K, Montealegre-Gallegos M, et al. Echocardiography derived three-dimensional printing of normal and abnormal mitral annuli. *Ann Card Anaesth.* 2014;17(4):279−283.

28. Owais K, Pal A, Matyal R, et al. Three-dimensional printing of the mitral annulus using echocardiographic data: science fiction or in the operating room next door? *J Cardiothorac Vasc Anesth.* 2014;28(5):1393−1396.

29. Little SH, Vukicevic M, Avenatti E, Ramchandani M, Barker CM. 3D printed modeling for patient-specific mitral valve intervention: repair with a clip and a plug. *JACC Cardiovasc Interv.* 2016;9(9):973−975.

30. El Sabbagh A, Eleid MF, Matsumoto JM, et al. Three-dimensional prototyping for procedural simulation of transcatheter mitral valve replacement in patients with mitral annular calcification. *Cathet Cardiovasc Interv.* 2018;92(7):E537−E549.

31. Wang DD, Eng M, Greenbaum A, et al. Predicting LVOT obstruction after TMVR. *JACC Cardiovasc Imaging.* 2016; 9(11):1349−1352.

32. Laing J, Moore J, Vassallo R, Bainbridge D, Drangova M, Peters T. Patient-specific cardiac phantom for clinical training and preprocedure surgical planning. *J Med Imaging.* 2018;5(2):021222.

33. Kim MS, Hansgen AR, Wink O, Quaife RA, Carroll JD. Rapid prototyping: a new tool in understanding and treating structural heart disease. *Circulation.* 2008; 117(18):2388−2394.

34. Taramasso M, Maisano F. Transcatheter tricuspid valve intervention: state of the art. *EuroIntervention.* 2017; 13(AA):AA40−AA50.

35. Chung R, Taylor AM. Imaging for preintervention planning: transcatheter pulmonary valve therapy. *Circ Cardiovasc Imaging.* 2014;7(1):182−189.

36. Pluchinotta FR, Bussadori C, Butera G, et al. Treatment of right ventricular outflow tract dysfunction: a multimodality approach. *Eur Heart J Suppl.* 2016;18(suppl E): E22−E26.

37. Schievano S, Migliavacca F, Coats L, et al. Percutaneous pulmonary valve implantation based on rapid prototyping of right ventricular outflow tract and pulmonary trunk from MR data. *Radiology.* 2007;242(2):490−497.

38. Schievano S, Sala G, Migliavacca F, et al. Use of rapid prototyping models in the planning of percutaneous

pulmonary valved stent implantation. *Proc Inst Mech Eng H.* 2007;221(4):407−416.

39. Poterucha JT, Foley TA, Taggart NW. Percutaneous pulmonary valve implantation in a native outflow tract: 3-dimensional DynaCT rotational angiographic reconstruction and 3-dimensional printed model. *JACC Cardiovasc Interv.* 2014;7(10):e151−e152.

40. Phillips ABM, Nevin P, Shah A, Olshove V, Garg R, Zahn EM. Development of a novel hybrid strategy for transcatheter pulmonary valve placement in patients following transannular patch repair of tetralogy of fallot. *Cathet Cardiovasc Interv.* 2016;87(3):403−410.

41. Muraru D, Veronesi F, Romeo G, et al. Feasibility and relative accuracy of three-dimensional printing of normal and pathologic tricuspid valves from transthoracic three-dimensional echocardiographic data sets. *J Am Coll Cardiol.* 2016;67(13):1658.

42. Amerini A, Hatam N, Malasa M, et al. A personalized approach to interventional treatment of tricuspid regurgitation: experiences from an acute animal study. *Interact Cardiovasc Thorac Surg.* 2014;19(3):414−418.

43. O'Neill B, Wang DD, Pantelic M, et al. Transcatheter caval valve implantation using multimodality imaging: roles of TEE, CT, and 3D printing. *JACC Cardiovasc Imaging.* 2015; 8(2):221−225.

44. Holmes DR, Lakkireddy DR, Whitlock RP, Waksman R, Mack MJ. Left atrial appendage occlusion opportunities and challenges. *J Am Coll Cardiol.* 2014;63(4):291−298.

45. Wunderlich NC, Beigel R, Swaans MJ, Ho SY, Siegel RJ. Percutaneous interventions for left atrial appendage exclusion: options, assessment, and imaging using 2D and 3D echocardiography. *JACC Cardiovasc Imaging.* 2015;8(4):472−488.

46. Yu CM, Khattab AA, Bertog SC, et al. Mechanical antithrombotic intervention by LAA occlusion in atrial fibrillation. *Nat Rev Cardiol.* 2013;10(12):707−722.

47. Pison L, Potpara TS, Chen J, et al. Left atrial appendage closure—indications, techniques, and outcomes: results of the European Heart Rhythm Association Survey. *Europace.* 2015;17(4):642−646.

48. Masoudi FA, Calkins H, Kavinsky CJ, et al. 2015 ACC/HRS/SCAI left atrial appendage occlusion device societal overview: a professional societal overview from the American college of cardiology, heart rhythm society, and society for cardiovascular angiography and interventions. *Cathet Cardiovasc Interv.* 2015;86(5): 791−807.

49. Pellegrino PL, Fassini G, DIB M, Tondo C. Left atrial appendage closure guided by 3D printed cardiac reconstruction: emerging directions and future trends. *J Cardiovasc Electrophysiol.* 2016;27(6):768−771.

50. Otton JM, Spina R, Sulas R, et al. Left atrial appendage closure guided by personalized 3D-printed cardiac reconstruction. *JACC Cardiovasc Interv.* 2015;8(7): 1004−1006.

51. Hell MM, Achenbach S, Seong Yoo I, et al. 3D printing for sizing left atrial appendage closure device: head-to-head comparison with computed tomography and

transoesophageal echocardiography. *EuroIntervention.* 2017;13(10):1234–1241.

52. Goitein O, Fink N, Guetta V, et al. Printed MDCT 3D models for prediction of left atrial appendage (LAA) occluder device size: a feasibility study. *EuroIntervention.* 2017;13(9):e1076–e1079.

53. Li H, Qingyao, Bingshen, et al. Application of 3D printing technology to left atrial appendage occlusion. *Int J Cardiol.* 2017;231:258–263.

54. ClinicalTrialsgov. *Left Atrial Appendage Occlusion Guided by 3D Printing (LAA-PrintRegis).* ClinicalTrials.gov; 2017. Available from: https://clinicaltrials.gov/ct2/show/NCT03330210?term=3D+printing&draw=2&rank=7.

55. Robinson SS, Alaie S, Sidoti H, et al. Patient-specific design of a soft occluder for the left atrial appendage. *Nat Biomed Eng.* 2018;2(1):8–16.

56. Gianni C, Natale A. Personalized occluders for the left atrial appendage. *Nat Biomed Eng.* 2018;2(1):2–3.

57. Pepper J, Petrou M, Rega F, Rosendahl U, Golesworthy T, Treasure T. Implantation of an individually computer-designed and manufactured external support for the Marfan aortic root. *Multimedia Man Cardiothorac Surg.* 2013; 2013:mmt004.

58. Tam MD, Latham T, Brown JR, Jakeways M. Use of a 3D printed hollow aortic model to assist EVAR planning in a case with complex neck anatomy: potential of 3D printing to improve patient outcome. *J Endovasc Ther.* 2014; 21(5):760–762.

59. Izgi C, Nyktari E, Alpendurada F, et al. Effect of personalized external aortic root support on aortic root motion and distension in Marfan syndrome patients. *Int J Cardiol.* 2015;197:154–160.

60. Pepper J, Goddard M, Mohiaddin R, Treasure T. Histology of a Marfan aorta 4.5 years after personalized external aortic root support. *Eur J Cardiothorac Surg.* 2015;48(3): 502–505.

61. Treasure T, Takkenberg JJ, Golesworthy T, et al. Personalised external aortic root support (PEARS) in Marfan syndrome: analysis of 1-9 year outcomes by intention-to-treat in a cohort of the first 30 consecutive patients to receive a novel tissue and valve-conserving procedure, compared with the published results of aortic root replacement. *Heart.* 2014;100(12):969–975.

62. Sodian R, Schmauss D, Schmitz C, et al. 3-dimensional printing of models to create custom-made devices for coil embolization of an anastomotic leak after aortic arch replacement. *Ann Thorac Surg.* 2009;88(3):974–978.

63. Valverde I, Gomez G, Coserria JF, et al. 3D printed models for planning endovascular stenting in transverse aortic arch hypoplasia. *Cathet Cardiovasc Interv.* 2015; 85(6):1006–1012.

64. Schmauss D, Juchem G, Weber S, Gerber N, Hagl C, Sodian R. Three-dimensional printing for perioperative planning of complex aortic arch surgery. *Ann Thorac Surg.* 2014;97(6):2160–2163.

65. Ho D, Squelch A, Sun Z. Modelling of aortic aneurysm and aortic dissection through 3D printing. *J Med Radiat Sci.* 2017;64(1):10–17.

66. Chen N, Zhu K, Zhang H, Sun X, Wang C. Three-dimensional printing guided precise surgery for right-sided aortic arch associated with Kommerell's diverticulum. *J Thorac Dis.* 2017;9(6):1639–1643.

67. Maron BJ. Clinical course and management of hypertrophic cardiomyopathy. *N Engl J Med.* 2018;379(7): 655–668.

68. Gersh BJ, Maron BJ, Bonow RO, et al. 2011 ACCF/AHA guideline for the diagnosis and treatment of hypertrophic cardiomyopathy: A report of the American college of cardiology foundation/American heart association task force on practice guidelines developed in collaboration with the American association for thoracic surgery, American society of echocardiography, American society of nuclear cardiology, heart failure society of America, heart rhythm society, society for cardiovascular angiography and interventions, and society of thoracic surgeons. *J Am Coll Cardiol.* 2011;58(25):e212–e260.

69. Elliott PM, Anastasakis A, Borger MA, et al. 2014 ESC Guidelines on diagnosis and management of hypertrophic cardiomyopathy. The task force for the diagnosis and management of hypertrophic cardiomyopathy of the European Society of Cardiology (ESC). *Eur Heart J.* 2014;35(39):2733–2779.

70. Maron BJ, Yacoub M, Dearani JA. Benefits of surgery in obstructive hypertrophic cardiomyopathy: bring septal myectomy back for European patients. *Eur Heart J.* 2011;32(9):1055–1058.

71. Andrushchuk U, Adzintsou V, Nevyglas A, Model H. Virtual and real septal myectomy using 3-dimensional printed models. *Interact Cardiovasc Thorac Surg.* 2018; 26(5):881–882.

72. Hamatani Y, Amaki M, Kanzaki H, et al. Contrast-enhanced computed tomography with myocardial three-dimensional printing can guide treatment in symptomatic hypertrophic obstructive cardiomyopathy. *Esc Heart Failure.* 2017;4(4):665–669.

73. Yang DH, Kang JW, Kim N, Song JK, Lee JW, Lim TH. Myocardial 3-dimensional printing for septal myectomy guidance in a patient with obstructive hypertrophic cardiomyopathy. *Circulation.* 2015;132(4):300–301.

74. Hermsen JL, Burke TM, Seslar SP, et al. Scan, plan, print, practice, perform: development and use of a patient-specific 3-dimensional printed model in adult cardiac surgery. *J Thorac Cardiovasc Surg.* 2017;153(1): 132–140.

75. Guo HC, Wang Y, Dai J, Ren CW, Li JH, Lai YQ. Application of 3D printing in the surgical planning of hypertrophic obstructive cardiomyopathy and physician-patient communication: a preliminary study. *J Thorac Dis.* 2018;10(2):867–873.

76. Leja MJ, Shah DJ, Reardon MJ. Primary cardiac tumors. *Tex Heart Inst J.* 2011;38(3):261–262.

77. Hoffmeier A, Sindermann JR, Scheld HH, Martens S. Cardiac tumors—diagnosis and surgical treatment. *Dtsch Ärztebl Int.* 2014;111(12):205–211.

78. Bartel T, Rivard A, Jimenez A, Mestres CA, Müller S. Medical three-dimensional printing opens up new

opportunities in cardiology and cardiac surgery. *Eur Heart J.* 2018;39(15):1246–1254.

79. Jacobs S, Grunert R, Mohr FW, Falk V. 3D-Imaging of cardiac structures using 3D heart models for planning in heart surgery: a preliminary study. *Interact Cardiovasc Thorac Surg.* 2008;7(1):6–9.

80. Son KH, Kim KW, Ahn CB, et al. Surgical planning by 3D printing for primary cardiac Schwannoma resection. *Yonsei Med J.* 2015;56(6):1735–1737.

81. Schmauss D, Gerber N, Sodian R. Three-dimensional printing of models for surgical planning in patients with primary cardiac tumors. *J Thorac Cardiovasc Surg.* 2013;145(5):1407–1408.

82. Al Jabbari O, Abu Saleh WK, Patel AP, Igo SR, Reardon MJ. Use of three-dimensional models to assist in the resection of malignant cardiac tumors. *J Card Surg.* 2016;31(9):581–583.

83. Moore RA, Taylor MD. Cardiac tumors. In: Farooqi KM, ed. *Rapid Prototyping in Cardiac Disease*. Springer International Publishing AG; 2017.

84. Mügge A, Daniel WG, Angermann C, et al. Atrial septal aneurysm in adult patients: a multicenter study using transthoracic and transesophageal echocardiography. *Circulation.* 1995;91(11):2785–2792.

85. Ba'albaki HA, Clements Jr SD. Left ventricular aneurysm: a review. *Clin Cardiol.* 1989;12(1):5–13.

86. Ruzza A, Czer LSC, Arabia F, et al. Left ventricular reconstruction for postinfarction left ventricular aneurysm: review of surgical techniques. *Tex Heart Inst J.* 2017;44(5):326–335.

87. Burger AJ, Sherman HB, Charlamb MJ. Low incidence of embolic strokes with atrial septal aneurysms: a prospective, long-term study. *Am Heart J.* 2000;139(1):149–152.

88. Wahl A, Krumsdorf U, Meier B, et al. Transcatheter treatment of atrial septal aneurysm associated with patent foramen ovale for prevention of recurrent paradoxical embolism in high-risk patients. *J Am Coll Cardiol.* 2005;45(3):377–380.

89. Treasure T. False aneurysm of the left ventricle. *Heart.* 1998;80(1):7–8.

90. Giannopoulos AA, Mitsouras D, Yoo SJ, Liu PP, Chatzizisis YS, Rybicki FJ. Applications of 3D printing in cardiovascular diseases. *Nat Rev Cardiol.* 2016; 13(12):701–718.

91. Arnaoutakis GJ, Zhao Y, George TJ, Sciortino CM, McCarthy PM, Conte JV. Surgical repair of ventricular septal defect after myocardial infarction: outcomes from the society of thoracic surgeons national database. *Ann Thorac Surg.* 2012;94(2):436–444.

92. Thiele H, Kaulfersch C, Daehnert I, et al. Immediate primary transcatheter closure of postinfarction ventricular septal defects. *Eur Heart J.* 2009;30(1):81–88.

93. Lazkani M, Bashir F, Brady K, Pophal S, Morris M, Pershad A. Postinfarct VSD management using 3D computer printing assisted percutaneous closure. *Indian Heart J.* 2015;67(6):581–585.

94. Norozi K, Wessel A, Alpers V, et al. Incidence and risk distribution of heart failure in adolescents and adults with congenital heart disease after cardiac surgery. *Am J Cardiol.* 2006;97(8):1238–1243.

95. Farooqi KM, Saeed O, Zaidi A, et al. 3D printing to guide ventricular assist device placement in adults with congenital heart disease and heart failure. *JACC Heart Fail.* 2016; 4(4):301–311.

96. Giannopoulos AA, Steigner ML, George E, et al. Cardiothoracic applications of 3D printing. *J Thorac Imaging.* 2016;31(5):253–272.

97. Porras D, Mitsouras D, Steigner M, et al. Transcatheter mustard revision using endovascular graft prostheses. *Ann Thorac Surg.* 2017;103(6):e509–e512.

98. Duan B. State-of-the-Art review of 3D bioprinting for cardiovascular tissue engineering. *Ann Biomed Eng.* 2016; 45(1):195–209.

99. Duan B, Hockaday LA, Kang KH, Butcher JT. 3D bioprinting of heterogeneous aortic valve conduits with alginate/gelatin hydrogels. *J Biomed Mater Res A.* 2013; 101(5):1255–1264.

100. Hockaday LA, Kang KH, Colangelo NW, et al. Rapid 3D printing of anatomically accurate and mechanically heterogeneous aortic valve hydrogel scaffolds. *Biofabrication.* 2012;4(3):035005.

101. Lueders C, Jastram B, Hetzer R, Schwandt H. Rapid manufacturing techniques for the tissue engineering of human heart valves. *Eur J Cardiothorac Surg.* 2014; 46(4):593–601.

CHAPTER 7

3D Modeling as a Tool for Structural Heart Interventions

MARIJA VUKICEVIC, PHD • STEFANO FILIPPINI, MS • STEPHEN H. LITTLE, MD

STRUCTURAL HEART INTERVENTIONS

Structural heart disease comprises noncoronary congenital and acquired heart disorders. With the advancement of clinical imaging and noninvasive percutaneous procedures, structural heart interventions offer potentially life-saving treatment for patients with advanced age and prohibitive surgical risks. The introduction of a large number of percutaneous devices has fueled the need for superior imaging tools to view and appreciate complex cardiac structures. These imaging methods are now relied upon to predict device–tissue interactions and for preprocedural planning of structural heart interventions. Different from surgical interventions, catheter-based structural procedures do not allow for the excision of abnormal native cardiac tissue. Consequently, for such procedures to be successful, the imaging must be sufficiently detailed and robust to allow at least some prediction of the interaction between the newly inserted percutaneous device and dynamic anatomical elements of the beating heart. In particular, interventionalists must consider device deformation under interactive stress with the native tissue and blood flow dynamics. Thus, use of patient-specific three-dimensional (3D) modeling is a critical step toward more comprehensive understanding of possible intraoperative and postoperative complications and outcomes during structural heart interventions.

3D Modeling Techniques for Planning Structural Heart Interventions

Three-dimensional modeling uses mathematical equations that define surface shapes and govern underlying mechanics to create realistic 3D replicas of cardiac structures. These objects can remain as digital-only constructs or can be translated into physical objects using 3D printing methodologies as described in previous chapters. Cardiovascular applications of 3D modeling include the digital reconstruction of patient-specific anatomies, computational simulation of blood flow and anatomical structures, and physical 3D-printed modeling.

Digital modeling

Generating a patient-specific digital cardiac model starts with collecting high-quality medical imaging datasets including, computed tomography (CT), magnetic resonance imaging, and 3D transesophageal echocardiography (TEE). Clinical data are then exported into the Digital Imaging and Communications in Medicine (DICOM) format into an image processing software platform. There are several image processing applications used for image display and processing, including open-source platforms (e.g., OsiriX, InVesalius, ITK SANP, Seg3D, 3D Slicer, De Vide, Turtle Seg) and commercially available applications (e.g., Mimics, Philips Intell, Singovia, 3mensio). A commonly used commercial software platform (Mimics, Materialize, Leuven, Belgium) was recently approved by the Food and Drug Administration (FDA) for the manipulation and refinement of stereolithography (STL) digital files of anatomical models before 3D printing. This comprises the identification of target anatomical elements, the exclusion of undesired surrounding organs and tissues, and the delineation of anatomical elements of interest (Fig. 7.1), a process that can be automatic, semiautomatic, or manual.

Large cardiac chambers and vessels can be extracted using automatic segmentation tools. However, segmentation of finer and softer tissue elements, such as the heart valves and chordae tendineae, requires additional semiautomatic or manual editing. Automatic segmentation is based on brightness of the clinical images. The variation of brightness in CT images depends on tissue density, where the hard structures such as calcium appear brighter and soft tissues appear darker. TEE

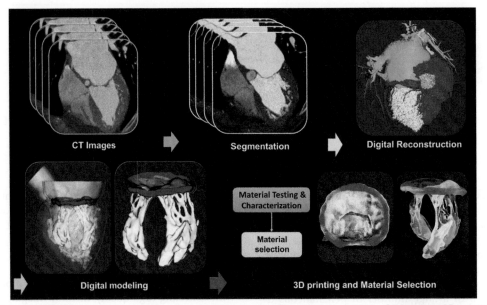

FIG. 7.1 Development of a multimaterial, patient-specific 3D-printed model from CT images. 3D-printed modeling starts with clinical imaging acquisition, followed by the segmentation, 3D digital modeling and STL file generation, material selection, and 3D printing using a blend of different materials. (Lower panels adapted with permission from Vukicevic et al.[1])

images include focused tissue regions and are ideal for the extraction of detailed heart valve geometries. Using the coregistration technique, the entire left ventricle (LV), with mitral leaflets and papillary muscles, can be reconstructed from two datasets acquired from en-face and long-axis view.[1] After the segmentation step, 3D digital models are created through a 3D digital rendering process. However, the resulting 3D digital geometries are often incomplete and require smoothing, hollowing, and wall creation or exclusion of surrounding anatomical elements to qualify for the extraction to the final STL file. Final 3D digital models can be exported as an STL file that can be used for further computational analysis and simulations or be translated into a 3D physical model. Although 3D physical models combined with the clinical imaging are an unparalleled visualization tool for inspecting cardiovascular anatomies, digital 3D models can be instrumental during the clinical team discussions to enhance communication and procedural planning. 3D models can be presented within 3D PDF documents that can be exported from image processing applications. 3D PDF is useful not only for digital 3D models visualization, but also for observation of target geometry from different angles, transparent visualization, digital dissection, selective visualization, and color and illumination variation (Fig. 7.2).

Computational modeling and simulations

Computational simulations incorporate both patient-specific modeling and mathematical equations to model the biomechanical behavior of living tissue, devices, and fluid flow under approximated hemodynamic conditions. Such tools have the potential to revolutionize the way structural heart interventions are practiced and performed. In particular, this methodology can be useful for estimating relevant parameters that are not measureable in clinical practice but that can be calculated using 3D computational methods; these parameters help to predict potential complications, such as the device-induced stress exerted on living tissue, that can lead to a rupture. However, computational models are not broadly used in current clinical practice because the proof-of-concept developmental stage requires further validation and utilization testing that could be difficult to perform for such complex, multistaged treatment approaches.[2]

3D-printed modeling for planning structural heart interventions

The 3D printing techniques most commonly used in medicine currently are stereolithography, PolyJet technology, fused deposition modeling (FDM), and selective laser sintering (SLS). Stereolithography and PolyJet technology build objects through polymerization, whereas

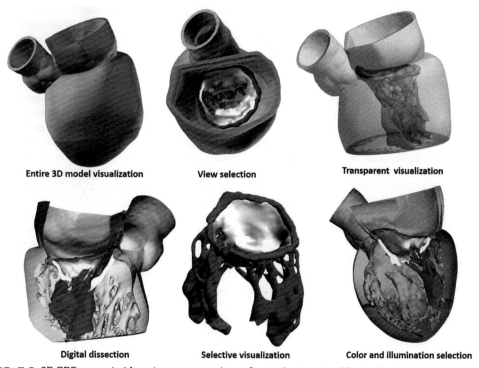

Entire 3D model visualization   **View selection**   **Transparent visualization**

Digital dissection   **Selective visualization**   **Color and illumination selection**

FIG. 7.2   3D PDF generated from image processing software that permits 3D visualization of digital models and its manipulation including angle visualization, transparent visualization, digital dissection, selective visualization of target anatomy, and color and illumination selection.

FDM and SLS build models through material melting. Sterolithography is a laser-based manufacturing technique that builds solid objects by focusing the ultraviolet (UV) light on a digitally defined map of the liquid resin layer. Sterolithography offers a very fast manufacturing process and allows fabrication of large physical objects with highly accurate and smooth surface characteristics. However, the objects printed with stereolithography have several disadvantages, including limited mechanical and thermal strength and required support structures that could restrict the range of printable geometries. PolyJet technology sprays thin layers of photopolymers, then cures them using UV light, which is ideal for manufacturing complex, patient-specific cardiovascular models with multiple color-coded anatomical elements that may have diverse material characteristics and textures. FDM technology is a relatively cheap and provides durable 3D models that do not require multiple materials with diverse qualities. Finally, SLS is an additive manufacturing technique that uses a high-power laser beam to fuse particles of plastic, glass, ceramic or metal powder and creates digitally designed 3D objects. This technique is ideal for producing high-quality prototypes.

Material selection for 3D printing patient-specific cardiac models

There is a wide range of 3D print materials that can be used for additive manufacturing of anatomical models. Early versions of patient-specific models were rigid and primarily functioned to facilitate anatomy visualization and doctor—patient communication. Because these first-generation models were used as visual aids, their construction did not mandate the use of tissue-like elastic materials and complex material composites. However, more recent applications of 3D-printed models for preprocedural planning,[3] device testing,[1,4,5] and functional analysis of clinical outcomes[6,7] require models to have tissue-like mechanical properties. Sylgard, TangoPlus, and HeartPrint Flex materials are the most popular for fabrication of patient-specific anatomical models. The rubber-like TangoPlus materials generally have mechanical properties most similar to some human tissues.[8] PolyJet technology has been instrumental in fabricating 3D-printed objects using the wide spectra of TangoPlus materials, which feature mechanical properties ranging from rubber-like and flexible to calcium-like and hard. Biglino and colleagues used TangoPlus materials to fabricate compliant arterial phantoms, showing that this material can approximate the physiological behavior of arterial vessels.[9] However, it was demonstrated that a single 3D print material cannot replicate the nonlinear mechanical behavior of cardiac tissue under large deformations. Thus, several groups made efforts to build 3D-print material composites to mimic mechanical properties of cardiac tissue. For instance, Vukicevic and colleagues developed the multilayer mitral valve (MV) structure, showing the feasibility of combining soft materials with different mechanical qualities to replicate the layered architecture of mitral leaflets and improve the mechanical behaviors of 3D-printed MV models.[8] They demonstrated that TangoPlus material composites could replicate valve tissue mechanics up to 15% of strain, where the uncramping of elastic fibers occurs. In addition, Wang et al. showed that incorporating wavy or helical structures of hard materials within soft materials could improve mechanical properties of 3D print composites and create metamaterials with improved mechanical capabilities more comparable to those of native tissue.[10]

Structural Heart Interventions
Aortic valve replacement
Transcatheter aortic valve replacement (TAVR) is a catheter-based intervention for the treatment of severe aortic stenosis (AS) in patients with increased surgical risks. Recent clinical trials suggest that TAVR procedures represent an attractive alternative to surgical aortic valve replacement for select patients.[11] CT imaging is used primarily to evaluate vascular anatomy and for sizing and selection of TAVR devices. Despite the large number of TAVR procedures globally (>200,000 cases), the most common postprocedural complication remains paravalvular regurgitation around the external frame of a TAVR device due to incomplete coaptation of the circular device frame against an irregular aortic root contour. Hence, more complete understanding of native aortic morphology and improved prediction of TAVR device interaction with surrounding tissue could lead to more effective preprocedural planning and improved clinical outcomes.

Mitral valve repair
Mitral regurgitation (MR) is one of the most prevalent MV diseases,[12,13] and surgical repair remains the gold standard for treating severe MR cases. However, many patients with multiple comorbidities and high surgical risk remain untreated. The recent development of percutaneous interventional techniques and advancements in intraprocedural imaging have promoted the rapid adoption of minimally invasive catheter-based MV repair with MitraClip (Abbott Vascular, Santa Clara, CA) and encouraged innovation in the field of transcatheter MV replacement (TMVR) devices. The MitraClip procedure is a catheter-based approach that represents an alternative for surgical edge-to-edge repair of MV with degenerative or functional mitral regurgitation. The MitraClip system incorporates a catheter-based delivery system and a clip device with two arms wrapped with fabric and graspers that are capable of approximating the MV leaflets at the site of regurgitation. A MV repair could include one or multiple MitraClip devices, creating double or multiple diastolic mitral orifices. After more than 52,000 MitraClip implantations globally, the MitraClip procedure has become a routine repair technique. However, the selection of patients with anatomy most appropriate for this procedure, and the evaluation of acceptable residual MR remain problematic. Although well established, MitraClip interventions can be challenging due to the complexity of abnormal lesions within mitral leaflets, which in turn can lead to insufficient grasping, loss of leaflet insertion, and partial detachment of MitraClip devices.[14] Careful preoperative observations of mitral anatomy can play a key role in successful MitraClip performance, thereby reducing the need for remedial procedures and minimizing the risk of poor outcomes.[14]

TMVR procedures are another promising percutaneous alternative for treating MR in patients at high or prohibitive surgical risk. After the wide adoption of TAVR, it was anticipated that the emerging TMVR approach could be an equally efficient solution to completely and reproducibly eliminate MR.[15] Different from the aortic valve, the MV has a particularly complex, dynamic nature that makes applying less invasive techniques more difficult. Implantation of TMVR devices in mitral annuli with extended calcification has proven to be very challenging. In addition, TMVR devices that are currently FDA approved and under clinical trials incorporate large frame profiles, varied anchoring solutions, and large delivery systems that require transapical approaches. Obstruction of the LV outflow tract (LVOT) and paravalvular MV leaks are common concerns after implantation of TMVR devices.[16,17]

Left Atrial (LA) closure
Atrial fibrillation (AF) is a common cardiac arrhythmia that affects roughly 33.5 million people worldwide.[18] In this arrhythmia, the left atrium (LA) no longer contracts, which permits blood stasis within specific low-flow regions of the LA (e.g., the LA appendage [LAA]). This markedly increases the risk of intracardiac thrombus formation and associated thromboembolic clinical events such as stroke.[18,19] Accordingly,

anticoagulation therapy remains the gold-standard treatment for stroke prevention in patients with AF. However, anticoagulation therapy may be contraindicated in patients with increased risk of bleeding.[20] Thus, percutaneous exclusion of the LAA structure represents an attractive alternative treatment for patients with contraindication for anticoagulation therapy and a high risk for stroke.[21] Successful stroke prevention using percutaneous occluding devices has driven the ongoing development and refinement of catheter-based LAA exclusion devices.[20] Commonly used LAA occluder devices include the Watchman device (Boston Scientific, Natick, Massachusetts), the first-generation LAA Amplatzer Cardiac Plug (St. Jude Medical, Inc., St. Paul, Minnesota), and the flexible LAA occlusion device Coherex WaveCrest (Coherex Medical, Inc., Salt Lake City, Utah).[19] Although these devices exhibit good results regarding stroke prevention, the sheer variety of LAA morphologies makes selecting the appropriate device design and size very challenging. Fortunately, 3D computational simulation and 3D-printed modeling can optimize both device and patient selection, thereby minimizing complications such as device embolization, para-device leakage (PVL), and incomplete LAA sequestration from the blood pool.

Atrial septal defect closure

Atrial septal defect (ASD) is a common congenital anomaly that can appear in a few different variations: ostium secundum, ostium primum, sinus venosus, coronary sinus defect, and patent foramen ovale.[22,23] Patent foramen ovale is present at birth, but the opening normally fuses shut during infancy. Nevertheless, patent foramen ovale occurs in about 25% of the worldwide population.[22] Left untreated, ASD can degrade over time, leading to a series of complications including stroke, atrial fibrillation, and pulmonary hypertension.[22] Patients with untreated ASD have lower life expectancies.[24] Approximately 50% of adult patients undergo surgical or percutaneous ASD closure.[22] There are several FDA-approved occluding devices that are commonly used for percutaneous ASD closure (Amplatzer Septal Occluder (ASO), Amplatzer Cribriform device, and Gore HELEX device). The percutaneous ASD closure device implantations are often guided by 3D TEE imaging, which when operated correctly, provides an excellent real-time visualization of the interatrial septum and ASD defect.[23] As assessment of ASD size can be overestimated using only echocardiographic images, the use of 3D modeling and physical replicas of defects can provide additional visual information and may optimize implantation outcomes.

Computational Modeling Applications in Planning Structural Heart Interventions

Computational simulation incorporates patient-specific modeling and mathematical equations to model the biomechanical behavior of living tissue, cardiovascular devices, and fluid—structure interactions. One of the most frequently studied percutaneous interventions using computational methods is TAVR implantation. Successful TAVR implantation is directly related to proper patient selection and predictive alleviation of paravalvular regurgitation. The necessity for an accurate estimation of the potential paravalvular regurgitation and intraprocedural risks led to the increase of computational modeling endeavors to predict and resolve these acute complications.[25-32] Many studies have been dedicated to simulation of TAVR device implantation, mechanics, and residual interaction with surrounding aortic leaflets and calcific structures that are not excised during TAVR intervention.

Bosmans and colleagues developed and validated the workflow for the implantation of TAVR devices, seeking to predict the amount of residual aortic regurgitation and risks of severe complications (Fig. 7.3A). The stent was modeled using the finite element method while the aortic root geometry was reconstructed from CT images.[33] Their simulation results compared favorably with post-TAVR constructs extracted from postprocedural CT images.

Initial computational modeling studies focused on an accurate simulation of aortic valve mechanics and the interaction of aortic leaflets with blood flow, incorporating fluid—structure interaction solutions.[36-41] A series of studies have investigated and simulated TAVR procedures in patient-specific settings,[25-28] but their estimation of patient-specific parameters of aortic leaflets and aortic wall material quality remained uncertain.[42] Bosi et al. developed a computational framework to simulate TAVR device implantation (Edwards Sapien XT device) in CT-based patient-specific aortic geometry (Fig. 7.3B). They modeled the aortic leaflets with linear elastic properties and the calcium as elastoplastic structures.[34] They showed that prediction of paravalvular regurgitation incidence, and its location in specific cases, is feasible using only geometric considerations (Fig. 7.3). Comparing the relevant parameters obtained from finite element simulations of TAVR device implantation with those obtained from clinical measurements, they found that the most significant cause of divergence rested in the variation of prescribed aortic leaflet thickness and mechanical properties (Young's modulus) of the aortic root and leaflets.[34]

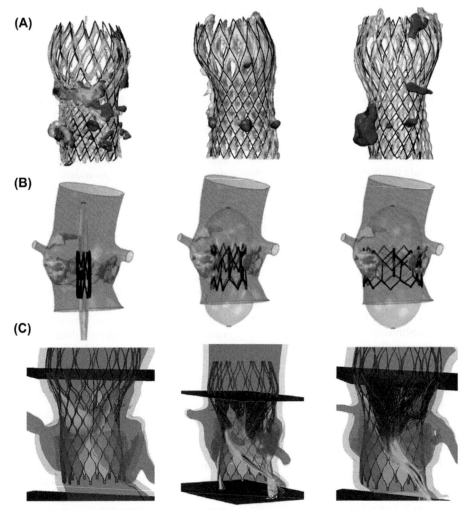

FIG. 7.3 Computational simulation of TAVR implantation. **(A)** Verification of simulated deformation of the TAVR stent by superimposing it over the stent and calcium model reconstructed from post-TAVR images. **(B)** Computational simulation of TAVR device implantation within patient-specific aortic arch geometry for the geometrical-based analysis of potential paravalvular regurgitation. **(C)** Computational simulation of blood flow across the TAVR device showing the device with and without the presence of paravalvular leaks. (**(A)** Adapted with permission from Bosmans et al.[33] **(B)** Adapted with permission from Bosi et al.[34] **(C)** Adapted with permission from de Jaegere et al.[35])

In addition, de Jaegere and colleagues developed a proof-of-concept modeling algorithm that simulated mechanical deformation of virtual TAVR device and its interactions with native aortic leaflets.[35] They utilized computational fluid dynamics methods to simulate aortic flow and predict eventual post-TAVR regurgitation (Fig. 7.3C).

The need to better understand the interaction between newly developed TMVR devices and patient-specific mitral anatomy has inspired the development of LV computational models. Such models are used to assess the effect of TMVR device (Tendyne artificial valve) implantation on LVOT obstruction and related pressure gradients. Work by Alharbi et al. incorporated Navier–Stokes equations and the mass continuity equation for blood flow characterization, and included ventricular wall motion. Although the model was able to simulate intraventricular flow features and post-TMVR LVOT pressure gradients, the modeling approach disregarded the presence of mitral leaflets and their interaction with the TMVR device.[43] Given that mitral leaflets and associated dynamics can further exacerbate the obstruction of fluid flow within the LVOT, omission of this structure from input parameters can lead to inaccurate predictions of procedural outcomes.

Another application of computational modeling included simulation of WATCHMAN device implantation and sizing. Otton and colleagues used 3D digital patient-specific LAA models to virtually implant three sizes of WATCHMAN devices (Fig. 7.4). In addition, they calculated LAA wall deformations after deployment of each device.[44] The associated color-coded LAA maps depicted engagement of the occluding device on LAA walls and the corresponding degree of LAA tissue deformations (Fig. 7.4).

Sturla and colleagues used finite element methods to simulate MitraClip implantation in MV leaflets. The MitraClip device was simplified to two rigid rectangular plates that represented the MitraClip arms implanted into optimal and suboptimal positions of the MV. This work was a step forward in patient-specific simulations of percutaneous MitraClip device implantation; however, the modeling method did not include the realistic thickness of native mitral leaflets or any of the subvalvular apparatus.[45]

3D-Printed Modeling for Planning Structural Heart Interventions

Several studies have demonstrated the utility of 3D-printed models as tools for planning TAVR procedures, device sizing, and predictions of possible pre- and post-procedural risks.[6,7,46–48] First-generation 3D-printed models were used for initial training of the transapical TAVR procedure.[49] Hernandez-Enriquez and colleagues created a patient-specific digital model of the aortic root using CT angiography images. They inserted digitally

designed TAVR devices (23 mm, 26 mm, 29 mm) into aortic root models to perform device sizing and visually evaluate paravalvular regurgitation (Fig. 7.5A). However, the digital model did not show realistic device–anatomy interaction and deformation of the construct. In addition, the group 3D printed the model of aortic root and TAVR devices for visual observation before the procedure.[47]

Ripley and colleagues developed CT-based flexible aortic models and rigid TAVR device replicas to plan interventional procedures and observe the TAVR device's interaction with surrounding anatomical morphology (Fig. 7.5B).[46] Their results suggest that this methodology has a potential to accurately visualize anatomy–device interactions and improve device-sizing accuracy. In addition, they showed that 3D-printed aortic models may be instrumental in identifying potential paravalvular regurgitation locations.[46]

The next generation of patient-specific aortic models were developed for functional evaluation of hemodynamic features across the stenotic aortic valve.[6,7] Maragiannis and colleagues built a series of patient-specific aortic valve models using a blend of materials to mimic calcified aortic tissue quality. They fabricated aortic leaflets and aortic wall tissue using flexible, rubber-like materials, while hard calcific structures were printed from hard, calcium-like materials. They proved that flexible aortic models, when subjected to tailored hemodynamic conditions, can accurately replicate flow features across the stenotic aortic valve and closely mimic echocardiographic parameters assessed in patients during systole.[6,7] The same group of researchers created a functional multimaterial model of the left ventricle with aortic root and aortic valve to replicate pressure and flow waveforms found in individual patients (Fig. 7.6A). Moreover, the authors used patient-specific 3D-printed aortic models to implant the TAVR

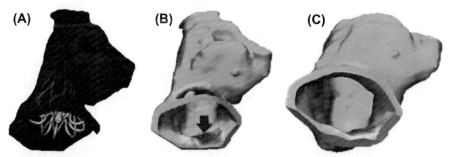

FIG. 7.4 Virtual LAA occluder implantation in a patient-specific anatomical model reconstructed from CT images. **(A)** Implanted Watchman device within digital model for sizing. **(B and C)** Color-map representation of anatomical distortion caused by the Watchman device computationally calculated, showing increased radial force exerted by the device bearing's LAA walls. (**(A–C)** Adapted with permission from Otton et al.[44])

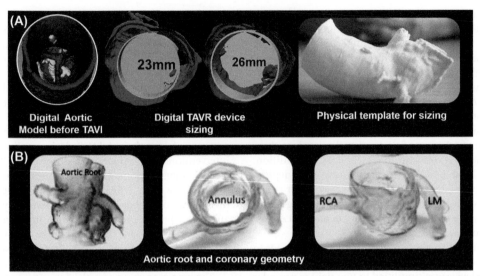

FIG. 7.5 Aortic anatomy observation for TAVR procedure planning. **(A)** Digital patient-specific model of aortic valve used for the virtual sizing of TAVR device and 3D printed for visual inspection and sizing before the procedure. **(B)** 3D-printed models of aortic root with coronary arteries used for anatomical observations and the inspection of aortic arch geometry. (**(A)** Adapted with permission from Hernandez-Enriquez et al.[47] **(B)** Adapted with permission from Ripley et al.[46])

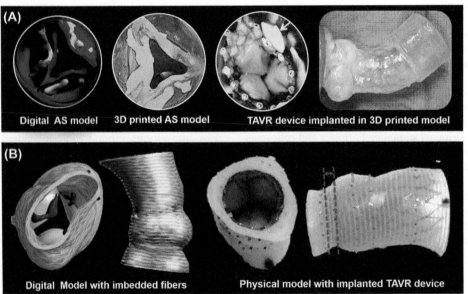

FIG. 7.6 Planning of TAVR procedure using patient-specific 3D-printed models. **(A)** Multimaterial, patient-specific digital and 3D-printed model of flexible aortic cusps and rigid calcium used for the functional analysis of hemodynamic parameters and TAVR device implantation within the aortic root for the observation of deformation (*yellow arrow*) and interaction of the device with calcified tissue. **(B)** Digital patient-specific model of aortic root with imbedded fiber reinforcements for tissue-mimicking effect were converted into a physical multimaterial model for TAVR device implantation and quantitative prediction of potential paravalvular leakes. (**(A)** Adapted with permission from Maragiannis et al. and Vukicevic et al.[1,6,7] **(B)** Adapted with permission from Quian et al.[48])

device and observed the interplay between anatomical elements and the percutaneous device (Fig. 7.6A). Different from nondeformable digital models whose primary utility rested in device sizing,[47] these flexible aortic replicas could be physically implanted with TAVR devices allowing for real, as opposed to merely virtual, TAVR procedure simulations. With flexible 3D replicas, calcified aortic cusps were able to deform under device expansion, and the resulting device deformation occurred in contact with the calcified structures. The models proved useful in the evaluation of post-TAVR PVL and sizing.

Qian and colleagues developed aortic 3D model with imbedded fiber reinforcements to approximate aortic tissue mechanical properties. They investigated the feasibility of using such patient-specific aortic root models to predict the occurrence, location, and severity of potential paravalvular leaks after TAVR procedures. Using patient-specific models, they performed in vitro analysis of post-TAVR aortic root strain (Fig. 7.6B). Their results showed that post-TAVR annular strain unevenness and annular bulge index are promising parameters for accurate prediction of potential paravalvular leak risks.[48] In vitro simulation of percutaneous MV repair and replacement interventions can be performed using anatomically accurate 3D-printed models with physiologically realistic material properties. It has been demonstrated that 3D-printed patient-specific models can be instrumental in complex anatomy observation, preprocedural planning, and optimization of structural interventions on the MV apparatus.

Models of the MV apparatus can be reconstructed from multimodality imaging data, including CT and 3D echocardiographic images.[8] 3D-printed modeling of mitral elements started with simple mitral annulus models using 3D TEE images.[50] Those models were fabricated from rigid materials to demonstrate the feasibility of generating normal and abnormal patient-specific geometries of saddle-shaped MV annuli.[50] The next series of MV models were reconstructed using 3D TEE images and included flexible leaflets and annulus.[51] They were useful replicas for the anatomical observation of the MV, but were unlikely to be suitable for percutaneous device testing. The next generation of MV models included the MV annulus, leaflets, LV, and papillary muscles.[8] The MV was reconstructed from en-face 3D TEE views, whereas the LV and papillary muscles were reconstructed from long-axis 3D TEE images. Using coregistration techniques, digital elements of the MV and the LV with papillary muscles were fused into a unique model. Mitral elements were color-coded and 3D printed using a blend of different 3D-print material textures.[1,8] The next iteration of models extracted from 3D TEE images involved the entire subvalvular MV apparatus, including the branch of chordae, which have an anatomical arrangement that could have an important impact on percutaneous device position.[1] More detailed 3D digital reconstruction of the entire subvalvular apparatus is possible using CT images because of the superior spatial resolution of this modality. Little and colleagues demonstrated that flexible, multimaterial 3D-printed models could be useful for planning MV repair interventions using the plug and MitraClip devices for positioning, device selection, and sizing (Fig. 7.7A).[3] Vukicevic and colleagues reconstructed the entire MV apparatus (annulus, leaflets, chordae, and papillary muscles within the LV with LVOT) using CT images to perform in vitro simulation percutaneous MV repair.[52] They demonstrated that their MV apparatus models were fabricated from sufficiently flexible materials that allowed MitraClip implantation and conformal deformations of leaflets under device closure (Fig. 7.7B). Moreover, it has been shown that 3D-printed patient-specific models could be powerful tools for planning MitraClip implantation in complex and challenging valve geometries.[3] Another group used 3D-printed LV models for preoperative preparation of percutaneous mitral annuloplasty using the Mitralign repair system.[53] Advancing the Mitralign catheter through the aortic root to the LV and placing it between the papillary muscles near the mitral annulus could be challenging. However, it has been clinically shown that training on a patient-specific 3D-printed heart model before the procedure can facilitate maneuvering the catheter around the papillary muscles and annulus.[53]

Functional MV models could be instrumental in replicating hemodynamic conditions observed in patients after interventional procedures. Mashari and colleagues generated echo-derived post-MitraClip anatomical morphology using a combination of 3D-printed mold and cast fabrication techniques. They integrated the post-MitraClip silicone-based replica into pulse duplicator under pressurized flow conditions, replicating continuous-wave Doppler tracings found at the mitral inflow in diastole.[54] Such hemodynamic information can be useful for predicting postprocedural risks that arise when anatomical features are altered by implanted devices and optimization of percutaneous MV repair procedures.

Novel TMVR devices and corresponding percutaneous procedures can be challenging due to the complexity of the mitral subvalvular apparatus and TMVR device interaction with functional MV elements,

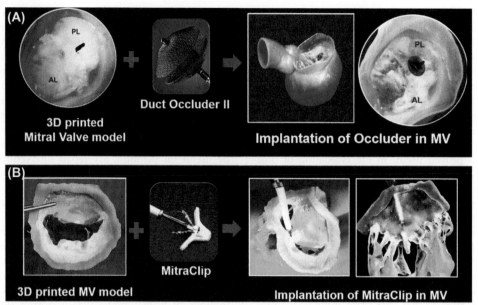

FIG. 7.7 3D-printed modeling for preprocedural planning of percutaneous MV repair and replacement procedures. **(A)** Patient-specific, multimaterial 3D-printed model of MV with P2 perforation used for the preprocedural planning of MV repair using the Amplatzer occluder II and MitraClip devices. **(B)** Multimaterial, 3D-printed model of the MV apparatus (left) as a useful tool for planning of MitraClip device implantation. (**(A)** Adapted with permission from Little et al.[3] **(B)** Adapted with permission from Vukicevic et al.[52])

including the mitral annulus, chordae tendineae, and papillary muscles. More comprehensive preparation for this novel percutaneous approach can be performed using compliant patient-specific 3D-printed models to analyze individual interactions of the TMVR device with intraventricular elements. 3D digital reconstruction of LV geometry and implantation of stylized cylindrical TMVR-like devices can be useful tools for planning TMVR procedures. Several studies have investigated a digital implantation of TMVR devices in virtual patient-specific anatomy[16,17,55,56] and consequent LVOT obstruction. However, digitally delineated tissue is unsuitable to conform under pressure of implanted devices, and digital devices cannot conform to tissue tension. A digitally implanted device does not realistically interact with MV leaflets; therefore, it does not realistically predict deflection of the anterior mitral leaflet that causes LVOT obstruction. Thus, using 3D-printed patient-specific phantoms with accurate anatomical geometry and mechanical properties that mimic mitral tissue quality could facilitate better patient selection and more precisely predict eventual LVOT obstruction risks.

Wang and colleagues have demonstrated the feasibility of using 3D digital models for planning TMVR procedures in patients with severe mitral calcification, mitral ring, or mitral bioprothesis. They showed how a computer-aided design-based stylized TMVR device can be virtually implanted into a digital 3D reconstruction of a patient-specific LV to evaluate eventual LVOT obstruction.[55] Digital models illustrated possible risks of LVOT obstruction in these cases; however, different from 3D-printed models, they are unable to depict the deformation of calcified elements and previously implanted devices. This methodology was further validated using 3D-printed patient-specific models.[55,56]

MV replacement in patients with mitral annular calcification (MAC) can be particularly difficult. The device most commonly used for MV replacement with prominent MAC is the SAPIEN balloon expandable valve (Edwards Lifesciences). Appropriate device sizing, anchoring, LVOT obstruction, and eventual device under expansion can be very difficult to predict. Thus, El Sabbagh and colleagues showed that multimaterial 3D-printed left ventricle models with prominent MAC can facilitate more accurate preprocedural planning and identify potential pitfalls of interaction between the SAPIEN device and the complex subvalvular MV apparatus. Various sizes of computationally designed SAPIEN valve models were inserted into 3D digital models of the LV with calcified structures around the mitral annulus; these were used for visual inspection of the device and sizing, appropriate anchoring, potential paravalvular gaps, and LVOT obstruction. They showed that digital models were able to predict accurate device sizing and LVOT obstruction to a certain extent, but could not predict under expansion and migration of the device.[57] An additional limitation of these models was the lack of mitral leaflets and chordae branches, which could cause LVOT obstruction if deflected during TMVR device implantation.

Vukicevic and colleagues have developed patient-specific, multimaterial, 3D-printed models of the entire MV apparatus, including the annulus, leaflets, chordae tendineae, and papillary muscles (Fig. 7.8). They proved that including the entire subvalvular apparatus led to a more accurate prediction of LVOT obstruction and estimation of eventual intraprocedural risks. They also showed how the TMVR device deforms within the D-shaped annulus, while MV tissue conforms under pressure of the TMVR device.[52] CT scans of such device–3D-model constructs allow for analysis of deformations and measurements within commonly used clinical software (3mensio, Pie Medical Imaging), suggesting that 3D-printed modeling is a useful tool for more accurate prediction of the LVOT.

CT-based 3D-printed models proved useful in planning of the percutaneous implantation of a Hybrid Melody valve (Medtronic) in a low-weight pediatric patient with multiple previous surgical reconstructions.[58] To avoid LVOT obstruction and ensure good device anchoring in such a small heart, the surgical team performed a benchtop preprocedural implantation in the patient's 3D-printed model. After predicting optimal device sizing and positioning without LVOT obstruction, the interventional procedure was executed in the patient using the planned transseptal interventional strategy.[58]

High-risk patients with multiple previous sternotomies are often referred for percutaneous interventional valve procedures. Their altered native anatomy caused by previous valve repairs requires thorough observation of anatomy and more comprehensive preprocedural preparation. Such individualized preprocedural planning using a patient-specific 3D-printed model has been performed in a patient with previously implanted aortic mechanical valve, aortomitral curtain reconstruction, and mitral ring and deemed suitable for valve-in-ring replacement with a TIARA valve (Neovasc Inc.). Oversizing of the TIARA valve was not required because accurate device positioning and anchoring at the fibrous trigons was simulated using the 3D-printed LV model with LVOT and the mechanical aortic valve during preprocedural planning.[59]

Patient-specific 3D-printed models derived from high-quality CT images may be particularly significant for optimal planning of percutaneous LAA closures. Individual variation in LAA geometry and the complexity of LAA morphology can make accurate selection of closure devices difficult (Fig. 7.9B). More detailed investigation of LAA geometry can be performed using patient-specific 3D-printed models (Fig. 7.9A).[60] 3D-printed LAA models can be reconstructed from both CT and 3D TEE images (Fig. 7.9C).[61] It has been shown that flexible, patient-specific 3D-printed models can enhance LAA closure device sizing and design selection and allow for testing of different occluding device shapes (Fig. 7.9B

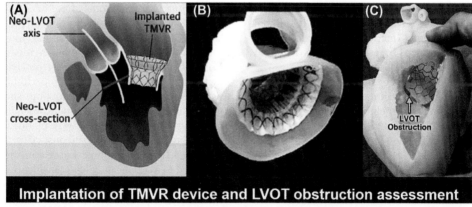

Implantation of TMVR device and LVOT obstruction assessment

FIG. 7.8 Patient-specific 3D-printed modeling can facilitate TMVR preprocedural planning. **(A)** Schematic representation of LVOT obstruction after TMVR device implantation. **(B)** TMVR device implanted into a patient-specific MV apparatus for observation of possible LVOT obstruction due to surrounding tissue deformation under TMVR device expansion. **(C)** 3D-printed model to assess LVOT obstruction after TMVR implantation. ((A) Adapted with permission from Vukicevic et al.[52] **(B)** Adapted with permission from Vukicevic et al.[52] **(C)** Adapted with permission from Eleid et al.[5])

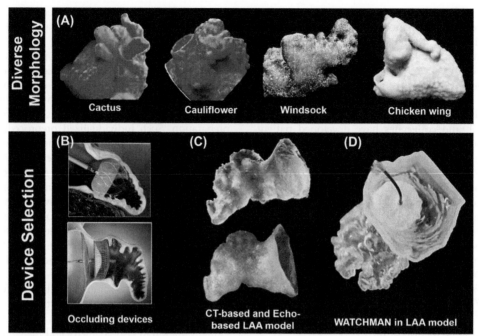

FIG. 7.9 3D-printed models can facilitate device selection and sizing for LAA exclusion. **(A)** Four different 3D-printed models depicting most commonly encountered anatomical shapes of LAA. **(B)** Commonly used percutaneous devices for exclusion of LAA in patients with AF. **(C)** 3D-printed models from CT and 3D echo images. **(D)** Watchman device implantation in patient-specific 3D-printed LAA model. (**(A)** Adapted with permission from Hachulla et al.[60] **(C)** Adapted with permission from Obasare et al.[61] **(D)** Adapted with permission from Liu et al.[62])

and D).[62,63] 3D-printed models generated to guide LAA closure procedures should include the entire atrium and LAA morphology to allow for planning and more accurate optimization of the sheath approach, angulation, and landing zone during the interventional team's benchtop preprocedural trial. Observing 3D-printed model before the actual intervention increased procedural efficacy, optimized safety, decreased operation time, and led to a more complete LAA closure.[63]

Accurate sizing of the LAA ostium is very challenging and LAA size can be underestimated when analyzed using only clinical imaging methodologies.[44] Therefore, using rubber-like patient-specific 3D models of the LAA to optimize device sizing is crucial.[44] It was shown that 3D-printed models enhanced accurate selection among three different WATCHMAN device sizes (Boston Scientific, Natick, Massachusetts). Occluding devices have been deployed into patient-specific 3D-printed models of LAA, showing that selection based on TEE imaging leads to undersized devices. Device selection based on models were optimal when later implanted into the patient. The study suggests that the selection of an oversized device could have led to

postprocedural pericardial effusion and intraoperative complications of the percutaneous closure, while the device selected based on 3D-printed modeling was implanted without incidence.[44]

3D-printed cardiac models have been shown to be beneficial, not only as a visualization and preprocedural planning tool, but also for training interventional teams.[4] Training on 3D-printed LAA models instead of on patients provides a smoother procedural workflow and lowers the number of occluding devices wasted.[64] Three-month CT follow-up showed that more accurate device sizing was performed in the series of patients whose procedures were planned based on both clinical imaging and patient-specific 3D-printed modeling. Use of 3D-printed models in the planning process led to a significantly lower incidence of reoccurring leakage from occluded LAA (15% less) compared to that in patients whose procedures were planned based only on TEE and CT imaging.[64] Another example of a 3D-printed model enhancing procedural planning in a patient with unusual double ostium LAA is shown in Fig. 7.10 (upper panel).[65] Two Watchman devices were tested within 3D-printed models and later

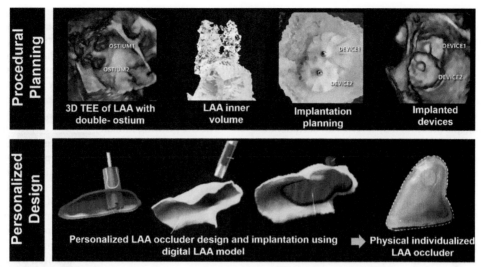

FIG. 7.10 Individualized LAA closure device selection. **(A)** Preprocedural planning of LAA occluder implantation in double ostium LAA and demonstration of postoperative configuration of the implanted device showing agreement with the 3D print-device construct used for planning purposes. **(B)** Digitally designed personalized occluder generated to fit the patient-specific geometry of LAA (left panels). It was fabricated using the molding technique for a proof-of-concept canine study and in vitro simulation. (**(A)** Adapted with permission from Song et al.[65] **(B)** Adapted with permission from Robinson et al.[66])

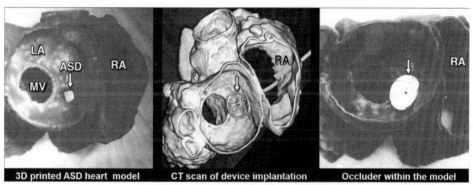

FIG. 7.11 Process of preprocedural planning of ASD repair using occluder device implantation in a 3D-printed model. Patient-specific 3D-printed model of the heart with an ASD defect generated from CT images (left panel). The 3D-printed model proved useful for procedural simulation and imaging of occluding device positioning, sizing, and selection (middle panel). Implanted occluding device in the 3D-printed patient-specific model showing interaction of the device with the surrounding valve elements and the defect (right panel). (Adapted with permission from Vukicevic et al.[52])

implanted in the actual patient (Fig. 7.10). This preprocedural planning process led to an efficient interventional procedure.[65]

Additionally, 3D-printed models can be used as templates to individualize novel percutaneous devices. Robinson and colleagues developed an individualized LAA occluding device prototype using a patient-specific model derived from CT images (Fig. 7.10, lower panel).[66] They used patient-specific LAA volume as a template to design molds of the occluder, which was 3D printed to fabricate a personalized occluder using the molding technique (Fig. 7.10). This device was tested in a LAA occluder model and a canine model for proof of concept.

Another useful application of 3D-printed models is preprocedural planning of percutaneous ASD repair (Fig. 7.11). The team at Houston Methodist Hospital has developed a patient-specific heart model of left and right atria with ASD defect, bioprosthetic valve ring, and parts of ventricular chambers (Fig. 7.11, left panel).[1] In this patient, the ASD was particularly close to the prosthetic MV, raising the risk of its obstruction from an incorrectly sized device. Consequently, the interventional team used the 3D-printed model to simulate the procedure and size the device (Fig. 7.11, middle panel). Using this method, they selected an occluder device that would effectively repair the ASD while assuring optimal interaction with the bioprosthetic valve and allowing its unrestricted performance (Fig. 7.11, right panel).

Challenges and Future Directions in 3D Modeling Structural Heart Interventions

The development of clinical imaging and visualization tools has fueled the rapid expansion of percutaneous structural heart interventions. In a world where medical care is increasingly individualized, computational and 3D-printed modeling are critical tools used by practitioners to tailor patient-specific structural heart interventions. 3D modeling can vastly improve the understanding of complex cardiac anatomies, thereby optimizing preprocedural planning and patient outcomes. 3D modeling can also result in step-changing improvements in the teaching of clinicians and facilitate communication with patients and their families.

Technology-driven improvements in digital visualization and computational modeling have already transformed these processes into important tools for simulation of interventional outcomes. However, these digital predictive tools are still a work in progress. A lack of both validation data and realistic computational modeling of the interplay between cardiac tissue and implantable percutaneous devices impedes the transition of these powerful virtual instruments from research laboratories into everyday clinical practice.

3D-printed modeling establishes a new paradigm in how we plan and practice structural heart interventions. Sophisticated patient-specific models can accurately replicate patient-specific geometry and complex defects, thereby facilitating the implantation and realistic interaction of percutaneous devices with native morphology to enhance the success of percutaneous procedures. Rehearsal of structural heart interventions can save time in the catheterization laboratory and prevent potential risks and trauma in patients. This results in significant procedural cost savings. 3D-printed models are also useful in the innovation of novel percutaneous devices and can accelerate their translation in clinical practice.

Emerging 3D print materials are becoming more analogous to cardiovascular tissues, making patient-specific models ever more realistic. Moreover, advancements in biocompatible 3D print materials and bioprinting research has the potential to transform medical devices production and may soon become an alternative for the treatment of structural heart disorders.

The 3D printing industry is vastly improving printer performance. Faster and more cost effective printers will augment the application rate of 3D-printed models in medical practice. Future efforts in patient-specific, multimaterial 3D-printed modeling research should be directed toward the improvement of image data processing, automatic segmentation, and generation of novel 3D-printed materials with improved biomechanical characteristics. In addition, the impact of individualized modeling should be documented by those who are practicing structural heart interventions.

REFERENCES

1. Vukicevic M, Vekilov DP, Grande-Allen J, Little SH. Patient-specific 3D valve modeling for structural intervention. *Struct Heart*. 2017;1(5–6):236–248.
2. Neal ML, Kerckhoffs R. Current progress in patient-specific modeling. *Briefings Bioinf*. 2010;11(1):111–126.
3. Little SH, Vukicevic M, Avenatti E, Ramchandani M, Barker CM. 3D printed modeling for patient-specific mitral valve intervention: repair with a clip and a plug. *JACC Cardiovasc Interv*. 2016;9(9):973–975.
4. Izzo RL, O'Hara RP, Iyer V, et al. 3D printed cardiac phantom for procedural planning of a transcatheter native mitral valve replacement. *Proc SPIE-Int Soc Opt Eng*. 2016;9789. https://doi.org/10.1117/12.2216952.
5. Eleid MF, Foley TA, Said SM, Pislaru SV, Rihal CS. Severe mitral annular calcification: multimodality imaging for therapeutic strategies and interventions. *JACC Cardiovasc Imaging*. 2016;9(11):1318–1337.
6. Maragiannis D, Jackson MS, Igo SR, Chang SM, Zoghbi WA, Little SH. Functional 3D printed patient-specific modeling of severe aortic stenosis. *J Am Coll Cardiol*. 2014;64(10):1066–1068.
7. Maragiannis D, Jackson MS, Igo SR, et al. Replicating patient-specific severe aortic valve stenosis with functional 3D modeling. *Circ Cardiovasc Imaging*. 2015;8(10):e003626.
8. Vukicevic M, Puperi DS, Jane Grande-Allen K, Little SH. 3D printed modeling of the mitral valve for catheter-based structural interventions. *Ann Biomed Eng*. 2017;45(2):508–519.
9. Biglino G, Verschueren P, Zegels R, Taylor AM, Schievano S. Rapid prototyping compliant arterial phantoms for in-vitro studies and device testing. *J Cardiovasc Magn Reson*. 2013;15, 2-429X-15-2.
10. Wang K, Wu C, Qian Z, Zhang C, Wang B, Vannan MA. Dual-material 3D printed metamaterials with tunable

mechanical properties for patient-specific tissue-mimicking phantoms. *Addit Manuf.* 2016;12(Part A): 31–37.

11. Reardon MJ, Van Mieghem NM, Popma JJ, et al. Surgical or transcatheter aortic-valve replacement in intermediate-risk patients. *N Engl J Med.* 2017;376(14):1321–1331.

12. Nkomo VT, Gardin JM, Skelton TN, Gottdiener JS, Scott CG, Enriquez-Sarano M. Burden of valvular heart diseases: a population-based study. *Lancet.* 2006;368(9540): 1005–1011.

13. Kheradvar A, Groves EM, Simmons CA, et al. Emerging trends in heart valve engineering: Part III. novel technologies for mitral valve repair and replacement. *Ann Biomed Eng.* 2015;43(4):858–870.

14. Kreidel F, Frerker C, Schluter M, et al. Repeat MitraClip therapy for significant recurrent mitral regurgitation in high surgical risk patients: impact of loss of leaflet insertion. *JACC Cardiovasc Interv.* 2015;8(11): 1480–1489.

15. Regueiro A, Granada JF, Dagenais F, Rodes-Cabau J. Transcatheter mitral valve replacement: insights from early clinical experience and future challenges. *J Am Coll Cardiol.* 2017;69(17):2175–2192.

16. Blanke P, Naoum C, Webb J, et al. Multimodality imaging in the context of transcatheter mitral valve replacement: establishing consensus among modalities and disciplines. *JACC Cardiovasc Imaging.* 2015;8(10): 1191–1208.

17. Blanke P, Naoum C, Dvir D, et al. Predicting LVOT obstruction in transcatheter mitral valve implantation: concept of the neo-LVOT. *JACC Cardiovasc Imaging.* 2017; 10(4):482–485.

18. Vaidya VR, Asirvatham R, Tri J, Asirvatham SJ. Left atrial appendage exclusion for atrial fibrillation: does the protection from stroke prevail in the long-term? *J Thorac Dis.* 2016;8(10):E1260–E1267.

19. Wunderlich NC, Beigel R, Swaans MJ, Ho SY, Siegel RJ. Percutaneous interventions for left atrial appendage exclusion: options, assessment, and imaging using 2D and 3D echocardiography. *JACC Cardiovasc Imaging.* 2015;8(4): 472–488.

20. Suradi HS, Hijazi ZM. Left atrial appendage closure: outcomes and challenges. *Neth Heart J.* 2017;25(2):143–151.

21. Sakellaridis T, Argiriou M, Charitos C, et al. Left atrial appendage exclusion-where do we stand? *J Thorac Dis.* 2014;6(suppl 1):S70–S77.

22. Rao PS, Harris AD. Recent advances in managing septal defects: atrial septal defects. *F1000Res.* 2017;6:2042.

23. Saric M, Perk G, Purgess JR, Kronzon I. Imaging atrial septal defects by real-time three-dimensional transesophageal echocardiography: step-by-step approach. *J Am Soc Echocardiogr.* 2010;23(11):1128–1135.

24. Konstantinides S, Geibel A, Kasper W, Just H. The natural course of atrial septal defect in adults-a still unsettled issue. *Klin Wochenschr.* 1991;69(12):506–510.

25. Bianchi M, Ghosh RP, Marom G, Slepian MJ, Bluestein D. Simulation of transcatheter aortic valve replacement in patient-specific aortic roots: effect of crimping and positioning on device performance. *Conf Proc IEEE Eng Med Biol Soc.* 2015;2015:282–285.

26. Capelli C, Bosi GM, Cerri E, et al. Patient-specific simulations of transcatheter aortic valve stent implantation. *Med Biol Eng Comput.* 2012;50(2):183–192.

27. Gunning PS, Vaughan TJ, McNamara LM. Simulation of self expanding transcatheter aortic valve in a realistic aortic root: implications of deployment geometry on leaflet deformation. *Ann Biomed Eng.* 2014;42(9):1989–2001.

28. Morganti S, Conti M, Aiello M, et al. Simulation of transcatheter aortic valve implantation through patient-specific finite element analysis: two clinical cases. *J Biomech.* 2014. JID - 0157375.

29. Sirois E, Mao W, Li K, Calderan J, Sun W. Simulated transcatheter aortic valve flow: implications of elliptical deployment and under-expansion at the aortic annulus. *Artif Organs.* 2018;42(7):E141–E152.

30. Sturla F, Ronzoni M, Vitali M, et al. Impact of different aortic valve calcification patterns on the outcome of transcatheter aortic valve implantation: a finite element study. *J Biomech.* 2016;49(12):2520–2530.

31. Wang Y, Quaini A, Canic S, Vukicevic M, Little SH. 3D experimental and computational analysis of eccentric mitral regurgitant jets in a mock imaging heart chamber. *Cardiovasc Eng Technol.* 2017;8(4):419–438.

32. Wu W, Pott D, Mazza B, et al. Fluid-structure interaction model of a percutaneous aortic valve: comparison with an in vitro test and feasibility study in a patient-specific case. *Ann Biomed Eng.* 2016;44(2):590–603.

33. Bosmans B, Famaey N, Verhoelst E, Bosmans J, Vander Sloten J. A validated methodology for patient specific computational modeling of self-expandable transcatheter aortic valve implantation. *J Biomech.* 2016;49(13):2824–2830.

34. Bosi GM, Capelli C, Cheang MH, et al. Population-specific material properties of the implantation site for transcatheter aortic valve replacement finite element simulations. *J Biomech.* 2018;71:236–244.

35. de Jaegere P, De Santis G, Rodriguez-Olivares R, et al. Patient-specific computer modeling to predict aortic regurgitation after transcatheter aortic valve replacement. *JACC Cardiovasc Interv.* 2016;9(5):508–512.

36. Carmody CJ, Burriesci G, Howard IC, Patterson EA. An approach to the simulation of fluid-structure interaction in the aortic valve. *J Biomech.* 2006;39(1):158–169.

37. Nicosia MA, Cochran RP, Einstein DR, Rutland CJ, Kunzelman KS. A coupled fluid-structure finite element model of the aortic valve and root. *J Heart Valve Dis.* 2003. JID - 9312096.

38. De Hart J, Baaijens FP, Peters GW, Schreurs PJ. A computational fluid-structure interaction analysis of a fiber-reinforced stentless aortic valve. *J Biomech.* 2003; 36(5):699–712.

39. Ranga A, Bouchot O, Mongrain R, Ugolini P, Cartier R. Computational simulations of the aortic valve validated by imaging data: evaluation of valve-sparing techniques. *Interact Cardiovasc Thorac Surg.* 2006;5(4): 373–378.
40. Weinberg EJ, Kaazempur Mofrad MR. A multiscale computational comparison of the bicuspid and tricuspid aortic valves in relation to calcific aortic stenosis. *J Biomech.* 2008;41(16):3482–3487.
41. Weinberg EJ, Kaazempur Mofrad MR. Transient, three-dimensional, multiscale simulations of the human aortic valve. *Cardiovasc Eng.* 2007;7(4):140–155.
42. Tang AY, Chung WC, Liu ET, et al. Computational fluid dynamics study of bifurcation aneurysms treated with pipeline embolization device: side branch diameter study. *J Med Biol Eng.* 2015;35(3):293–304.
43. Alharbi Y, Otton J, Al Abed A, Muller D, Lovell N, Dokos S. Computational modelling of transcatheter mitral valve replacement to predict Post–Procedural haemodynamics. *Heart Lung Circ.* 2018;27:S229.
44. Otton JM, Spina R, Sulas R, et al. Left atrial appendage closure guided by personalized 3D-printed cardiac reconstruction. *JACC Cardiovasc Interv.* 2015;8(7): 1004–1006.
45. Sturla F, Vismara R, Jaworek M, et al. In vitro and in silico approaches to quantify the effects of the mitraclip((R)) system on mitral valve function. *J Biomech.* 2017;50: 83–92.
46. Ripley B, Kelil T, Cheezum MK, et al. 3D printing based on cardiac CT assists anatomic visualization prior to transcatheter aortic valve replacement. *J Cardiovasc Comput Tomogr.* 2016;10(1):28–36.
47. Hernandez-Enriquez M, Brugaletta S, Andreu D, et al. Three-dimensional printing of an aortic model for transcatheter aortic valve implantation: possible clinical applications. *Int J Cardiovasc Imaging.* 2017;33(2): 283–285.
48. Qian Z, Wang K, Liu S, et al. Quantitative prediction of paravalvular leak in transcatheter aortic valve replacement based on tissue-mimicking 3D printing. *JACC Cardiovasc Imaging.* 2017;10(7):719–731.
49. Abdel-Sayed P, Kalejs M, von Segesser LK. A new training set-up for trans-apical aortic valve replacement. *Interact Cardiovasc Thorac Surg.* 2009;8(6):599–601.
50. Mahmood F, Owais K, Montealegre-Gallegos M, et al. Echocardiography derived three-dimensional printing of normal and abnormal mitral annuli. *Ann Card Anaesth.* 2014;17(4):279–283.
51. Mahmood F, Owais K, Taylor C, et al. Three-dimensional printing of mitral valve using echocardiographic data. *JACC Cardiovasc Imaging.* 2015;8(2):227–229.
52. Vukicevic M, Mosadegh B, Min JK, Little SH. Cardiac 3D printing and its future directions. *JACC Cardiovasc Imaging.* 2017;10(2):171–184.
53. Dankowski R, Baszko A, Sutherland M, et al. 3D heart model printing for preparation of percutaneous structural interventions: description of the technology and case report. *Kardiol Pol.* 2014;72(6):546–551.
54. Mashari A, Knio Z, Jeganathan J, et al. Hemodynamic testing of patient-specific mitral valves using a pulse duplicator: a clinical application of three-dimensional printing. *J Cardiothorac Vasc Anesth.* 2016;30(5):1278–1285.
55. Wang DD, Eng M, Greenbaum A, et al. Predicting LVOT obstruction after TMVR. *JACC Cardiovasc Imaging.* 2016; 9(11):1349–1352.
56. Wang DD, Eng MH, Greenbaum AB, et al. Validating a prediction modeling tool for left ventricular outflow tract (LVOT) obstruction after transcatheter mitral valve replacement (TMVR). *Cathet Cardiovasc Interv.* 2018;92(2).
57. El Sabbagh A, Eleid MF, Matsumoto JM, et al. Three-dimensional prototyping for procedural simulation of transcatheter mitral valve replacement in patients with mitral annular calcification. *Cathet Cardiovasc Interv.* 2018.
58. Jalal Z, Seguela P, Iriart X, et al. Hybrid melody valve implantation in mitral position in a child: usefulness of a 3-dimensional printed model for preprocedural planning. *Can J Cardiol.* 2018;34(6):812.e5–812.e7. https://doi.org/10.1016/j.cjca.2018.02.011.
59. Bagur R, Cheung A, Chu MWA, Kiaii B. 3-dimensional-printed model for planning transcatheter mitral valve replacement. *JACC Cardiovasc Interv.* 2018;11(8): 812–813.
60. Hachulla AL, Noble S, Guglielmi G, Agulleiro D, Muller H, Vallee JP. 3D-printed heart model to guide LAA closure: useful in clinical practice? *Eur Radiol.* 2018.
61. Obasare E, Mainigi SK, Morris DL, et al. CT based 3D printing is superior to transesophageal echocardiography for pre-procedure planning in left atrial appendage device closure. *Int J Cardiovasc Imaging.* 2018;34(5):821–831.
62. Liu P, Liu R, Zhang Y, Liu Y, Tang X, Cheng Y. The value of 3D printing models of left atrial appendage using real-time 3D transesophageal echocardiographic data in left atrial appendage occlusion: applications toward an era of truly personalized medicine. *Cardiology.* 2016;135(4):255–261.
63. Iriart X, Ciobotaru V, Martin C, et al. Role of cardiac imaging and three-dimensional printing in percutaneous appendage closure. *Arch Cardiovasc Dis.* 2018.
64. Bieliauskas G, Otton J, Chow DHF, et al. Use of 3-dimensional models to optimize pre-procedural planning of percutaneous left atrial appendage closure. *JACC Cardiovasc Interv.* 2017;10(10):1067–1070.
65. Song H, Zhou Q, Zhang L, et al. Evaluating the morphology of the left atrial appendage by a transesophageal echocardiographic 3-dimensional printed model. *Medicine (Baltim).* 2017;96(38):e7865.
66. Robinson SS, Alaie S, Sidoti H, et al. Patient-specific design of a soft occluder for the left atrial appendage. *Nat Biomed Eng.* 2018;2(1):8–16.

CHAPTER 8

The Role of 3D Modeling in the Treatment of Advanced Heart Failure

PLASENCIA JONATHAN, PHD • RYAN JUSTIN, PHD • STEPHEN POPHAL, MD

BACKGROUND

Heart Failure

Heart failure (HF) is the inability of the heart to keep up with the body's needs, or more specifically, a condition where the heart generates inadequate output to meet the metabolic needs of the body. Over 26 million people worldwide, 6 million in the United States, have been diagnosed with HF. Advanced heart failure (AHF) is the final stage of HF in which conventional medical therapies are no longer adequate; this later stage represents 10% of the HF population.[1,2] Approximately 250,000 people are diagnosed as having AHF in the United States per year, with 10% representing the pediatric population.[3,4] These statistics suggest 1% of HF patients are children with AHF. The prevalence of HF is increasing and the prognosis from AHF is still poor. As medical breakthroughs continue, the median age for patients in HF rises. Moreover, the prevalence of HF across all populations continues to increase as the population ages.[5]

Even as medical breakthroughs continue, the prognosis for patients with AHF continues to remain unchanged. Mortality rates are as high as 10% and 50% at 5 years and 10 years, respectively, for patients admitted for the first time with AHF.[6–9] These mortality rates increase in elderly patients. In fact, patients over 70 years of age have >35% 1-year mortality when admitted for AHF.[10] Over half of the adults with AHF die within 5 years, despite maximal medical and pharmacological therapies.[5]

There are numerous causes of HF, but these causes can be subcategorized into HF with reduced ejection fraction (HFrEF) or HF with preserved ejection fraction (HFpEF). HFrEF and HFpEF populations are fairly evenly distributed but, as risk factors for HF are reduced, and with aggressive early revascularization, the percentage of patients with HFpEF is increasing. This may also be a factor of the aging population.[2,11] HFpEF can be subdivided further based on two criteria: proper pump filling or inadequate pump filling with diastolic dysfunction. Patients may have appropriate filling and ejection mechanics of their hearts and still have HF due to the increased metabolic needs of the body. Increased needs include overwhelming sepsis or anemia and will not be covered in this chapter. HFpEF may not be a myocardial function issue but an ineffective valve issue, as commonly seen with aortic or mitral valve disease. Valve abnormalities can certainly lead to chronic or acute HF and will be covered in the structural and congenital sections of this book. Pump failure will be covered in this chapter and include HFpEF with inadequate pump performance due to inadequate filling (diastolic dysfunction) or HFrEF with inadequate pumping (systolic dysfunction). Hypertension or hypertrophic cardiomyopathy is an example of inadequate filling where there is significant diastolic dysfunction creating a scenario where the pump cannot fill appropriately to keep up with the body's needs. Postischemic or dilated cardiomyopathy is an example where the pump can fill, but cannot generate enough cardiac output to keep up with the body's metabolic needs. Congenital heart disease (CHD) has its own complexities in which the pump has predictable early failure rates.

While HF therapies, possibly supported by 3D modeling, may palliate a patient's chronic condition, the definitive solution for a patient with AHF has historically been heart transplantation. However, current availability of donor hearts in the United States is a significant limitation of this first-rate treatment option for the AHF patient. Only 2200 donor hearts are available annually with around 45% of those hearts used for pediatric heart transplants (HTxs).[3,4] One in ten adults die while on the wait list.[12–15] Due to a large deficit of appropriately sized allografts being available for children listed for heart transplantation, these patients

3-Dimensional Modeling in Cardiovascular Disease. https://doi.org/10.1016/B978-0-323-65391-6.00008-9

have the highest waiting list mortality in solid-organ transplant in the United States. In fact, 17% of pediatric patients died while waiting for an appropriate donor heart in the United States.[16] Waitlist mortality is highest in the smallest of pediatric patients (24% and 20% for body weights $\leq 5kg$ and $\leq 20kg$, respectively) while the mortality in the largest of pediatric patients (11% for body weights $> 65kg$) is comparable to the adult population.[12,16]

Mechanical circulatory support (MCS) devices are a series of engineering solutions designed to address limitations of cardiac allograft transplantations—including donor shortage—and even an attempt to allow diseased hearts a chance to recover before resorting to an orthotropic HTx. These devices are medical pumps designed to either aid or fully replace a patient's cardiac flow needs for their pulmonary circulation, systemic circulation, or both. After many design iterations over the last 30 years, MCS devices are becoming an increasingly popular option to address the donor shortage as a "bridge-to-transplant" or even as a feasible alternative to the allograft HTx (bridge-to-destination).

Finding appropriately sized MCS devices and allografts is a clinical challenge—particularly in small adults, children, and the overall CHD patient population. The challenge is that the treatment must meet the patient's cardiac output needs while not significantly oversizing the implantable portion of the device or allograft. Oversizing is concern for compressing clinically significant anatomical structures—usually in the cardiothoracic space. It is important to (1) identify available MCS options for a patient and (2) improve the available donor population for a given patient, in order to best treat for AHF. Clinical standards for both MCS device and allograft fit assessments are limiting due to the metrics being far removed from cardiac anatomy and/or fail to fully realize the complex anatomy of the congenital patient.

Mechanical Circulatory Support

The first MCS device was implanted into a human in 1969, but it was not until the early 1980s that the first permanent MCS device was implanted.[17] MCS devices work to move approximately 6 L of blood every minute in the adult patient. These cardiac pumps can further be divided into several more subgroups that include ventricular assist devices (VADs) and artificial hearts. The use of the MCS terminology in this chapter refers to VADs and artificial hearts. Extracorporeal membrane oxygenation and cardiopulmonary bypass machines are technically further subgroups of MCS devices but, unless otherwise stated, these additional device classes

are not encompassed in this chapter's use of "MCS." The setbacks and successes of all MCS device designs in the 1980s demonstrate the engineering and clinical complexity of these modern devices used today. The first generation of MCS devices developed for human implantation was designed over 30 years ago. The increased frequency of heterotopic HTxs and the desire for a reliable, permanent MCS device was driven, in part, by the high rate of allograft rejections during this time period as this was in the era before effective immunosuppressive agents became available.[18–20]

The first-generation VADs were large, bulky, displacing devices with limited durability. They were placed below the diaphragm in the abdominal cavity leading to additional organ dysfunction.[21] In addition, the power supply was limited, and patients required bulky drive lines tethered to the power source. The drive lines frequently became infected.[22] The success of immunosuppressive agents reducing allograft rejection, engineering limitations of the time, and the short survivability durations while on the first-generation devices, pushed MCS designs from trying to provide a permanent solution to a bridge-to-transplant option in the late 1980s.[17]

Over the past several decades, MCS devices have continued to improve. VAD and artificial heart designs have been refined for less displacement in average to large size adults. Larger systems have been replaced with smaller flow systems that can be placed inside the thorax with much smaller and reliable energy supplies. Enhanced durability and reliability of modern MCS devices have greatly reduced the morbidity and mortality of patients awaiting HTx.[23] The relatively recent Randomized Evaluation of Mechanical Assistance for the Treatment of Congestive Heart Failure (REMATCH) study further energized the clinical and engineering communities that MCS devices can be an alternative, permanent bridge-to-destination solution for the AHF patient.[17]

Today, MCS devices can be used as a stopgap measure to extend the patient's survival, either for the return of organ function necessary for successful heart transplantation (bridge-to-candidacy), or for increasing chances of an available donor heart (bridge-to-transplantation).[24] Older patients with AHF and patients with multiple organ failure may not be HTx candidates but can be candidates to MCS devices for destination therapy (bridge-to-destination). These designs, regardless of their smaller size relative to older device generations, are generally only approved for use in individuals with average or above average adult size. The size of modern device designs is still a critical consideration for implantation in small adults and children, even though MCS devices have been used in the pediatric population since the late 1980s as a bridge-to-transplantation.[25] However, the International Heart Lung Transplant Society (ISHLT) provides evidence that MCS use is increasing, especially in pediatric medicine.[26] At present, nearly one-fifth of pediatric patients, prior to heart transplantation, are first bridged with an MCS device. These scenarios support a clinical need for understanding MCS use and novel implantation techniques. This is especially important for pediatric patients due to the few devices approved for pediatric implantation.

Complex congenital anatomies further restrict the use of this technology in the congenital heart population who are prone to developing AHF at an early age. Over 25% of CHD patients will progress to AHF by 30 years of age.[27] This continues to be an issue in the adult survivors of CHD, who with improved childhood survival, now outnumber children with CHD.[28,29] This adult congenital patient population may be the most significant subset of all those with cardiovascular disease due to the difficulties in customizing standard MCS therapy into their unique, patient-specific spaces. Frequently, the cardiac mass of the CHD patient is displaced and inverted, making MCS insertion difficult or impossible. The potential for other comorbidities and often history of multiple previous surgeries are additional challenges for advanced MCS therapy options in this population.

Heart Transplantation

Heart transplantation is considered the ultimate therapy for AHF patients with no evidence of recovery after pharmacologic measures or VAD support; even with the currently increasing acceptance of MCS therapy as a bridge-to-destination. The first human cardiac allograft transplant was an orthotopic HTx performed in 1967 with the first recognized successful infant HTx being performed in 1984.[30] Although the first human transplantation was an orthotopic HTx, physicians shifted toward heterotopic HTx due to the high rate of allograft rejection. With an orthotopic HTx the native heart is replaced with the allograft while a heterotopic HTx preserves the native heart by attaching the secondary heart to the first heart. A key clinical justification for the heterotopic procedure in the early years of HTx was the hope that the native heart could take over if a second allograft was needed due to allograft rejection.

Immunosuppressive agents became available in the 1980s to prevent allograft rejection, nearly 2 decades after the first human HTx. Since immunotherapy became available, orthotopic HTxs became the clinical standard with only a few justifications warranting heterotopic HTx, e.g., undersized donor and/or high pulmonary pressure. Despite advancements in transplantation with immunotherapy, it is worth pointing out that the 1, 3, and 5 year survival rates post HTx are 85%, 75%, and 70%, respectively.[31] Half-life for patient and graft survival is 14 years, only slightly improved from previous eras. The success of immunotherapies in the mid-1980s began a shift in the clinical concern from overcoming allograft rejections to addressing donor shortage. As previously discussed, it was this increasing focus on donor shortage and waitlist mortality, along with MCS device challenges of the time, that shifted MCS designs from providing a permanent solution in the AHF patient to creating a bridge-to-transplant device.

Today, the donor shortage continues to be a concern in the United States, making allograft procurement a "waiting game." Waitlist mortality is approximately 1 in 10 in the adult population due to the gap between the needed for allografts and the donor supply. Quality of life and the duration patients can survive before an allograft becomes available has steadily increased since the 1980s—short- and long-term MCS have contributed to this success. The need for organs in the United States will continue to exceed the donor supply with an aging adult population and current clinical and donor enrollment practices. In fact, the gap between recipient needs and donor availability may increase rapidly with the usage of MCS devices solely, or largely, as bridge-to-transplant keeps sicker patients alive longer.

On the other end of the spectrum, the pediatric waitlist mortality is greater than in adults; the smallest of patients needing a cardiac allograft having the highest mortality for any solid-organ waitlist. Allograft shortages for the young pediatric population have pushed clinicians to aggressively expand donor pools.[16,32]

A major focus in expanding donor pools is finding ways to safely accept allografts that are traditionally seen as a size mismatch; this is particularly true with the oversized donor in pediatrics. Allograft size matching is considered a clinically relevant factor in HTx success.[33,34] In matching an ideal-sized allograft, clinicians heavily rely on a donor-to-recipient body weight ratio.[33] Focusing on allograft morphology, undersized allografts are at risk for cardiac output insufficiency, while oversized allografts are at risk for compression-related complications and limit the safety of chest closure post-op.

Historically, an HTx center will establish a donor-recipient body weight ratio criterion that is used when listing their patient for need of a donor organ. This body weight ratio criterion might be modified based on the specific clinical history of a patient. For example, clinical teams are often willing to accept oversized allografts for patients with cardiomyopathy due to their oversized native hearts. Some centers have expanded their donor-recipient body weight ratio criterion by expanding the upper and lower listing ranges for infants. Recent literature has suggested measurements and/or ratios other than body weight may better help expand a patient's donor pool—particularly focusing in the pediatric and congenital realms.[33,35,36] These publications suggest potential for optimally pushing donor size mismatch with the advent of newer imaging methods to acquire total cardiac volume and linear measurements with comparative 2D echo, CT, or MR measurements. The ultimate challenge with the body weight ratio (and medical imaging measurements avoids) is the metric is susceptible to sudden water retention, due to end-stage HF, and overweight. With complex congenital anatomies, clinical teams are often more conservative in accepting an allograft that is traditionally seen as oversized when compared to a "typical" or cardiomyopathy patient.

The waste of approximately 800 well-functioning donor organs—while there is a donor shortage in the United States—highlights the need to safely expand donor pools. There are several modern practices being implemented today to help procure a donor for the AHF patient—with an appropriately aggressive effort for obtaining an allograft for the pediatric and congenital AHF patient. The current challenge is further reducing the waste of well-functioning donor organs. Modern advancements in medical imaging and computer computational power has paved the way for 3D modeling techniques to help expand donor pools with the intent to reduce allograft waste and the ultimate goal of reducing the gap in the donor shortage and waitlist mortality rate.

3D Modeling and Its Use in Advance Heart Failure

In recent years, the innovative use of computer 3D modeling techniques has become increasingly popular in personalizing medicine to help physicians provide patient-specific therapies. Patient anatomy and medical devices can now be replicated as 3D computer modeled objects. Even preliminary device designs that are yet to be built can be modeled for in silico studies. These models can provide advanced visualizations of anatomy and guide preoperative device placement planning in the clinical environment. In engineering, 3D models

are used by industry to simulate fluid mechanics, i.e., computational fluid dynamic simulations, and drive anatomical fit during device development for AHF patient populations. These 3D models can be visualized by themselves or fused onto medial image datasets.

A computer 3D model is fundamentally a set of points describing an in silico object. For clinical and research applications, these models are generally described as a 3D Euclidian space that might include a fourth dimension to describe the relative position of the object's points in time. These computer models can be "surface meshes" to describe only the surface of the object or "volumetric meshes" to include points within the object. Surface meshes are computer resource friendly and therefore are the preferred mesh to use for basic task needing a model to describe only the surface of an object. Volumetric meshes are computationally expensive but are generally necessary for computer simulations, e.g., computational fluid dynamic simulations.

Cardiologist, interventionists, and surgeons have benefited from 3D modeling when personalizing medicine for their congenital, structural, acquired, and AHF patients. 3D visualization has allowed surgeons and interventionalists to see inside the thorax and inside the heart prior to critical procedures as described elsewhere in this book (Fig. 8.1). Virtual surgery including virtual VAD, total artificial heart (TAH), and heart transplantation is now a reality. As the size of MCS devices becomes smaller, more patients will be eligible for this type of support. Small adults, children, and patients born with CHDs will benefit from personalized virtual surgery. Surgeons, using 3D visualization techniques, will have added confidence in choosing the appropriate device or allograft to support all patients with AHF.

3D MODELING FOR MECHANICAL CIRCULATORY SUPPORT PLANNING
Background

Advanced imaging and 3D modeling may provide an outlook for potential complications associated to ill fit or complex morphology. Moreover, 3D modeling may even broaden utilization of MCS devices by opening devices to patients previously failing to meet eligibility criteria. For patients with CHD and structural heart disease, 3D printing has been shown to be useful for planning complex surgical and/or interventional procedures. Computer-based techniques of placing computational models of MCS devices into patient reconstructions (known colloquially as "virtual implantations") have been documented for over 5 years.[37,38]

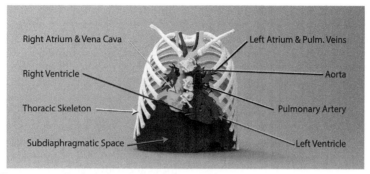

FIG. 8.1 A 3D reconstruction featuring skeletal and cardiac anatomy. Diaphragm location was achieved by reconstructing organ volume beneath the lungs (seen in brown).

Virtual implantation enables a surgical team to visualize the potential fit of a device and to preplan the orientation of the inflow and outflow cannulas (Fig. 8.2).

The size of current generation MCS devices effectively establishes an eligibility criterion regardless of cardiac output. The history of these MCS devices clearly shows that most of these devices were developed for the adult US population. Accordingly, these devices have an inherent size appropriate for that demographic. With a majority of women in the United States under the 1.7 m^2 body surface area measurement, it is understandable that a critical deficit of many of these devices is their barrier-to-use in smaller adult or pediatric patients. These barriers are delineated in the instructions-for-use of these devices as rigid thresholds for weight, height, BSA, BMI, and/or other gross patient parameters. These gross metrics do not directly take into account the specific regions of interest: the internal

thoracic space and the space available for an MCS device. 3D modeling, through a combination of patient image reconstruction and CAD modeling, can provide a pathway for considering patient-to-patient variation when determining fit.

Over two-thirds of patients with L-transposition (congenital heart condition where the right and left ventricles are in opposing positions) and other associated lesions (pulmonary stenosis, ventricular septal defect, Ebstein's anomaly) typically develop AHF by 45 years of age.[39] The complexities of the systemic right ventricle presently limit the utility of MCS implantation in this setting. With 20%−30% of patients with either simple or L transposition of the great arteries already developing AHF in early adulthood,[40] novel MCS use will become standard of care. In these patients, the right ventricle fails as a systemic ventricular pump and becomes heavily trabeculated, hypertrophic, and dysfunctional. Placement of VADs in this complex anatomy can lead to inflow obstruction, thrombosis, and hemolysis.

Proper positioning can be assessed with 3D visualization or 3D printing to minimize these complications. Understanding, preoperatively, the complexities of the right ventricular trabeculations and the septal and anterior leaflets of the tricuspid valve allows for more precise positioning of the inflow cannula. Extracardiac anatomy is also modeled to minimize compression of vital organs displaced by MCS systems. It is not uncommon to place a VAD in the right upper quadrant due to the positioning of the systemic ventricle in complex CHD. 3D modeling is uniquely suited to tackle these morphological challenges posed by complex or undersized cardiac and thoracic anatomy. MCS support in CHD is increasing rapidly but the complexities of CHD cannot be understated. The ventricle and cardiac mass may be misplaced to the right side of the chest in dextrocardia. The right and left ventricles may be

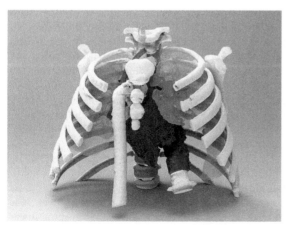

FIG. 8.2 A 3D model of a potential ventricular assist device recipient. Inflow and outflow cannulas are simulated (seen in white).

inverted in l-transposition of the great arteries. The atria may be surgically baffled to the opposite ventricle in Mustard or Senning repairs of d-transposition of the great arteries. Single ventricle physiology with hypoplastic right of left ventricle creates an even more challenging MCS/VAD support environment as there is an absence of small ventricle that may require mechanical support. Cases of 3D printing for presurgical VAD planning have shown great promise.[27] Advances in 3D modeling may take the place of 3D printing for select VAD planning for complex CHD.

Methods

The following methods are intended to represent a common approach for using 3D modeling for MCS device planning. It is not intended as complete overview of all 3D modeling methods found in contemporary literature.

Given the critical state of the patient with HF, it is expected that medical images (CT or MR) will be obtained, per standard of care, for a patient in or near organ failure. The resulting images may have poor spatial resolution and may have limited or no contrast. For patients with congenital anatomy, the unusual cardiac pathways may further complicate imaging of blood volumes. An ideal scenario would be isometric voxels as small as possible (typically less than 1 mm) with adequate differentiation of blood volumes. For the purpose of emergent MCS planning, a noncontrast scan can still provide critical information in device selection or optimal approach planning.

The image datasets can be imported into medical imaging software suites that enable segmentation: the process of differentiating an image into discrete subsets. The differentiation is typically achieved through intensity value changes in an image. For MCS planning, an ideal reconstruction may result in a 3D model featuring the thoracic skeleton, airway, and cardiac structures. Additional anatomical structures such as the diaphragm and thoracic wall (soft tissue) may yield additional critical information in the planning process. The resulting segmented structures can be used to generate 3D computer mesh files. A common example of this is a stereolithographic file or STL. Additional use of computer-aided design (CAD) software packages can help to remove noise and imaging artifacts from the mesh files. The same or similar software packages can also add color information to differentiate the components of a 3D model. The color differentiation can help with communication between interdisciplinary teams or to aid in visual differentiation on a screen or workstation.

In advanced medical image processing software, the patient computation mesh files can be registered to the original medical images. A computational mesh of a potential MCS device can be imported and registered into the same hybrid imaging dataset. This device mesh can be acquired by 3D scanning a medical device, reverse engineering the exterior of a medical device, or openly provided by a medical device company. Once the mesh for the device is in the same computational environment as the patient mesh files, an interdisciplinary team can move, rotate, and position the device in a manner similar to an actual surgery.

For instance, in the case of an artificial heart, the ventricles and native valves are removed. An operator of the medical software would replicate this process by removing the ventricular myocardium and/or the ventricular blood volume. He or she would then orient the artificial heart inflows and outflows in coordination with a surgical team member. If fit is a concern of this device, then the mesh can be compared to the original medical images. It is common for medical imaging software to overlay contours of a 3D geometry onto a 2D orthogonal medical image. This leaves the impression of the potential placement of the MCS device. If the contour is over a critical structure, this could imply significant displacement or obstruction of said structure (Fig. 8.3).

Recent Findings

Virtual surgery as a mean for procedural planning is a developing field. AbioMed released a software platform (AbioFit, ABIOMED, Danvers, MA) to assist clinical teams in evaluating the potential fit of the AbioCor device.[41] This software platform utilized computational rendering to build an image of patient geometry and allowed a virtual AbioCor to be superimposed in the 3D environment. Several centers have similarly explored virtual applications of this technology with similar methods.[37,38,42,43] These studies illustrate cases whereby an undersized patient received an adult-sized MCS device following virtual implantation. These types of cases are not unique. While virtual implantation is not always used to help determine fit, there are numerous other cases of patients with smaller thoracic dimensions, such as adolescent and small adult patients with advanced, biventricular HF awaiting transplant.[42,44,45]

A recent study reviewed the perceived use of 3D modeling to predict TAH device fit when compared to traditional eligibility criteria. In this analysis, a false acceptance of a medical device occurred in over 20% of cases where the criteria was a sternal-to-spine linear dimension at T10, suggesting that potentially 20% of cases could receive a device according to traditional

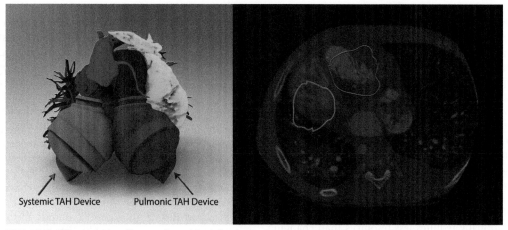

Systemic TAH Device   Pulmonic TAH Device

FIG. 8.3 3D reconstruction and a virtual implant of a Total Artificial Heart (TAH) in a patient with dextroposition.

criteria when virtual results question the safety of such an implantation. Interestingly, false device omission rates also approached 20%, suggesting that a significant number of potential cases where the MCS device would actually fit would have been rejected. In other words, these cases also had conflicting results between traditional criteria and the virtual result.[45] Examples of these patients, who should have received a device and did not include patients with dilated cardiomyopathy and pectus deformity.

That being said, virtual implantation has some significant limitations. Most importantly, there is a lack of validation of this entire virtual process. The only corroborating evidence in literature appears to be case studies supporting MCS device use in smaller patients following a virtual study. Animal models or cadaveric studies are needed to properly validate that virtual implantation is a viable planning tool.

Future work required for this technology includes the need for finite element analysis of tissue displacement in conjunction with virtual implantation. Currently finite element modeling is done on advanced workstations, often run by engineers or scientists. However, novel technologies in the field of 3D modeling can put similar tools in the hands of clinicians. Virtual, mixed, and augmented realities are already being used by clinicians to plan procedures in a computational environment. The incorporation of these technologies in device fit analysis is in development.[46] In addition, there are similar developments to "virtual" implantation by 3D printing patient-specific anatomy and performing mock operations and mock implantations. 3D print–guided procedures give clinicians an

opportunity to place devices multiple times, or in multiple orientations, before performing the ultimate procedure on the patient.[27]

3D MODELING FOR MECHANICAL CIRCULATORY SUPPORT DESIGN
Background
While 3D modeling can help better utilize available MCS devices in undersized or complex patients, the technology is also well suited to address the needs for future device design and development.

While some device manufacturers are researching and developing pediatric and small adult-specific MCS devices, at present, clinical teams using currently available MCS devices must fully appreciate patient-specific thoracic morphology when deciding on a specific device for an individual patient. 3D modeling can assist in establishing more accurate eligibility criteria for fit.

Methods
The methods for research and development using 3D modeling follows a similar pathway to planning as describe previously. A medical image reconstruction would take place over a patient population targeted by the medical device.

In cases where a biventricular device was considered, the devices would be computationally translated and rotated to the region of interest, likely being where the cardiac mass currently resides. In addition, the inflow and outflow structure(s) or cannula(s) would be computationally guided by a cardiothoracic surgeon. Advanced medical image software packages allow for real-time placement and distortion of cannula structures; however, there are computational limitations which may impact accuracy. Finite element modeling is seen as an accurate measure to approximate structure deformation, but this process requires a great amount of computational resources.

Following placement of the device and inflow and outflow cannulas, the research team may begin analysis. From contemporary literature on MCS trials, regions of interest include linear distance to the native valves and gross analysis of any structures that may extend beyond the region of implantation (such as extracorporeal parts of a device). The information gleaned from these virtual studies may assist in redesigning the shape and structures of an MCS device. Changing aspects of a device computationally requires less resources than changing a physical prototype.

Recent Findings

A recent use of 3D modeling in MCS device planning can be observed in the NIH-funded PumpKIN (Pumps for Kids, Infants, and Neonates) trial. The trial is geared toward the development of a pediatric-focused VAD. Trial coordinators utilized 3D modeling to computationally implant the VAD into a series of patient reconstructions that varied in age, weight, and height. Researchers placed the devices in a series of orientations using comparatively novel approaches (including placing the device inferior to the diaphragm). This information gave the VAD company an opportunity to review implantation orientations as well as understand possible impediments to the technology. With regards to the clinical trial, the information was used to justify the eligibility criteria for safe and effective deployment of a pediatric MCS device (Fig. 8.4).[45,47]

3D MODELING FOR HEART TRANSPLANTATION

Background

The geometric-related considerations a HTx team need to evaluate at the time of donor offer are whether an allograft can (1) effectively provide the patient's cardiac output needs (i.e., is not undersized) and (2) not compress critical anatomy (i.e., oversized), such as pulmonary veins and airway. With respect to the undersized allograft, the complex physiological interaction of a transplanted allograft and patient anatomy is one likely reason that 3D modeling techniques, e.g., with computational fluid dynamic simulations, have yet to be presented in the literature. While geometric volume of the heart dictate gross cardiac output, factors such as the electrical firing rate and muscle contractility percentage also contribute to minor flow rate adjustments. Future work would need to develop methods of using 3D modeling techniques—such as fluid simulations and associated of minor flow rate adjustments—to assess the performance of undersized allografts in meeting an individual patient's cardiac output needs efficiently.

On the other hand, volume measurements and 3D modeling have been increasingly used to assess oversized allograft fits. Donor-recipient body weight ratio is the clinical standard overwhelmingly used as the stand-alone metric in evaluating allograft size matching in the current era. This stand-alone metric may be unnecessarily limiting a patient's donor pool by suggesting an allograft is oversized. As previously discussed, body weight is far removed from cardiac anatomy and accounts neither for sudden recipient weight gains in the AHF patient due to fluid retention nor body type due to overweight. CHD patient anatomies often result

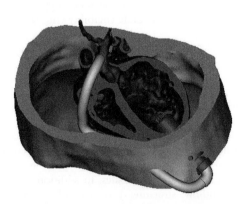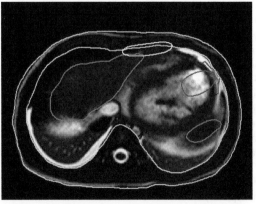

FIG. 8.4 A 3D reconstruction of a patient with dilated cardiomyopathy. A virtual device is placed in the reconstruction to gauge potential fit of the device in the patient-specific anatomy.

in heightened caution when accepting an oversized allograft offer. Nonlinear growth patterns and inconsistent growth rates in pediatric patient may further exacerbate the utility of body weight in the pediatric patient.

Building off of developments in the virtual MCS fit assessment space, virtual HTx fit assessments have undergone development in recent years. Echocardiographic measurements, including total cardiac volume measurements, have been suggested by several groups as potential solutions to overcome the limitations of the aforementioned body weight ratio. Similarly, basic, linear regression models have been used to compare total cardiac volume ratios. These recent activities by transplant teams point to a shift in the clinical community to using geometric assessment of the heart and/or surrounding anatomy to determine appropriate allograft fit.

Another challenge in the development of a tool for virtual HTx assessment is the infinite variability of donor allografts. With MCS devices there are a finite set of designs that can be considered. Additionally, MCS devices are generally rigid while a heart has some compliance. With all of these challenges yet to overcome, it can be said that at the current time, virtual HTx fit assessment methods are in their infancy and will need to evolve to become consistently clinically useful.

Methods

Virtual HTx fit assessments follow similar methodology to virtual MCS device assessments. An allograft, 3D computer model is strategically fused onto a volumetric medical CT or MR image by an interdisciplinary team. Geometry of the total cardiac volume, including great vessel anatomy and blood volume deep to the extracardiac myocardium tracing, is included. Placement considering atrium and ventricle locations of the recipient and donor are taken into account when translating and rotating the allograft onto patient geometry. The team has the opportunity during the translate-and-rotate procedure to evaluate the donor anatomy within the confines of the recipient's anatomy. Overlap of rigid structures, e.g., sternum and vertebral column, and compliant (but critical) structures, e.g., pulmonary veins and airways, are typical concerns for transplant surgeons evaluating virtual fits. During the virtual placement it is the obstacles observed and overall challenge of attempting to find an ideal fit for the model, through translations and rotations, that a surgeon will get an overall impression of the fit for an offered allograft.

Fusing an allograft geometry to a volumetric medical image is typically sufficient for surgical evaluation of fit. However, in selected complex cases, virtual 3D model reconstructions of recipient bones, airway, great vessels, and atria (both recipient and donor) have been found to be helpful for surgical evaluation. The added benefit of evaluating the allograft model in the potential recipient's 3D modeled anatomy is surgeons can evaluate the final fit in a virtual 3D space. Furthermore, a 3D model of a recipient's total cardiac volume can be measured and compared to the donor total cardiac volume—in a similar fashion to how the donor-recipient body weight ratio was made.

Two additional clinical challenges of developing and implementing a virtual HTx assessment tool exist. First, clinicians often have an hour or less to provisionally accept an allograft necessitating that any virtual assessment tool would need to be expedient in delivering decision support. Second, not all donors receive diagnostic volumetric images (CT or MRI). One academic approach at overcoming these limitations was the development of an advanced statistical model to predict allograft total cardiac volume.[48,49] The model was developed with consideration of noninvasive, donor parameters that would be readily available at donor offer. The predictive total cardiac volume model assumed donor allografts are normal, healthy hearts, i.e., the predictive model was developed using measurements from healthy heart individuals. The 3D total cardiac volume models of the healthy hearts were also stored in a library to be used later for fit assessments that relied on the total cardiac volume prediction model.

The virtual HTx pipeline that was ultimately developed consisted of taking a listed patient's CT or MR images and making an initial 3D modeling of patient anatomy. Total cardiac volume was also measured from the computer model and archived. Once an offer was made, the ideal situation would be to get the donor images electronically transferred and a total cardiac volume model made and measured. With a donor image in hand, a total cardiac volume can be generated within minutes. The computer model would then be fused onto the listed patient's archived dataset and the anatomy could be evaluated for fit. If a donor image set is not available, donor gross parameters could be used to predict the allograft total cardiac volume and a library model could be fused and evaluated for fit.

These statistical models to predict total cardiac volume generally rely on the theory that human growth proceeds such that different anatomical structures grow at different rates; that is, a scaling of anatomy from a newborn to an adult would not necessarily be on a linear scale. To understand this nonlinear scale, advanced statistical learning methods can be utilized to understand how cardiac volume relates to noninvasive parameters (parameters available at donor listing). To perform this learning algorithm, multiple 3D datasets are necessary for complex analysis. A large dataset of normal cardiac volumes is reconstructed (as surface mesh datasets) and utilized to train the computer algorithm. An example implementation is well described in which power law concepts from the field of allometry are used to account for the nonlinear growth patterns seen during animal development.

The result of this statistical learning process is a regression model that may yield a closer morphological match than simple donor-to-recipient body weight comparisons. However, it is worth noting that this technology is still undergoing validation.

Recent Findings

As noted, the donor-to-recipient body weight ratio is the current gold standard for allograft size matching. The main limitation of this ratio is that cardiac anatomy is not directly proportional and related to body weight. A comparison of recipient and donor weight may not yield accurate information on potential allograft. Furthermore, the ratio does not account for cardiomyopathy or complex CHD lesions. Aggressively expanding donor pool acceptance ranges out of perceived clinical necessity, without an objective tool to predict acceptability, may expose patients to additional risk or lead physicians to decline otherwise acceptable organs due to uncertainty. The objective of this chapter's transplant subsection is to demonstrate that virtual transplant fit assessments are a feasible method to account for patient-specific morphology with present-day technology which may help in reducing ambiguity in clinical decision-making.

Recent literature supports statistical learning-based approaches—generally referred in the current era as machine learning—which can model, more accurately, the size of the cardiac volume from noninvasive imaging and nonimaging parameters such as the information made available to clinicians at allograft availability. This formula may provide a better approach to assessing optimal fit than body weight ratio; however, regression models do have limitations.

First, regression models work best with a relatively large amount of training data (ideally, much greater than 100 datasets). Capturing normal images, especially images derived using ionizing radiation, of a large sample size may be challenging. Patients do not typically receive a CT for normal cardiac anatomy, so medical images are typically repurposed from trauma or other illness. Researchers would work with the assumption that the images are illustrating a normal anatomy despite whatever medical problem necessitates the image acquisition. CT images are generally better volumetric datasets because they capture more out-of-plane image slices than MRI due to the poor temporal resolution of the latter and the fact that the heart is beating during the scan. ECG gating, if feasible, can reduce motion artifact. Functional MR scans may limit the total number of slices creating less ideal volumetric datasets. Second, regression models only predict or help describe the sample data population, and do not describe an actual donor's total cardiac volume or geometry.

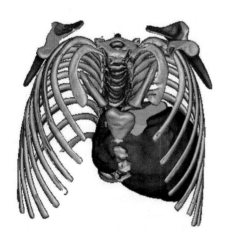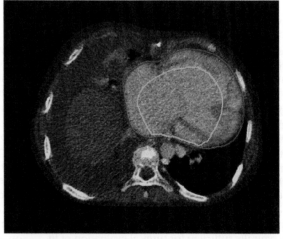

FIG. 8.5 A 3D reconstruction of a patient with dilated cardiomyopathy. A virtual allograft (green) can be observed against recipient anatomy (red).

Increasing subject size will allow for even more advance statistical learning techniques to be implemented to better address human development and variability.

While regression modeling has its deficits, it is important to restate that acquisition of donor images may circumvent the need to use a regression model and will likely yield a virtual transplant with greater accuracy. A virtual HTx when donor images were preoperatively available and assessed before transplant and the benefits of donor images to a regression model is already described in the literature.[49,50] Besides direct intraoperative comparison of cardiac volume, medical image reconstruction of donor and recipient anatomy will be the next best viable option as seen in Fig. 8.5. With the advent of low-dose CT scans, we may see a need from the medical community to consistently acquire medical images from donor patients and make them available to recipient institutes).

In addition to cardiac allografts, it is feasible to expect the translation of this process to develop into other allograft domains. 3D modeling therefore holds great potential to deliver patient-specific treatment plans for patients with AHF being evaluated for HTx.

CONCLUSION

3D modeling has and will continue to improve therapies for AHF patients. Innovations in this field are timely as the prevalence of HF is increasing, and the prognosis for patients with advance heart failure with standard therapies remains far from optimal. As novel CHD and AHF patients therapies evolve, patients will live longer, but their overall care will become more complex. MCS devices are becoming an increasingly popular option, but finding appropriate size match MCS devices for all populations remains a clinical challenge. In contrast to the increasing use and new designs of MCS devices, there is a limited number of donor allografts available for heart transplantation. Despite this limitation in organ supply, all quality donor organs are still not utilized. 3D modeling and computational matching techniques will help expand donor pools by reducing unnecessary allograft waste with the ultimate goal of reducing the gap in the donor shortage and wait-list mortality rate. Infants, small patients, and those with complex CHD pose unique challenges with MCS implantation and transplantation. Virtual implantation enables surgical teams to visualize the potential fit of devices and/or donor organs to preplan surgical techniques as well as gain confidence and practical experience prior to high-risk implantations.

As MCS designs improve and continue to get smaller, 3D modeling will assist HF teams in personalized MCS implantation. Machine learning and artificial intelligence may assist HF teams in perfecting imaging and customizing care pathways to utilize all available MCS devices and donor organs appropriately. Finite element analysis may help better predict outcomes in placing devices in complex spaces. Printing 3D models of customized grafts, replacement parts, and even organs will play an important role in improving future outcomes for patients with AHF.

REFERENCES

1. Savarese G, Lund LH. Global public health burden of heart failure. *Card Fail Rev.* 2017;3(1):7−11. https://doi.org/10.15420/cfr.2016:25:2.
2. Ponikowski P, Voors AA, Anker SD, et al. 2016 ESC Guidelines for the diagnosis and treatment of acute and chronic heart failure: The Task Force for the diagnosis and treatment of acute and chronic heart failure of the European Society of Cardiology (ESC)Developed with the special contribution of the Heart Failure Association (HFA) of the ESC. *Eur Heart J.* 2016;37(27):2129−2200. https://doi.org/10.1093/eurheartj/ehw128.
3. Givertz MM. Ventricular assist devices important information for patients and families. *Circulation.* 2011;124(12):e305−e311. https://doi.org/10.1161/CIRCULATIONAHA.111.018226.
4. Alboliras E. *Atlas of Neonatal Cardiology.* Hoboken, NJ: John Wiley & Sons; 2014.
5. Roger VL. Epidemiology of heart failure. *Circ Res.* 2013;113(6):646−659. https://www.ahajournals.org/doi/abs/10.1161/circresaha.113.300268.
6. Benjamin EJ, Virani SS, Callaway CW, et al. Heart disease and stroke statistics-2018 update: a report from the American heart association. *Circulation.* 2018;137(12):e67−e492. https://doi.org/10.1161/CIR.0000000000000558.
7. MacIntyre K, Capewell S, Stewart S, et al. Evidence of improving prognosis in heart failure: trends in case fatality in 66 547 patients hospitalized between 1986 and 1995. *Circulation.* 2000;102(10):1126−1131.
8. Mosterd A, Cost B, Hoes AW, et al. The prognosis of heart failure in the general population: the Rotterdam Study. *Eur Heart J.* 2001;22(15):1318−1327. https://doi.org/10.1053/euhj.2000.2533.
9. Chugh SS, Reinier K, Teodorescu C, et al. Epidemiology of sudden cardiac death: clinical and research implications. *Prog Cardiovasc Dis.* 2008;51(3):213−228. https://doi.org/10.1016/j.pcad.2008.06.003.
10. Rigatelli G, Santini F, Faggian G. Past and present of cardiocirculatory assist devices: a comprehensive critical review. *J Geriatr Cardiol.* 2012;9(4):389−400. https://doi.org/10.3724/SP.J.1263.2012.05281.

11. Ohlmeier C, Mikolajczyk R, Frick J, Prütz F, Haverkamp W, Garbe E. Incidence, prevalence and 1-year all-cause mortality of heart failure in Germany: a study based on electronic healthcare data of more than six million persons. *Clin Res Cardiol.* 2015;104(8):688–696. https://doi.org/10.1007/s00392-015-0841-4.

12. Singh TP, Milliren CE, Almond CS, Graham D. Survival benefit from transplantation in patients listed for heart transplantation in the United States. *J Am Coll Cardiol.* 2014;63(12):1169–1178. https://doi.org/10.1016/j.jacc.2013.11.045.

13. Lietz K, Miller LW. Improved survival of patients with end-stage heart failure listed for heart transplantation: analysis of organ procurement and transplantation network/U.S. United Network of Organ Sharing data, 1990 to 2005. *J Am Coll Cardiol.* 2007;50(13):1282–1290. https://doi.org/10.1016/j.jacc.2007.04.099.

14. Singh TP, Almond CS, Taylor DO, Graham DA. Decline in heart transplant wait list mortality in the United States following broader regional sharing of donor hearts. *Circ Heart Fail.* 2012;5(2):249–258. https://doi.org/10.1161/CIRCHEARTFAILURE.111.964247.

15. Khush KK, Menza R, Nguyen J, Zaroff JG, Goldstein BA. Donor predictors of allograft use and recipient outcomes after heart transplantation. *Circ Heart Fail.* 2013;6(2):300–309. https://doi.org/10.1161/CIRCHEARTFAILURE.112.000165.

16. Almond CSD, Thiagarajan RRM, Piercey GE, et al. Waiting list mortality among children listed for heart transplantation in the United States. *Circulation.* 2009;119(5):717–727. https://doi.org/10.1161/CIRCULATIONAHA.108.815712, 2009.

17. Culjat M, Singh R, Lee H. *Medical Devices: Surgical and Image-Guided Technologies.* 1 edition. Hoboken, N.J: Wiley; 2012.

18. Kadner A, Chen RH, Adams DH. Heterotopic heart transplantation: experimental development and clinical experience. *Eur J Cardiothorac Surg.* 2000;17(4):474–481.

19. Cooper DK, Novitzky D, Becerra E, Reichart B. Are there indications for heterotopic heart transplantation in 1986? A 2- to 11-year follow-up of 49 consecutive patients undergoing heterotopic heart transplantation. *Thorac Cardiovasc Surg.* 1986;34(5):300–304. https://doi.org/10.1055/s-2007-1022159.

20. Bellumkonda L, Bonde P. Ventricular assist device therapy for heart failure–past, present, and future. *Int Anesthesiol Clin.* 2012;50(3):123–145. https://doi.org/10.1097/AIA.0b013e31826233a9.

21. Costantini TW, Taylor JH, Beilman GJ. Abdominal complications of ventricular assist device placement. *Surg Infect.* 2005;6(4):409–418. https://doi.org/10.1089/sur.2005.6.409.

22. Prinzing A, Herold U, Berkefeld A, Krane M, Lange R, Voss B. Left ventricular assist devices-current state and perspectives. *J Thorac Dis.* 2016;8(8):E660–E666. https://doi.org/10.21037/jtd.2016.07.13.

23. Kirklin JK, Naftel DC, Pagani FD, et al. Seventh INTERMACS annual report: 15,000 patients and counting.

J Heart Lung Transplant. 2015;34(12):1495–1504. https://doi.org/10.1016/j.healun.2015.10.003.

24. Fang JC, Stehlik J. Moving beyond "bridges.". *JCHF.* 2013;1(5):379–381. https://doi.org/10.1016/j.jchf.2013.08.003.

25. Fuchs A, Netz H. Ventricular assist devices in pediatrics. *Images Paediatr Cardiol.* 2001;3(4):24–54.

26. The Registry of the International Society for Heart and Lung Transplantation: Nineteenth Pediatric Heart Transplantation Report–2016; Focus Theme: Primary Diagnostic Indications for Transplant – The Journal of Heart and Lung Transplantation. http://www.jhltonline.org/article/S1053-2498(16)30299-6/abstract.

27. Farooqi KM, Saeed O, Zaidi A, et al. 3D printing to guide ventricular assist device placement in adults with congenital heart disease and heart failure. *JACC Heart Fail.* 2016;4(4):301–311. https://doi.org/10.1016/j.jchf.2016.01.012.

28. Webb CL, Jenkins KJ, Karpawich PP, et al. Collaborative care for adults with congenital heart disease. *Circulation;* 2002. https://www.ahajournals.org/doi/abs/10.1161/01.cir.0000017557.24261.a7.

29. Greutmann M, Tobler D. Changing epidemiology and mortality in adult congenital heart disease: looking into the future. *Future Cardiol.* 2012;8(2):171–177. https://doi.org/10.2217/fca.12.6.

30. Chinnock RE, Bailey LL. Heart transplantation for congenital heart disease in the first year of life. *Curr Cardiol Rev.* 2011;7(2):72–84. https://doi.org/10.2174/157340311797484231.

31. Goldfarb SB, Hayes D, Levvey BJ, et al. The international thoracic organ transplant registry of the international society for heart and lung transplantation: twenty-first pediatric lung and heart–lung transplantation report-2018; focus theme: multiorgan transplantation. *J Heart Lung Transplant.* 2018;37(10):1196–1206. https://doi.org/10.1016/j.healun.2018.07.021.

32. Sorabella RA, Guglielmetti L, Kantor A, et al. Cardiac donor risk factors predictive of short-term heart transplant recipient mortality: an analysis of the united network for organ sharing database. *Transplant Proc.* 2015;47(10):2944–2951. https://doi.org/10.1016/j.transproceed.2015.10.021.

33. Camarda J, Saudek D, Tweddell J, et al. MRI validated echocardiographic technique to measure total cardiac volume: a tool for donor–recipient size matching in pediatric heart transplantation. *Pediatr Transplant.* 2013;17(3):300–306. https://doi.org/10.1111/petr.12063.

34. Reichart B. Size matching in heart transplantation. *J Heart Lung Transplant.* 1991;11(4 Pt 2):S199–S202.

35. Zuckerman WA, Richmond ME, Singh RK, Chen JM, Addonizio LJ. Use of height and a novel echocardiographic measurement to improve size-matching for pediatric heart transplantation. *J Heart Lung Transplant.* 2012;31(8):896–902. https://doi.org/10.1016/j.healun.2012.03.014.

36. Hahn E, Zuckerman WA, Chen JM, Singh RK, Addonizio LJ, Richmond ME. An echocardiographic measurement of superior vena cava to inferior vena cava distance in

patients<20 years of age with idiopathic dilated cardiomyopathy. *Am J Cardiol.* 2014;113(8):1405–1408. https://doi.org/10.1016/j.amjcard.2014.01.416.

37. Moore RA, Madueme PC, Lorts A, Morales DL, Taylor MD. Virtual implantation of the 50cc total artificial heart. *J Heart Lung Transplant.* 2015;34(4):S89. https://doi.org/10.1016/j.healun.2015.01.236.

38. Park SS, Sanders DB, Smith BP, et al. Total artificial heart in the pediatric patient with biventricular heart failure. *Perfusion.* 2014;29(1):82–88. https://doi.org/10.1177/0267659113496580.

39. Graham TP, Bernard YD, Mellen BG, et al. Long-term outcome in congenitally corrected transposition of the great arteries: a multi-institutional study. *J Am Coll Cardiol.* 2000;36(1):255–261.

40. Piran S, Veldtman G, Siu S, Webb GD, Liu PP. Heart failure and ventricular dysfunction in patients with single or systemic right ventricles. *Circulation.* 2002;105(10): 1189–1194.

41. Dowling RD, Etoch SW, Gray LA. Operative techniques for implantation of the AbioCor total artificial heart. *Operat Tech Thorac Cardiovasc Surg.* 2002;7(3):139–151. https://doi.org/10.1053/otct.2002.36316.

42. Moore RA, Madueme PC, Lorts A, Morales DLS, Taylor MD. Virtual implantation evaluation of the total artificial heart and compatibility: beyond standard fit criteria. *J Heart Lung Transplant.* 2014;33(11):1180–1183. https://doi.org/10.1016/j.healun.2014.08.010.

43. Moore RA, Madueme P, Pietila T, Lorts A, Taylor M, Morales D. Abstract 14122: total artificial heart fit study: using 3-dimensional computer simulation to perform virtual implantation of the total artificial heart in adolescents and young adults to ensure spatial suitability. *Circulation.* 2013;128(suppl 22). A14122-A14122.

44. Leprince P, Bonnet N, Varnous S, et al. Patients with a body surface area less than 1.7 m2 have a good outcome with the CardioWest Total Artificial Heart. *J Heart Lung Transplant.* 2005;24(10):1501–1505. https://doi.org/10.1016/j.healun.2005.01.016.

45. Ryan JR, Teal J, Pophal S, et al. Virtual implantation of the infant Jarvik 2015 for eligibility criteria establishment. *J Heart Lung Transplant.* 2017;36(4):S13–S14. https://doi.org/10.1016/j.healun.2017.01.021.

46. EchoPixel. Echopixel. http://www.echopixeltech.com/. Published 2018.

47. Baldwin JT, Adachi I, Teal J, et al. Closing in on the PumpKIN trial of the Jarvik 2015 ventricular assist device. *Semin Thorac Cardiovasc Surg Pediatr Card Surg Annu.* 2017;20: 9–15. https://doi.org/10.1053/j.pcsu.2016.09.003.

48. Plasencia J, Arizona State University. Development of a novel virtual tool for donor heart fitting. In: *ASU Electronic Theses and Dissertations.* Arizona State University; 2018. http://hdl.handle.net/2286/R.I.49031.

49. Plasencia JD, Kamarianakis Y, Ryan JR, et al. Alternative methods for virtual heart transplant-Size matching for pediatric heart transplantation with and without donor medical images available. *Pediatr Transplant.* 2018;22(8): e13290. https://doi.org/10.1111/petr.13290.

50. Plasencia JD, Ryan JR, Park SS, et al. The virtual heart transplant – the next step in size matching for pediatric heart transplantation. *J Heart Lung Transplant.* 2017;36(4): S165. https://doi.org/10.1016/j.healun.2017.01.433.

FURTHER READING

1. Ojo AO, Heinrichs D, Emond JC, et al. Organ donation and utilization in the USA. *Am J Transplant.* 2004;4:27–37. https://doi.org/10.1111/j.1600-6135.2004.00396.x.

2. Koomalsingh K, Kobashigawa JA. The future of cardiac transplantation. *Ann Cardiothorac Surg.* 2017;7(1):135–142. https://doi.org/10.3978/16430, 142.

CHAPTER 9

Current Challenges to the Use of 3D Modeling as a Standard Clinical Tool

REENA MARIA GHOSH, MD • ELIZABETH SILVESTRO, MSE • KEVIN K. WHITEHEAD, MD, PHD

INTRODUCTION

There are challenges that remain with incorporating 3D modeling into standard clinical practice. Though its utility has been demonstrated across a wide spectrum of adult and pediatric diseases, it is still an unfamiliar modality to most practitioners. Moreover, there is much practice variability in the multistep process of generating 3D models. The challenges faced in the widespread adoption of this new imaging technology can be approached at each step in that process: image acquisition, virtual reconstruction, and physical modeling. Finally at an institutional level there are specific challenges within the logistics of running a 3D modeling and/or printing lab.

IMAGE ACQUISITION

As mentioned previously but worth restating, the ability to generate 3D models is entirely reliant on excellent image acquisition. Without this, the rest of the process is impossible. Limitations in image acquisition involve the need for sedation/anesthesia, potential use of contrast, limiting radiation exposure, artifact obscuring a region of interest, use of images obtained without 3D modeling in mind, varying spatial and temporal resolutions of the imaging modalities, and the subsequent limitations on the level of detail it is possible to acquire.

Use of Sedation

Image acquisition in all modalities requires a patient to remain still for a certain period of time and ideally cooperate in breath-held sequences. As such, the need for sedation extends from pediatric patients and those with developmental delays, to patients with claustrophobia or altered mental state who are unable to follow directions. CT is the quickest method of image acquisition and in the abovementioned populations it is often able to be performed without sedation. However, in infants and young children, it still may require sedation or risk movement during acquisition. Furthermore, despite recent advances in radiation dose reduction, there are still concerns over minimizing radiation exposure in young and vulnerable populations. Adequate Cardiac MRI (CMR) image acquisition requires a patient to remain still for multiple extended periods of time, with high-resolution 3D sequences taking up to 10 min and a full study lasting at least 1 h.[1] Especially in pediatric patients, the degree of sedation required often causes enough respiratory depression that the safest option is to administer general anesthesia with mechanical ventilation.[2] 3D echocardiography also requires minimal patient and sonographer motion. Therefore many patients undergoing 3D transesophageal echocardiogram require sedation and intubation as well. Adequate 3D transthoracic echocardiography images can usually be acquired without sedation as long as a patient can participate in breath-held sequences. Eliminating respiratory variation in the image allows for multibeat acquisition and minimizes stitch artifact.[3,4]

Use of Contrast

Adequate visualization of a region of interest may require contrast administration. CT requires the use of iodinated contrast. Though rare, there is a risk of adverse reactions to contrast agents. Idiosyncratic reactions mimic signs and symptoms of anaphylaxis (i.e., hives, angioedema, wheezing, and hypotension) though the exact mechanism of action is unknown. Nonidiosyncratic reactions can lead to nausea, vomiting, pulmonary edema, or arrhythmia. Contrast-induced nephropathy can occur within 72 h of contrast administration and manifests with an increase in serum creatinine by at least 25%. Prestudy risk of nephropathy can be decreased by hydration.[5,6]

Once a decision is made to proceed with CT and expose a patient to contrast, the administration of a contrast bolus must be timed appropriately. This requires a good understanding of the anatomy and physiology of an individual patient and is extremely important in patients with congenital heart disease. Patients in low flow states, such as severe heart failure or passive pulmonary blood flow due to cavopulmonary anastomoses, may require a large bore IV or slower rate of contrast injection. If there is contrast washout or a poorly timed bolus, there will not be adequate contrast opacification of the structure of interest.[7] Additionally speckling within pools of contrast inside a chamber can lead to noise and result ultimately in segmentation error.[8]

Image acquisition using MRI for the purpose of segmentation and 3D modeling may or may not require the use of contrast. 3D steady-state free precession (SSFP) is advantageous because it is a noncontrast T2 weighted sequence that is ECG and respiratory gated. However, this sequence can have long acquisition times (7−10 min) during which a patient must remain completely still. Additionally, it is more susceptible to artifact generated from turbulent flow.[1] Contrast enhanced magnetic resonance angiography (CE-MRA) is a T1 sequence that utilizes the administration of gadolinium-based contrast which leads to increased differentiation between the myocardium and the blood pool. It allows for evaluation of myocardial perfusion and viability and allows for excellent segmentation of the blood pool and the vasculature. It is nongated and has the advantage of rapid acquisition (<1 min). However, administration of gadolinium-based contrast can lead to nephrogenic fibrosis and may not be possible in patients with existing evidence of renal injury.[1,9]

Image Artifact

Certain models of pacemakers and implantable cardioverter-defibrillators are contraindications to performing an MRI. However, even devices that are not absolutely contraindicated can still cause significant artifact and obscure a region of interest.[4] Typical objects which may result in important image artifact include stainless steel stents, coils, and wires previously placed in the cardiovascular system, or any other indwelling metal objects (i.e., orthodontics, spinal hardware).[10] Newer isotropic 3D dark blood sequences are less susceptible to metallic artifact but are not always available at all sites, and may not be employed unless a study is performed with 3D modeling in mind. It is more challenging and time consuming to segment the blood pool on these images, but it is an important alternative when metal artifact limits the quality of traditional MRA sequences.

The notable artifact present in echocardiograms is lung artifact, which despite otherwise adequate acoustic windows can prevent a skilled sonographer from obtaining adequate images. Metal artifact can also cause artifacts and streaking on CT images, though these tend to be more localized. High concentrations of contrast can also cause beam hardening artifact. Because 3D modeling may require details not always considered important in standard imaging (such as superior vena cava anatomy in a complex single ventricle), particular attention needs to be given to contrast bolus concentration and timing to ensure that the areas of interest are not degraded.

Use of Previously Acquired Images

Images obtained for the purpose of virtual or physical reconstruction ideally optimize spatial resolution and minimize temporal blurring (using cardiac gating), focus on the regions of interest, and are conducted using the appropriate amount of contrast and sedation (if necessary). The challenge in using images that were obtained prior to the decision to perform a 3D reconstruction is that the above factors may not have been addressed during image acquisition. The most frequent limitation is that slice thickness in cross-sectional imaging may be >1 mm leading to significant pixilation in other views during reconstruction.

Resolution of Imaging Modalities
CT

CT allows for excellent spatial resolution, with a typical slice thickness of less than 1 mm. It processes images in the form of a square matrix of voxels, which lends itself to generating 3D reconstructions. It is also excellent at detecting calcium deposition on valves. However, it has a lower temporal resolution than echocardiography and CMR. Temporal resolution is important because the heart is not a static structure. Unlike image acquisition for orthopedic or neuroanatomy, the heart is constantly in motion while obtaining images.

3D echocardiography

3D echo has excellent temporal resolution, which makes it particularly useful when imaging especially dynamic structures such as valve leaflets and chordal apparatus. However, its spatial resolution is best along the axial imaging plane which limits the ability of 3D echo to have adequate spatial resolution of two structures that are perpendicular to each other. Clinically this manifests as the inability to image the entire atrioventricular (AV) valve apparatus with a single dataset. Two sets of images need to be combined in the image processing software to generate the entire apparatus (i.e., a combination of the short and long axis images of the mitral valve).[11] Adequate spatial resolution is dependent on the need for breath-held acquisitions and four to six beat clips.[12] R wave–gated imaging enhances echocardiography spatial resolution but can only be used in patients with regular rhythm and minimal patient and probe motion.[13] Another limitation to good spatial resolution with echocardiography is that the images are represented in a narrow range of Hounsfield units that decrease its accuracy for smaller structures.[7]

MRI

Cardiac MRI has both adequate spatial and temporal resolution, with spatial resolution similar to but slightly inferior to that of CT. Traditional MRI slice thickness is often larger than CT which limits its utility in evaluating smaller vascular structures such as coronary arteries or the choral apparatus of AV valves. Slice thickness should be at most 1 mm thick to generate a high-quality segmentation.[8,14]

There is less artifact and more homogeneity when obtaining images on a 1.5T as compared to a 3T scanner, especially in the SSFP sequences that are commonly used for segmentation.[8,15] However, regardless of the strength of the magnet, there is some susceptibility to turbulent flow in MRI that can obscure critical anatomy. In the case of certain cardiac lesions, blood flow may be extremely turbulent and that flow may be governed by higher derivatives of motion other than velocity. This can cause phase dispersion and signal loss. As a result critical anatomic structures may not be well visualized.[10] This can often be overcome by imaging in diastole where velocities are lower, or using dark blood imaging which does not have this limitation. Despite these limitations, using respiratory navigated, cardiac gated sequences often provides high-quality images suitable for segmentation and 3D reconstruction across a wide range of anatomies. The use of newer intravascular contrast agents such as ferumoxytol along with novel sequences promise to provide multiphase 3D datasets that rival CT in their spatial resolution.

VIRTUAL RECONSTRUCTION

Segmentation of the acquired images and selecting the structures of interest is a very deliberate process.[16] Some segmentation is semiautomated, but standardization of the process is challenging because it is inherently very operator dependent.[17,18] As previously mentioned, the heart and particularly the valves are not static structures. The first decision to be made in this process is to choose the part of the cardiac cycle that will be used for segmenting the region of interest. For very dynamic structures such as the right ventricular outflow tract or the semilunar and AV valves, the decision may be to create two separate models, one mid-systole and the other in diastole.[11] Another challenge that hinders standardization of 3D modeling is that the operator chooses the range of units for thresholding. This can be a source of much variability, even when using the same source image. This challenge is demonstrated most clearly when attempting to print thin or tortuous structures. Choosing a narrow window minimizes the probability of including structures or tissue external to the region of interest, but it is a more laborious process and is prone to operator error.[19]

Another significant limitation in virtual reconstruction is the predominance of blood pool modeling. Existing methods for segmenting the myocardium are suboptimal. Dark blood sequences in MRI can be utilized,[15] but it can still be quite challenging to differentiate between myocardium and fat. Currently, hollow models are created by wrapping the blood pool. The operator chooses the thickness of the shell, which is added outside the blood pool interface, and the shell is applied uniformly. It likely does not accurately represent the wall of the great vessels or the myocardium.

ADDITIVE MANUFACTURING
Accuracy of Models

Generation of a physical model has proven to be quite useful across a wide spectrum of diseases. However, lack of evidence regarding the fidelity and accuracy of those models has limited its adoption as a clinical tool. Currently, there is no standard method for additive manufacturing (AM) of cardiac models in part due to limited evidence regarding validation of accuracy across different imaging modalities and printing methods. One of the few studies that exist is a recent international case-crossover study by Valverde et al. which demonstrated that 3D models accurately replicated cardiac anatomy with a mean bias of -027 ± 0.73 mm.[20] An agreement was determined between caliper measurements on the 3D model and on the MRI and CT images. They found that reliability in repeated measurements was extremely high with an intraobserver, intraclass correlation coefficient of 0.998 and interobserver variability of 0.996. These findings suggest that printed models can quite accurately represent patient anatomy, but the dearth of such studies currently limits its adoption as a standard clinical tool.

Material and Machine Limitations

Another challenge in standardizing the use of printed models is that the wide range of materials available for AM still has limitations for the creation of microstructures such as chordae tendineae. While some machines can print with a resolution of 25–50 microns, these minute structures are often too thin to remain intact post printing cleaning when the support material must be removed from the model through mechanical or chemical means. For a similar reason, the thin and delicate leaflet structure of in vivo valves is challenging to replicate in printed models, especially for neonatal patients. These materials have been rapidly expanding to meet the various mechanical properties such as hardness and strength but are still a distance away from simulating biological materials. There remains a need to balance the durability and pliability of models, particularly in the applications intended to be utilized for surgical and stitching practice.

An alternative for creating thin, compliant structures is casting, in which the printer is used to create a mold in which the parts are cast out of materials with more desirable mechanical properties. These parts can be added to the printed model. It is particularly useful for modeling valves. However, these techniques require increased expertise in creating and using molds and are more time intensive. Access to fume hoods is often required depending on the molding materials chosen.

Technological Opportunity

With every new technology, there is a strong drive to push it to its extreme to allow for maximum benefit. This creates a challenge to consider the benefits of a model or adjustment versus the potential to mislead or miscommunicate aspects. Examples of this can be seen in the consideration to enlarge models to provide a better view. Additionally, there can be a challenge to focus on models and project on what is truly needed to convey the condition without leading to overwhelming design iteration to include every potential option or features. This can be a challenging skill to learn how to properly balance medical need and more aesthetics wishes to ensure efficient work follow.

LOGISTICS OF RUNNING A 3D PRINTING/ ADDITIVE MANUFACTURING LAB

In addition to the physical limitations surrounding printing and modeling, another major concern is the obstacles faced in operating an in-house 3D printing lab. An onsite lab offers faster turnaround and stronger integration of clinicians in the modeling process resulting in a growing interest in the creation of these labs.

However, creation and maintenance of such a lab involves significant planning as well as important logistical, staffing, and financial issues that will vary from institution to institution.

Cost

There is currently no method for reimbursement for printing, but there have been several groups working on such applications. This will leave the burden of most costs to hospitals or companies. To this end there can be several aspects that need to be considered; machine selection, segmentation software, where the lab will be located, and who will create the model and run the machine. Each of these considerations can come with a multitude of options and trade-offs. Money can be saved on machine and software selection but could create a limitation on print options and challenge the accuracy of the models. To make 3D modeling and printing a standard clinical tool, additional staff may become necessary, including engineers to ensure top conditions and utilization of the machine.

Time

In addition to the cost of integration of 3D printing as a standard clinical tool, time can become a significant challenge. This can include the time spent segmenting, printing, cleaning parts, and machine maintenance. Each of these aspects requires a substantial amount of time to address and is not easily squeezed into an already tight schedule experienced in most imaging and cardiology departments. While time constraints must be considered a major factor in the creation of an in-house 3D lab and utilization of 3D modeling as a clinical tool, thoughtful and efficient planning can effectively address many of these issues.

VIRTUAL AND AUGMENTED REALITY

Along with AM, there has been an increasing interest in utilizing virtual and augmented reality. These platforms allow for the use of virtual headsets or projections to allow for a three-dimensional representation of models. This offers the benefits of more rapid turnaround and no need for printers and materials. However, this technology currently has a steep learning curve and typically requires significant equipment investment for ideal use. While this option may offer cost savings compared to 3D printed models, it lacks the tactile hands-on feel that many clinicians prefer. More time will be needed to determine the ultimate role these emerging technologies play in the 3D assessment of the heart and circulatory system.

CONCLUSION

While much progress has been made, 3D printing in cardiovascular imaging is still a new and growing field, and as such continues to have challenges. Currently these challenges include additional imaging considerations above that of a typical diagnostic scan, considerations on segmentation techniques, printer and material selection, and how to accommodate the additional burdens of time and cost required to run an effective 3D modeling lab. Despite these challenges, however, 3D modeling and printing has the potential to offer significant benefits to clinicians and with careful planning can be a powerful tool which will hopefully improve clinical workflow and patient outcomes.

REFERENCES

1. Fratz S, Chung T, Greil GF, et al. Guidelines and protocols for cardiovascular magnetic resonance in children and adults with congenital heart disease: SCMR expert consensus group on congenital heart disease. *J Cardiovasc Magn Reson.* 2013;15(1):1. https://doi.org/10.1186/1532-429X-15-51.
2. Mitchell FM, Prasad SK, Greil GF, Drivas P, Vassiliou VS, Raphael CE. Cardiovascular magnetic resonance: diagnostic utility and specific considerations in the pediatric population. *World J Clin Pediatr.* 2016;5(1):1–15. https://doi.org/10.5409/wjcp.v5.i1.1.
3. Mahmood F, Owais K, Taylor C, et al. Three-dimensional printing of mitral valve using echocardiographic data. *JACC Cardiovasc Imaging.* 2015;8(2):227–229. https://doi.org/10.1016/j.jcmg.2014.06.020.
4. Olivieri LJ, Krieger A, Loke Y-H, Nath DS, Kim PCW, Sable CA. Three-dimensional printing of intracardiac defects from three-dimensional echocardiographic images: feasibility and relative accuracy. *J Am Soc Echocardiogr.* 2015;28(4):392–397. https://doi.org/10.1016/j.echo.2014.12.016.
5. Wang Y, Alkasab TK, Narin O, et al. Incidence of nephrogenic systemic fibrosis after adoption of restrictive gadolinium-based contrast agent guidelines. *Radiology.* 2011;260(1):105–111. https://doi.org/10.1148/radiol.11102340.
6. Hellman RN. Gadolinium-induced nephrogenic systemic fibrosis. *Semin Nephrol.* 2011;31(3):310–316. https://doi.org/10.1016/j.semnephrol.2011.05.010.
7. Wang DD, Gheewala N, Shah R, et al. Three-dimensional printing for planning of structural heart interventions. *Interv Cardiol Clin.* 2018;7(3):415–423. https://doi.org/10.1016/j.iccl.2018.04.004.
8. Abudayyeh I, Gordon B, Ansari MM, Jutzy K, Stoletniy L, Hilliard A. A practical guide to cardiovascular 3D printing in clinical practice: overview and examples. *J Interv Cardiol.* 2017;31(3):375–383. https://doi.org/10.1111/joic.12446.
9. Reiter T, Ritter O, Prince MR, et al. Minimizing risk of nephrogenic systemic fibrosis in cardiovascular magnetic resonance. *J Cardiovasc Magn Reson.* 2012;14(1):31. https://doi.org/10.1186/1532-429X-14-31.
10. Ferreira PF, Gatehouse PD, Mohiaddin RH, Firmin DN. Cardiovascular magnetic resonance artefacts. *J Cardiovasc Magn Reson.* 2013;15(1):1–39. https://doi.org/10.1186/1532-429x-15-41.
11. Vukicevic M, Puperi DS, Grande-Allen KJ, Little SH. 3D printed modeling of the mitral valve for catheter-based structural interventions. *Ann Biomed Eng.* 2016:1–12. https://doi.org/10.1007/s10439-016-1676-5.
12. Scanlan AB. Comparison of 3D echocardiogram-derived 3D printed valve models to molded models for simulated repair of pediatric atrioventricular valves. *Pediatr Cardiol.* 2018;39(3):538–547. https://doi.org/10.1007/s00246-017-1785-4.
13. Mashari A, Montealegre-Gallegos M, Knio Z, et al. Making three-dimensional echocardiography more tangible: a workflow for three-dimensional printing with echocardiographic data. *Echo Res Pract.* 2016;3(4):R57–R64. https://doi.org/10.1530/ERP-16-0036.
14. Farooqi KM, ed. *Rapid Prototyping in Cardiac Disease.* Cham: Springer International Publishing; 2017:1–196. https://doi.org/10.1007/978-3-319-53523-4.
15. Rajiah P, Tandon A, Greil GF, Abbara S. Update on the role of cardiac magnetic resonance imaging in congenital heart disease. *Curr Treat Options Cardiovasc Med.* 2017:1–24. https://doi.org/10.1007/s11936-017-0504-z.
16. Bartel T, Rivard A, Jimenez A, Mestres CA, Müller S. Medical three-dimensional printing opens up new opportunities in cardiology and cardiac surgery. *Eur Heart J.* 2017;39(15):1246–1254. https://doi.org/10.1093/eurheartj/ehx016.
17. Tandon A, Byrne N, Nieves Velasco Forte M de L, et al. Use of a semi-automated cardiac segmentation tool improves reproducibility and speed of segmentation of contaminated right heart magnetic resonance angiography. *Int J Cardiovasc Imaging.* 2016;32(8):1273–1279. https://doi.org/10.1007/s10554-016-0906-0.
18. Pace DF, Dalca AV, Geva T, Powell AJ, Moghari MH, Golland P. Interactive whole-heart segmentation in congenital heart disease. *Med Image Comput Comput Assist Interv.* 2015;9351:80–88. https://doi.org/10.1007/978-3-319-24574-4_10 [Chapter 10].
19. Tack P, Victor J, Gemmel P, Annemans L. 3D-printing techniques in a medical setting: a systematic literature review. *Biomed Eng Online.* 2016:1–21. https://doi.org/10.1186/s12938-016-0236-4.
20. Valverde I, Gomez-Ciriza G, Hussain T, et al. Three-dimensional printed models for surgical planning of complex congenital heart defects: an international multicentre study. *Eur J Cardiothorac Surg.* 2017;52(6):1139–1148. https://doi.org/10.1093/ejcts/ezx208.

CONCLUSION

CHAPTER 10

Does 3D Modeling Alter Clinical Outcomes? What Are the Data?

ISRAEL VALVERDE, MD

INTRODUCTION

Clinical outcomes are measurable changes in quality of life that result from any healthcare intervention. In congenital heart defects (CHDs) they are usually measured as morbidity, mortality, hospital stay, hospital's readmissions, staff perspective, and patient satisfaction scale.

As 3D printing is relatively new to the cardiac space, there are little data to support with robust evidence the claimed benefits that 3D printing results in improved clinical outcomes. However, emerging reports from other surgical subspecialties appear promising. Recent data from craniofacial reports suggest that 3D printing can improve outcomes, including saving time in the operating room and thus translating to direct cost savings.[1,2]

In order to find out if 3D model alter clinical outcomes in CHD, research articles must be read and evaluated thoughtfully, otherwise we may be dazzled when a shiny new technology is presented that may not truly add clinical benefit.[3]

The purpose of this chapter is to provide a guide on how to critically evaluate a clinical paper about 3D printing and review the current evidence about how 3D printing influences clinical outcomes.

WHAT IS THE LEVEL OF EVIDENCE OF THE CLINICAL STUDY?

Evidence-based medicine is about finding evidence and using that data to make clinical decisions. Large randomized and blinded studies are on top of the hierarchical system of classifying evidence. Unfortunately, given the relatively recent use of 3D printing in the field of congenital heart defect (CHD), the level of evidence remains low and most published literature consists of case report studies or small series. A summary of some of the most relevant 3D printed studies in CHD are summarized in Table 10.1.

However, while potentially relevant, a single patient anecdote should not be extrapolated with a generalized and unsubstantial statement. There are several reasons that prevent the development of large evidence-based studies for 3D printing in CHD, such as ethical considerations when dealing with the pediatric population and huge anatomic variability which makes finding a matched control difficult. Additionally, when coupled with the relative paucity of complex cases of CHD, the high variance in metrics of operative performance (such as cross-clamp or bypass time) often necessitates multicenter study design.

Thus, although scientifically weak, there is a large body of reports claiming benefits of 3D models in surgical and interventional planning. Therefore, randomization raises ethical issues concerning the assignment of children to a hypothetical inferior care pathway without the potential advantage of a 3D model.[37] This may explain the lack of published prospective randomized control group studies. Retrospectively matched controls may be a preferable alternative to gather stronger, albeit imperfect evidence. Notably, the use of retrospectively matched controls within a multicenter study is hampered by variation in surgical practice between different hospitals. Even when selected from a single unit, cases matched on the basis of similar CHD anatomical features, weight, height, and clinical status are often drawn from different surgical eras and different teams (cardiac surgery, pediatric cardiology, intensive care units). Temporal variation in surgical practice is another potential confounding factor when considering a retrospectively controlled, multicenter study.

A case cross-over design study may be an elegant solution to overcome these methodological challenges. A case cross-over study design is a relatively new analytical epidemiological approach in which each case serves as its own control and it has been already used in

3-Dimensional Modeling in Cardiovascular Disease. https://doi.org/10.1016/B978-0-323-65391-6.00010-7

TABLE 10.1
Study Characteristics of 3D Printing in Congenital Heart Diseases Regarding Technical Details.

First Author/ Year of Publication	Study Design	Study Purpose	Sample Size	Main Study Findings	Imaging Modality	Segmentation Software	Segmentation Method	Segmentation Duration	Printing Material	Estimated Cost
Bhatla et al.[4] 2017	Case series	Preoperative planning, intraoperative orientation	6 printed models	3D printed models have helped in planning the surgical procedures for patients with double-outlet right ventricle and complex muscular ventricular septal defects (VSDs) by enhancing the understanding of the complex pathology.	CT, MRI	Mimics Innovation Suite software (Materialise HQ, Leuven, Belgium)	Thresholding, automatic segmentation, manual edition	N/A	N/A	N/A
Bhatla et al.[5] 2017	Case report	Surgical planning for a double outlet rightventricle	1 printed model	Surgical simulations based on 3D printed models improved understanding of complex anatomy, confirmed feasibility of operating procedure, and identified potential challenges of performing surgical approach.	CT	N/A	N/A	N/A	N/A	N/A
Biglino et al.[6] 2015	Randomized controlled trial (questionnaire-based)	Communication in medical practice	97 parents of congenital heart defect (CHD) patients	3D printed models have improved the parents-cardiologists communication.	MRI	Mimics Innovation Suite software (Materialise HQ, Leuven, Belgium)	Thresholding, region growing	0.5 h to 3 h	White nylon	£50 (USD64)
Biglino et al.[7] 2016	Cross-sectional	Medical education, preoperative planning, research, communication in medical practice	13 patients, 15 parents of patients, 14 clinicians, 11 nurses	3D printed models can have invaluable role in patient-doctor communication and teaching.	MRI	Mimics Innovation Suite software (Materialise HQ, Leuven, Belgium)	N/A	N/A	White nylon, stereolithography resin, thermoplastic, watershed resin, TangoPlus, powder print	N/A

Study	Design	Application	Sample	Findings	Modality	Software	Segmentation	Time	Material	Cost
Biglino et al.[8] 2017	Cross-sectional	Medical education	9 printed models, 100 cardiac nurses	3D printed models can be useful in training the cardiac nurses by demonstrating complex cardiac anatomy.	MRI	N/A	N/A	N/A	N/A	N/A
Biglino et al.[9] 2017	Cross-sectional	Communication in medical practice	20 adolescent patients with CHD	Patients' knowledge about their own condition can be improved with the use of 3D printed models during consultation.	MRI	Simpleware Ltd, Exeter, UK	N/A	1 h to 2 h	White nylon	£150 (USD163)
Costello et al.[10] 2014	Cross-sectional	Medical education	5 printed models, 29 premedical and medical students	It is feasible to create accurate 3D printed heart models. This technology is effective in teaching students about CHD.	MRI	Mimics Innovation Suite software (Materialise HQ, Leuven, Belgium)	N/A	N/A	PolyJet material (mixing transparent plastic material and rubberlike material)	N/A
Costello et al.[11] 2015	Cross-sectional	Medical education	5 printed models, 23 pediatric resident physicians	Use of 3D printed heart models as a tool for simulation-based education can improve residents understanding of CHD.	MRI	Mimics Innovation Suite software (Materialise HQ, Leuven, Belgium)	N/A	N/A	N/A	N/A
Farooqi et al.[12] 2016	Case series	Visualization of complex cardiac anatomy to aid surgical planning	6 printed models	Excellent correlation was found between 3D models and original source cardiac MR images in all of the measurements including aortic annulus diameters, VSD diameters and right ventricle long axis ($P = .57$–$.88$, $r = 0.74$–0.99).	MRI	Mimics Innovation Suite software (Materialise HQ, Leuven, Belgium)	Blood pool segmentation	2 h	Acrylonitrile butadiene styrene	N/A

Continued

TABLE 10.1
Study Characteristics of 3D Printing in Congenital Heart Diseases Regarding Technical Details.—cont'd

First Author/ Year of Publication	Study Design	Study Purpose	Sample Size	Main Study Findings	Imaging Modality	Segmentation Software	Segmentation Method	Segmentation Duration	Printing Material	Estimated Cost
Farooqi et al.[13] 2016	Case report	Preoperative planning	1 printed model	3D printed models are able to demonstrate intracardiac spatial information more comprehensively.	MRI	N/A	N/A	N/A	N/A	N/A
Garekar et al.[14] 2016	Case series	Preoperative planning	5 printed models, 1 radiologist, 1 cardiologist and 1 operating surgeon	3D printed models can boost the confidence level among the clinicians in planning the interventions.	CT, MRI	N/A	Thresholding, manual edition	N/A	Sandstone	N/A
Greil et al.[15] 2007	Case series	Feasibility and diagnostic accuracy	5 printed models	3D printed models of CHD using CT and MRI images enable reproduction of complex cardiac morphology and unique cardiac pathology, thus may serve as new ways for teaching and preoperative planning.	CT, MRI	N/A	Semiautomatic segmentation	1.5 h	Polyamide powder	N/A
Hadeed et al.[16] 2016	Case report	Preoperative planning	1 printed model	3D printed models allow better understanding of complex CHD and facilitate preoperative planning.	CT	Mimics Innovation Suite software (Materialise HQ, Leuven, Belgium)	N/A	N/A	HeartPrint flex material (Materialise)	N/A

Study	Study design	Application	Number	Findings	Imaging modality	Software	Segmentation	Time	Material	Cost
Jones et al.[17] 2017	Randomized controlled trial (questionnaire-based)	Medical education	36 participants	Incorporation of 3D printed models into teaching residents are shown to significantly improve their knowledge about congenital heart diseases (mainly vascular rings and pulmonary artery slings).	CT, MRI	Philips IntelliSpace Portal (Philips Healthcare, Best, The Netherlands)	NA	N/A	Polylactic acid	N/A
Kappanayil et al.[18] 2017	Case series	Surgical decision-making and preoperative planning	5 printed models	3D printed models improve understanding of complex cardiac anatomy, assist precise surgical planning and execution of all surgeries.	CT, MRI	Mimics Innovation Suite software (Materialise NV, Leuven, Belgium)	Semiautomatic heart segmentation tool	N/A	Power, polyamide and HeartPrint Flex	N/A
Kiraly et al.[19] 2016	Case report	Preoperative planning, presurgical simulation	1 printed model	3D printed models can be used as an effective tool to simulate the operative procedures.	CT	Mimics Innovation Suite software (Materialise HQ, Leuven, Belgium)	N/A	N/A	N/A	N/A
Loke et al.[20] 2017	Prospective randomized controlled trial (questionnaire-based)	Medical education	35 pediatric residents	3D printed models have increased the residents' satisfaction in learning CHD.	CT, MRI, echocardiogram	Mimics Innovation Suite software (Materialise HQ, Leuven, Belgium)	Delineation of heart wall	2 h	PolyJet photopolymer materials—Tango Black and Tango Clear	USD200
Ma et al.[21] 2015	Case control	Application of 3D printed models in CHD	35 printed models	3D printed models are accurate in replicating the anatomy of CHD, with significant differences in measuring VSD between 3D printed models and actual surgical measurements (mean _ SD: 14.98 _ 1.91 versus 15.11 _ 20.6, $P = .42$).	CT	Philips EBW Comp-cardiac post-processing software package	N/A	N/A	Selective laser sintering powder	N/A

Continued

TABLE 10.1
Study Characteristics of 3D Printing in Congenital Heart Diseases Regarding Technical Details.—cont'd

First Author/ Year of Publication	Study Design	Study Purpose	Sample Size	Main Study Findings	Imaging Modality	Segmentation Software	Segmentation Method	Segmentation Duration	Printing Material	Estimated Cost
Mottl-Link et al.[22] 2008	Case report	Demonstration of complex congenital cardiac pathologies for surgical intervention	1 case, 2 printed models	The 3D printed models have provided additional spatial information of CHD and can be an effective tool in guiding the surgical procedures intraoperatively.	MRI	Self-developed software tools	Semiautomatic segmentation	N/A	Plaster powder	USD364–810
Olejnik et al.[23] 2017	Case series	Operative planning of complex congenital heart diseases	8 printed models	High correlation was found between 3D printed models and original digital images and in vivo surgical measurements (+0.19 _ 0.38 mm, and +0.13 _ 0.26 mm respectively) by Bland–Altman analysis. Furthermore, 3D printed models facilitate surgical or interventional procedures.	CT	3D slicer	Extraction of the region of interest (cardiac chambers and vessel walls)	6–12 h	Plaster powder	Euro 300 (USD450)
Olivieri et al.[24] 2015	Case series	Feasibility and accuracy	9 printed models	3D printed models derived from 3D echocardiographic datasets show high accuracy in replicating congenital heart disease with excellent correlation between standard 2D and 3D model measurements (mean _ SD were 7.1 _ 6.2 mm vs. 7.5 _ 6.3 mm), with mean absolute error between	3D echocardiography	Mimics Innovation Suite software (Materialise, Leuven, Belgium)	Automatic, semiautomatic and hand segmentation methods.	N/A	N/A	N/A

Study	Study design	Application	No. of models	Findings	Imaging	Software	Segmentation	Time	Material	Cost
Olivieri et al.[25] 2016	Cross-sectional	Medical education	10 printed models, 70 clinicians	3D printed models are useful as simulation-based training tools for multidisciplinary intensive care teams. Overall average response was 8.4 out of 10 regarding whether 3D printed models were more effective in clinical management of cardiac surgery patients than standard hand off.	CT, MRI	Mimics Innovation Suite software (Materialise HQ, Leuven, Belgium)	N/A	N/A	Opaque, rigid plastic material	USD200
Riesenkampff et al.[26] 2009	Case series	Preoperative planning	11 printed models	3D printed models can provide extra diagnostic information to aid in surgical decision-making.	CT, MRI	Medical Imaging and Interaction Toolkit	Semiautomatic segmentation	0.67 h	Plaster powder	N/A
Shiraishi et al.[27] 2010	Case series	Preoperative planning, presurgical simulation	12 printed models	3D printed models are useful in preoperative planning and presurgical simulation.	CT	N/A	N/A	N/A	Photosensitive liquid epoxy or urethane, and solid resin	USD400–600
Sodian et al.[28] 2007	Case series	Preoperative planning, intraoperative	2 printed models	The 3D printed models were valuable for surgical decision-making and intraoperative orientation.	CT, MRI	N/A	N/A	N/A	N/A	N/A
Valverde et al.[29] 2015	Case report	Preoperative planning	1 printed model	The 3D printed models are very useful in planning corrective surgery of complex CHD cases.	MRI	AYRA (Ikiria, Spain)	Thresholding, region growing	4 h	Translucent polylactic acid polymer	USD350

Continued

TABLE 10.1
Study Characteristics of 3D Printing in Congenital Heart Diseases Regarding Technical Details.—cont'd

First Author/ Year of Publication	Study Design	Study Purpose	Sample Size	Main Study Findings	Imaging Modality	Segmentation Software	Segmentation Method	Segmentation Duration	Printing Material	Estimated Cost
Valverde et al.[30] 2015	Case report	Preoperative planning, presurgical simulation	1 case, 2 printed models	The 3D printed model shows high accuracy in measuring cardiac anatomical structures with no significant differences in diameter measurements compared to MRI and invasive angiography (measurement differences: 0.05 _ 0.17 mm, $P < .05$). Qualitative assessment shows that 3D printed model is very useful with a score of 8.5 out of 10 in terms of overall satisfaction.	MRI	AYRA (Ikiria, Spain)	Thresholding, region growing	6 h	Rigid and flexible polylactic acid polymers	N/A
Valverde et al.[31] 2017	Case report	Interventional simulation	1 case	First reported case using 3D printed model for simulation of "double stent" percutaneous pulmonary valve implantation technique by a solely percutaneous approach in large right ventricular (RV) outflow tract	MRI	ITK snap for image segmentation and Meshmixer 11.055 for computer-aided design	N/A	N/A	Polyurethane filament	N/A

Reference	Study type	Aim	Cases	Results	Imaging modality	Software		Time	Material	
Valverde et al.[32] 2017	Prospective multicentre study	Impact of 3D printed heart models on surgical planning of CHD	40 cases with 40 models involving 10 international centers	Excellent agreement in measurement of vascular diameters between 3D printed models and original CT and MRI images with a mean bias of _0.27 _ 0.73 mm for 3D models. Surgeons and pediatric cardiologist ranked models' satisfaction as 9.3 and 9.0 out of 10, respectively. In more than half the cases (52.5) 3D models did not change the surgical decision in CHD, but helped defining the surgical approach in 19 of 40 cases	CT (12 cases) and MRI (28 cases)	ITK snap for image segmentation and Meshmixer 11.055 for computer-aided design	N/A	Segmentation time: 75 ± 32 min Computer-aided design time: 89 ± 22 min	Polyurethane filament	N/A
Valverde et al.[33] 2018	Case report	Preoperative planning, presurgical simulation	1 case	Surgical decision planning in a complex case of multiple VSDs. The 3D model helped identifying the minimum number of septal bands to resect, the optimal patch size and morphology to completely close all VSDs without reducing significantly the RV cavity	CT	ITK snap for image segmentation and Meshmixer 11.055 for computer-aided design	N/A	N/A	Polyurethane filament	N/A

Continued

TABLE 10.1
Study Characteristics of 3D Printing in Congenital Heart Diseases Regarding Technical Details.—cont'd

First Author/ Year of Publication	Study Design	Study Purpose	Sample Size	Main Study Findings	Imaging Modality	Segmentation Software	Segmentation Method	Segmentation Duration	Printing Material	Estimated Cost
Velasco et al.[34] 2017	Case series	Interventional simulation	4 patients	In selected patients, using procedural simulation on a 3D printed model, percutaneous correction of sinus venosus atrial septal defect and partial anomalous pulmonary venous return is feasible and safe, and led to favorable short-term outcomes.	MRI, CT	Mimics Innovation Suite software (Materialise HQ, Leuven, Belgium)	Intensity thresholding, cropping and region growing tools	N/A	Tango Plus polyurethane filament	N/A
Velasco et al.[35] 2018	Case series	Interventional simulation	3 patients	In selected patients, using procedural simulation on a 3D printed model, percutaneous correction of sinus venosus atrial septal defect and partial anomalous pulmonary venous return is feasible and safe, and led to favorable short-term outcomes.	MRI	Mimics Innovation Suite software (Materialise HQ, Leuven, Belgium)	N/A	N/A	Tango Plus	N/A

CT, computed tomography; HQ, headquarters; MRI, magnetic resonance imaging; N/A, not available.
Reprint with permission from Lau et al.[36].

pediatric[38] and CHD[39] studies. Whereas cohort studies can be limited in power for rare disease outcomes, and case-control studies can be biased due to retrospective exposure assessment, case cross-over designs compare individuals to themselves (self-matched study) at different times. This removes bias associated with inconsistent surgical practice across centers and individuals, but maintains as source of objective and measurable statistical evidence. This approach was used by Valverde et al. in a multicenter study evaluating 3D printing and CHD.[32] However cross-over design studies have several important limitations. Namely, this methodology cannot be used when a subject receives only one intervention and this type of methodology cannot evaluate the long-term effects of an intervention.

DOES THE ARTICLE EVALUATE THE IMPACT ON PREOPERATIVE MANAGEMENT DECISION?

There is a large body of research papers evaluating the impact of 3D printed models for both surgical and interventional planning. For preoperative surgical planning, 3D models have been used in cases of arterial patch repair of the main pulmonary artery in tetralogy of Fallot,[40] Kommerell's diverticulum,[41] repair of pediatric atrioventricular valves,[42] double outlet right ventricle,[14,43,44] truncus arteriosus,[45] heart transplantation,[46,47] complex aortic arch surgery[28,48] including arch reconstruction postmodified Norwood-1,[19] aortic valve replacement,[49] septal myectomy in obstructive hypertrophic cardiomyopathy,[50] transposition of the great arteries (TGA)[51] including Nikaidoh procedure,[29] and complex cases of mixed CHD.[15,27,32,52,53]

For catheterization interventional planning, 3D models have been in cases of endovascular aortic interventions,[30,54,55] transcatheter aortic valve implantation,[56] percutaneous closure of secundum atrial septal defects,[57,58] stent angioplasty of pulmonary venous baffle obstruction in a Mustard repair of D-TGA,[59] transcatheter pulmonary valve placement in tetralogy of Fallot,[31,60,61] interventional correction of sinus venosus atrial septal defect and partial anomalous pulmonary venous drainage,[35] and coronary artery fistulae.[34]

The largest multicenter study to evaluate the impact of 3D printed models on surgical decision-making in patients with complex CHD involved 40 patients, 10 international centers, 80 pediatric cardiologists, and 20 cardiac surgeons.[32] The authors used a prospective, observational case, cross-over approach in which each patient served as its own case (surgical decision after evaluation of conventional imaging echocardiography,

CT, MRI) and its own control (surgical decision after evaluation of 3D printed model) in different surgical planning stages (Fig. 10.1).

At Stage-I, surgical management decision was based in the absence of 3D model, relying only on routine clinical practice observations and available conventional imaging data, including 2D and 3D echocardiography, MRI, and CT where virtual 3D image reconstructions of the anatomy were shown by imaging specialists.

At Stage-II, a 3D model was requested for surgical reassessment. Demographic, clinical, and imaging data (CT and MRI) were collected by participating centers, de-identified, and uploaded to a dedicated cloud server. Data were downloaded by a single center for consolidation and 3D printing. 3D printed models were sent by urgent delivery post to the referral center for surgical reevaluation by the same multidisciplinary team in order to know if the additional information from the 3D model changed the surgical decision. Surgeons were allowed to examine the model, cutting it with appropriate surgical instruments and planning potential strategies.

Finally, in Stage-III, in those cases undergoing surgery, after intraoperative inspection, it was evaluated if the surgical plan was changed compared to the 3D model—based plan.

The authors concluded that 3D printed models changed surgical decision-making in 19 out of the 40 cases (47.5% of the cases, confidence interval 29.6% —61.5%). In 9 cases, 3D models prompted only small modifications of the surgical approach. These included adjustment in biventricular repair (8 cases) and adaptation of univentricular heart (UVH) physiology approach (1 case). Remarkably in 10 cases (25%), inspection of the 3D model resulted in significant modifications of the surgical plan. It should be emphasized that in up to 3 cases, patients that were thought not to be surgical candidates were surgically corrected achieving a successful biventricular repair in two of them and one case palliated with UVH physiology. Also, importantly, in two cases initially considered for UVH physiologic palliation, evaluation of the 3D model changed the surgical decision to proceed with biventricular repair which was successfully achieved. It is also notable that in 3 cases, 3D models permitted the clinical team to reassess their initial plan, and adopt an approach perceived to reduce risk. In 2 cases considered initially for biventricular repair, UVH staged palliation was preferred after consideration of the 3D model. In these cases it was demonstrated that the ventricular septal defect was too large for septation. Had the

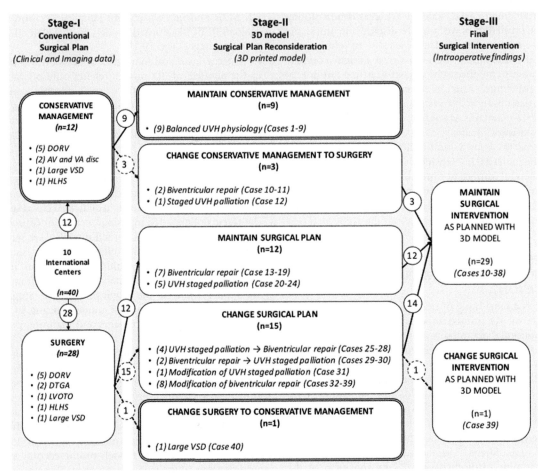

FIG. 10.1 Surgical management decision. Continuous arrow: no change in management decision. Dotted arrows: change in management decision. Conservative management showed in double line box. Surgery management showed in single line box. (Reprint with permission from Valverde et al.[32].)

3D model not been considered, this insight may have gone unnoticed and resulted in a difficult or unsuccessful biventricular repair.

Interestingly, in most of the cases, 21 cases (52.5% of the cases, confidence interval 38.5%–70.7%), the surgical decision was not objectively changed by consideration of a 3D model. This result must be considered in the context of complex case selection, as 3D models were only requested when significant differences in surgical pathway opinions were discussed at the local multidisciplinary meetings. It might be that the impact on surgical planning is lower in structurally simpler cases of CHD. The authors insinuated that in these instances, the added value of 3D models may not justify the time and expense invested in their fabrication.

Surgical planning and decision-making informed by 3D models were successfully accomplished in 29 out of the 30 cases undergoing surgery. This implicitly suggests that there was good geometrical agreement between a given 3D model and patient-specific anatomy. This is supported by the nonclinically significant diametric bias of only -0.27 ± 0.73 mm between medical images and the 3D models.[32]

While this study provided significant evidence of the contribution of 3D printed models to surgical planning and care, the approach of case cross-over study has several important limitations. A significant drawback of this approach is that it is only sensitive to the impact of 3D models on surgical planning, not on mid- and long-term surgical outcomes. Surgery is performed after experimental/control cross-over and data collection. Hence the effect of 3D models on morbidity, mortality, and reduced financial costs cannot be evaluated. Another limitation concerns the difficulty of blinding research participants. Having the same clinicians and surgeons assess each case either side of cross-over removes bias associated with variation in clinical practice. However, since the same group has requested the 3D model, this lack of blinding may exaggerate the positive effect recorded. To diminish the impact of individual bias, the complete multidisciplinary meeting team was involved in the surgical decision. Finally, another limitation is the wide variability of the complex CHD conditions that were included and the limited number of patients included (40 cases).

Therefore, larger randomized and blinded studies are required in order to produce better evidence. "3DHeart" is the first large-scale clinical trial to investigate the efficacy of 3D printing in medicine (www.opheart.org). So far, over 400 patients have been enrolled from 18 pediatric cardiac surgical centers in the United States. The results of this large study will surely shed more light and provide more answers regarding how 3D models alter clinical outcome.

DOES THE ARTICLE ASSESS THE REDUCTION IN OPERATING TIME?

How much does 1 min of operating room time cost? It is a question that has been widely pondered in the past.[62] Of course, there is no straight answer and it depends on factors such as the country where a procedure is being performed, the complexity of the surgical procedure, use of prosthesis, etc.

Operation room time has always been one of the major arguments for medical 3D printing. In a recent review article involving 227 articles in multiple surgical areas such as orthopedics, maxillofacial surgical, cranial surgery, and spinal surgery, 42 papers described the precise impact of using 3D printing technology on operating room time.[63] In most of the cases it resulted in time saving, with an average time saving in cases of cranial surgery of 69 min. However, in other cases such as orthopedic hip surgery, the time saving was not as relevant, and only saved 0.025 min.

In the field of congenital heart disease, a few reports have claimed that 3D models helped to shorten surgical intraoperative time.[16,19,23,29] However, in most published papers there is usually a lack of discussion of the quality of evidence to support the claimed benefits in operating room reduction time.

DOES THE ARTICLE ASSESS SURGICAL MORBIDITY AND MORTALITY?

A number of independent studies demonstrate that the risk of postoperative morbidity and mortality correlates significantly with the duration of general anesthesia, a trend that holds true across a wide range of surgical procedures and specialties and independent of most other surgical variables.[64,65] Therefore, time spent in the operating room is critical. Recent data from craniofacial reports suggest that 3D printing can improve outcomes, including saving time in the operating room and thus translating to direct cost savings.[1,2]

It is commonly stated that patient-specific presurgical and interventional planning in CHD may potentially reduce intraoperative duration and cross-clamp time and therefore it may result in fewer complications. In turn, this may lead to shorter postoperative stays, decreased reintervention rates, and lower healthcare costs. However, in most published papers there is usually a lack of discussion of the quality of evidence to support the claimed benefits of 3D printing and to date, there is no large statistical comparison with historical data or control group data to support these statements.

DOES THE ARTICLE ASSESS HEALTH PROFESSIONAL'S PERCEPTION?

Most studies in published current literature are successful cases in which the clinicians report that the 3D printed model was clinically useful. The usefulness is generally described as a rotund yes, and unfortunately those cases where 3D models were not useful are often not published. Only a few papers have properly evaluated the degree of usefulness for health professionals and medical academics. The evaluation method usually focusses on the perception of 3D printing in preoperative planning using Likert scale.

Biglinio et al. advised that evaluation of health professionals in the context of using 3D models of CHD in clinical practice should not be restricted to the cardiac surgeon but also involve the cardiologists, the imaging expert involved in acquisition of the imaging and 3D printing, and trainees.[45]

Lau et al. assessed the clinical value of 5 cases of complex CHD evaluated by 9 health professionals (two radiologists, two cardiologists, two cardiac surgeons, and three medical academic staff).[52] A total 66.7% of them strongly agreed that 3D models were helpful in planning interventions, and 50% strongly agreed that models were also helpful for testing devices for presurgical simulation. The remaining 33.3% and 50% were unsure about its usefulness. There were no participants who responded "no" to the questions in this category. The two surgeons involved in the study agreed that the 3D printed models would be able to provide additional information of the pathology compared to conventional imaging and computer simulation. They reported that the 3D printed cardiac model is helpful for them to appreciate potential procedural difficulties and hence will be able to increase the success rate of a surgery. Finally, participants reported an average satisfaction score of the model of 8.4 out of 10.

This agrees with a later study published by Valverde et al. which included a total of 43 health professionals (30 pediatric cardiologists, 13 cardiac surgeons) from 10 international centers,[32] see Fig. 10.2. For the purposes of surgical planning, 82% of the surgeons

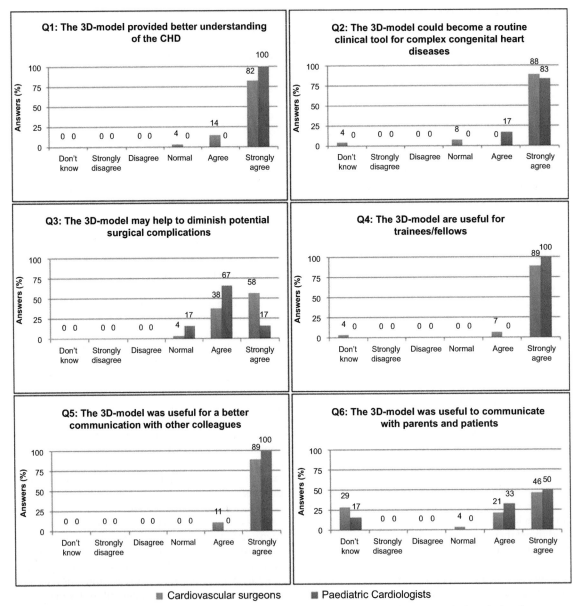

FIG. 10.2 Questionnaire evaluation of health professional's perception. (Reprint with permission from Valverde et al.[32].)

and 100% of the pediatric cardiologists strongly agreed that the 3D models provided better understanding of the lesion. A total 88% of the surgeons and 83% of the pediatric cardiologists strongly agreed that these models could become a routine tool for surgical planning in complex CHD. Only 17% of the pediatric cardiologists and 58% of the surgeons considered that 3D model may help to diminish potential surgical complications. A total 89% of the surgeons strongly agreed that the 3D model was useful for the education of trainees and fellows. Importantly, all of the surgeons and pediatric cardiologists agreed or strongly agreed that 3D models were useful for better communication with other colleagues. Overall, surgeons and pediatric cardiologists rated their satisfaction with 3D models as 9.3 and 9.0 out of 10, respectively.

DOES THE ARTICLE ASSESS PATIENT AND PARENT'S PERCEPTION?

Clinical outcome quality is often based on a patient's perception. Official and private organizations have developed quality standards and benchmarking programs using patient's and caretakers' opinions as a reliable source to measure quality.[66] Measure of treatment outcomes from a patient's perspective are an important part of outcomes measurement because they provide a patient-led assessment of health and health-related quality of life. It is also important to note that patient's trust in a healthcare professional is associated with improved health outcomes.[67]

Patient perception is also directly related to the degree of understanding of the specific disease state and proposed and/or performed procedure. In a recent

study, the impact of using patient-specific three-dimensional models of CHD during consultations with adolescent patients (15–18 years) was assessed.[9] This patient population group is key in successful transitioning to adult care. There is growing evidence to suggest that advances in the surgical treatment of CHD should be accompanied by assessments and interventions which attend to the psychosocial needs of adolescents.[68] Assuming responsibility for their health is part of the process, which necessitates a level of understanding and appreciation of what their condition entails and what their cardiac anatomy looks like.[68] Outcome measures were structured in several items: confidence in explaining their condition to others, knowledge of their CHD, impact of CHD on their lifestyle, satisfaction with previous/current visits, positive/negative features of the 3D model, and open-ended feedback. Significant improvements were registered in confidence in explaining their condition to others ($P = .008$), improvement in knowledge of CHD ($P < .001$) and patients' satisfaction following consultation with the 3D model ($P = .005$),[9] see Fig. 10.3.

The improvement in the level of participant satisfaction following the visit may result in improved patient adherence. Although this remains speculative in the absence of a cost-effectiveness analysis, the cost of a 3D model should be weighed against the cost of missing an appointment and nonadherence to other aspects of the treatment regimen.[9]

Descriptions of CHD and impact on lifestyle were more eloquent after seeing a 3D model. The majority of participants reported that models helped their understanding and improved their visit. Interestingly, a non-negligible 30% of participants indicated that the model

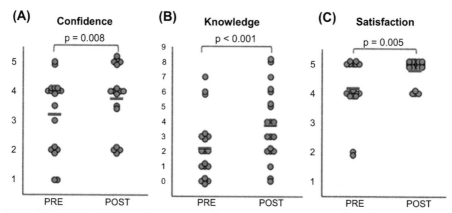

FIG. 10.3 Statistically significant changes were observed in confidence **(A)**, knowledge **(B)**, and satisfaction **(C)** among participants comparing responses before ("Pre") and after ("Post") their consultation. (Reprint with permission from Biglino et al.[9].)

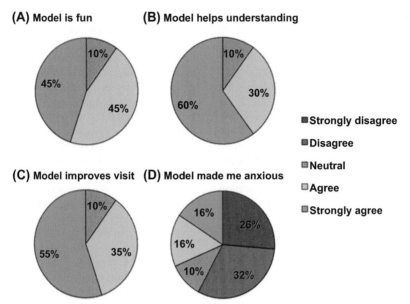

(A) Model is fun   **(B)** Model helps understanding

10%
45%
45%

10%
30%
60%

■ Strongly disagree

■ Disagree

■ Neutral

□ Agree

■ Strongly agree

(C) Model improves visit   **(D)** Model made me anxious

10%
55%
35%

16%
26%
16%
10%
32%

FIG. 10.4 Summary of participants' level of agreement to different statements on 3D models. (Reprint with permission from Biglino et al.[9].)

made them feel more anxious about their condition (Fig. 10.4).

However, the authors discussed that this is not necessarily a negative feature, as it may indicate an increased awareness as a result of the more in-depth conversation facilitated by the model. On the other hand, participants reported that they would want to have a 3D model for future visits and they would recommend it to a peer. The same group also evaluated patient's perception at younger ages. Biglinio et al. collected feedback from an 11-year-old male patient who had a right aortic arch, a repaired truncus arteriosus, pulmonary artery stenosis, as well as conduit stenosis, with a complex surgical plan being discussed.[45] The patient, although young, felt that the model helped him to understand why he needed the operation.

This study also investigated the usefulness of 3D printed models in parent's perception. For parents, there is an additional emotional component of distress and anxiety during a consultation. The parent's remarked the usefulness and the potential of the models for communicating with others, the advantages compared to conventional medical imaging and the potential of having follow-up models to highlight differences before/after surgeries/procedures.[45] Interestingly, the same group found that this increase in satisfaction and communication was not translated into an improved parental understanding of the

CHD.[6] Despite parental appreciation for the models, there was no objective evidence that parents' understanding of their child's heart condition was improved.

Other studies have tried to evaluate if 3D printed models are useful in enhancing communication from another point of view: the doctor's perspective. Several reports conclude that 3D models facilitate the consultation process with patients and parents.[6,9,45,52] Lau et al. reported that two cardiac surgeons and two cardiologists concluded that the 3D model may improve consultation experience as they would be able to explain the CHD to the patients more efficiently and that the patients could understand the condition much better.[52] Interestingly, when the health professionals were asked whether they prefer to use 3D printed model or medical images to communicate with the patients or other health professionals, four out of six indicated they prefer to use both of them as a medium in communication. This is in agreement with the largest multicenter study which included scale satisfaction questionnaires from 13 surgeons and 30 pediatric cardiologists. A total 67% of surgeons and 83% of the pediatric cardiologists agreed or strongly agreed that the model was useful to communicate with parents and patients.[32]

In summary, several elements will lead to translation of 3D printing technology into clinical practice: one is gathering evidence of the effectiveness of the models on large-scale studies, and the other is considering the perspective of all stakeholders in the technology.[45] Stakeholders must include not only clinicians but also other crucial elements including patients and their families.[45]

DOES THE ARTICLE ADEQUATELY DISCUSS THE COST OF THE 3D PRINTING PROCESS?

Congenital and structural heart disease place a high cost burden on our healthcare systems. Medical technology is often seen as an expensive luxury and proving efficiency saving is a challenge in 3D printing. The cost of 3D printing is considered one of the hurdles that impede the incorporation of this technology in routine clinical practice.[36,69,70]

As clinicians, we passionately believe that science and technology are the key enablers in increasing efficiency and quality of care, thus reducing healthcare costs. Now it is time to demonstrate it to our healthcare providers with solid scientific evidence, particularly since the cost and size of 3D printers have rapidly decreased over the last decade.

Unfortunately, cost-effectiveness analyses in the 3D printing research articles are sparse and vague. There are several literature review articles which discuss the cost of image-segmentation software[71] and 3D printing;[72] however, depicted costs are often missed in individual research articles.

Any study examining the clinical utility and practicality of 3D printing should examine how much the entire procedure costs which involve: cost of a 3D printer, material cost, software, clinician, and engineer cost per hour dedicated to segmentation of the images and computer-aided design. The latter costs may vary significantly across countries. The cost of 3D printers is summarized in Table 10.2.[72] This table is just a general indication as prices and new printers are continuously updated in the market. Another interesting point to keep in mind is the material cost associated with each kind of printer. This is also summarized in Table 10.3.[72]

In a recent systematic review article, Lau et al. could only identify eight studies reporting the cost to produce a life-size 3D printed model.[36] The cost ranged from USD 55 to USD 810.

There is a trend to produce low-cost printed models in order to save costs, while maintaining good quality and facilitating its adoption into clinical practice.[12,14,29,33,73] It has been verified that low-cost fused deposition modeling printers can produce low-cost but yet excellent accurate models with a mean bias compared to medical images of only -0.27 ± 0.73 mm.[32]

DOES THE ARTICLE COMPARE 3D PRINTING WITH EXISTING ALTERNATIVES?

Recently, there are several new technologies emerging as complementary tools to conventional imaging, some of which foresee replacing 3D printing. These include augmented reality (AR), virtual reality (VR), and 3D display (Fig. 10.5).[74]

AR is a technology that superimposes a computer-generated image on a user's view of the real world, thus providing a composite view. VR is defined as the 3D simulation of the real world allowing the user (cardiologist and surgeon) to have a direct immersive experience and interaction with the heart.[75] A 3D display is a device capable of conveying depth perception to the viewer by means of stereopsis for binocular vision.

The workflow is similar between these technologies. Both 3D printing, AR and VR, are based on patient-specific medical images. Raw medical images require to be segmented and refined using computer-aided design technologies. Once the 3D geometry of the heart (mesh) is obtained, instead of sending the file to the 3D printer to obtain a physical object in the hands (3D printed model), the file is loaded in a computer. The immersion into the virtual world is done using a VR headset, and the interaction with the simulation is performed using controllers. In the VR environment, the user can magnify, handle, rotate the 3D heart, and use the clipping plane for intracardiac anatomy inspection. To examine the heart from different angles, the user can even walk into the heart along its chambers.

A preliminary use of VR has been used in two complex cases of CHD to illustrate its feasibility and potential of this new technology compared to 3D printing.[76] VR was found to have some potential advantages when compared to 3D printing: Visualization of the cardiac anatomy is not limited to cutting plane or windows created on a physical 3D model, and there is no deterioration of the heart after manipulation and scalpel incisions. Second, VR is a cost-effective alternative to 3D printing in the long term. Start-up cost requires an investment which may vary widely depending on the quality of the VR equipment, but adequate equipment cost below $4000. There is no need to regularly purchase 3D printing material. Third, magnification and resolution of VR allows for better visualization of cardiac structures and are not limited by the capabilities of the 3D printer.

Although there was no quantitative or qualitative comparison between technologies, larger comparatives studies are warranted in order to demonstrate the advantages and limitations of this technology compared to 3D printed models.

TABLE 10.2
Summary of Commercially Available 3D Printers From Ten Leading 3D Printing Companies in the World.

Type	Name	Company	Cost (USD)	Print Area (cm)	Print Resolution (nm)	Printer Size (cm)	Printer Weight (kg)
SLA	Form 1 +	Formlabs	3999	12.5 × 12.5 × 16.5	25	30.0 × 28.0 × 45.0	8
SLA	Projet 1200	3D Systems	4900	4.3 × 2.7 × 15.0	30.5	22.9 × 22.9 × 35.6	9
SLA	Projet 6000	3D Systems	200,000	25.0 × 25.0 × 25.0	50	78.7 × 73.7 × 183.0	181
SLA	Projet 7000	3D Systems	300,000	38.0 × 38.0 × 25.0	50	98.4 × 85.4 × 183.0	272
SLA	ProX 950	3D Systems	950,000	150.0 × 75.0 × 55.0	50	220.0 × 160.0 × 226.0	1951
MJM	Objet 24 series	Stratasys	19,900	23.4 × 19.2 × 14.9	28	82.5 × 62.0 × 59.0	93
MJM	Objet 30 series	Stratasys	40,900	29.4 × 19.2 × 14.9	28	82.5 × 62.0 × 59.0	93
MJM	Projet 3510 series	3D Systems	69,500	29.8 × 18.5 × 20.3	16	29.5 × 47.0 × 59.5	43.4
MJM	Objet Eden	Stratasys	123,000	49.0 × 39.0 × 20.0	16	132.0 × 99.0 × 120.0	410
MJM	Projet 5000	3D Systems	155,000	53.3 × 38.1 × 30.0	32	60.3 × 35.7 × 57.1	53.8
MJM	Projet 5500X	3D Systems	155,000	53.3 × 38.1 × 30.0	29	80.0 × 48.0 × 78.0	115.7
MJM	Connex series	Stratasys	164,000	49.0 × 39.0 × 20.0	16	140.0 × 126.0 × 110.0	430
MJM	Objet Connex series	Stratasys	164,000	49.0 × 39.0 × 20.0	16	142.0 × 112.0 × 113.0	500
MJM	Objet 1000	Stratasys	614,000	100.0 × 80.0 × 50.0	16	280.0 × 180.0 × 180.0	1,950
SLS	sPro series	3D Systems	300,000	55.0 × 55.0 × 46.0	80	203.0 × 160.0 × 216.0	2,700
SLS	ProX series	3D Systems	500,000	38.1 × 33.0 × 45.7	100	174.4 × 122.6 × 229.5	1,360
BJT	Projet 160	3D Systems	40,000	23.6 × 18.5 × 12.7	100	74.0 × 79.0 × 140.0	165
BJT	Projet 260C	3D Systems	40,000	23.6 × 18.5 × 12.7	100	74.0 × 79.0 × 140.0	165
BJT	Projet 360	3D Systems	40,000	20.3 × 25.4 × 20.3	100	122.0 × 79.0 × 140.0	179
BJT	Projet 460 Plus	3D Systems	40,000	20.3 × 25.4 × 20.3	100	122.0 × 79.0 × 140.0	193
BJT	Projet 4500	3D Systems	40,000	20.3 × 25.4 × 20.3	100	162.0 × 80.0 × 152.0	272
BJT	Projet 660 Pro	3D Systems	40,000	25.4 × 38.1 × 20.3	100	188.0 × 74.0 × 145.0	340
BJT	Projet 860 Plus	3D Systems	40,000	50.8 × 38.1 × 22.9	100	119.0 × 116.0 × 162.0	363
FDM	Huxley Duo	RepRapPro	453	13.8 × 14.0 × 9.5	12.5	26.0 × 28.0 × 28.0	4.5
FDM	Mendel	RepRapPro	586	21.0 × 19.0 × 14.0	12.5	50.0 × 46.0 × 41.0	8
FDM	Ormerod 2	RepRapPro	702	20.0 × 20.0 × 20.0	12.5	50.0 × 46.0 × 41.0	6
FDM	Tricolor Mendel	RepRapPro	863	21.0 × 19.0 × 14.0	12.5	50.0 × 46.0 × 41.0	8

Technique	Printer	Manufacturer	Cost ($)	Largest print area (cm)	Print resolution (nm)	Largest printer size (cm)	Weight (kg)
FDM	Cube 3	3D Systems	999	15.3 × 15.3 × 15.3	70	33.5 × 34.3 × 24.1	7.7
FDM	Buccaneer	Pirate 3D	999	14.5 × 12.5 × 15.5	85	25.8 × 25.8 × 44.0	8
FDM	Original +	Ultimaker	1238	21.0 × 21.0 × 20.5	20	35.7 × 34.2 × 38.8	N/A
FDM	Replicator mini	MakerBot	1375	10.0 × 10.0 × 12.5	200	29.5 × 31.0 × 38.1	8
FDM	Creatr	Leapfrog	1706	20.0 × 27.0 × 20.0	50	60.0 × 50.0 × 50.0	32
FDM	Replicator 2	MakerBot	1999	28.5 × 15.3 × 15.5	100	49.0 × 42.0 × 38.0	11.5
FDM	LulzBot TAZ 4	Aleph Objects	2195	29.8 × 27.5 × 25.0	75	668.0 × 52.0 × 51.5	11
FDM	AW3D HDL	Airwolf 3D	2295	30.0 × 20.0 × 28.0	100	61.0 × 44.5 × 46.0	17
FDM	Creatr HS	Leapfrog	2373	29.0 × 24.0 × 18.0	50	60.0 × 60.0 × 50.0	40
FDM	Replicator 2x	MakerBot	2499	24.6 × 15.2 × 15.5	100	49.0 × 42.0 × 53.1	12.6
FDM	Ultimaker 2	Ultimaker	2500	23.0 × 22.5 × 20.5	20	35.7 × 34.2 × 38.8	N/A
FDM	Replicator 5th gen	MakerBot	2899	25.2.19.9 × 15.0	100	52.8 × 44.1 × 41.0	16
FDM	AW3D HD	Airwolf 3D	2995	30.0 × 20.0 × 30.0	60	61.0 × 44.5 × 46.0	17
FDM	Cube Pro	3D Systems	3129	20.0 × 23 × 27.0	100	57.8 × 59.1 × 57.8	44
FDM	AW3D HDX	Airwolf 3D	3495	30.0 × 20.0 × 30.0	60	61.0 × 44.5 × 46.0	17
FDM	AW3D HD2X	Airwolf 3D	3995	27.9 × 20.3 × 30.5	60	61.0 × 45.7 × 45.7	18
FDM	Creatr xl	Leapfrog	4988	20.0 × 27.0 × 60.0	50	75.0 × 65.0 × 126.0	37
FDM	Replicator Z18	MakerBot	6499	30.5 × 30.5 × 45.7	100	49.3 × 56.5 × 85.4	41
FDM	Xeed	Leapfrog	8705	35.0 × 27.0 × 60.0	50	101.0 × 66.0 × 100.0	115
FDM	Mojo	Stratasys	9900	12.7 × 12.7 × 12.7	178	63.0 × 45.0 × 53.0	27
FDM	uPrint	Stratasys	13,9C0	20.3 × 15.2 × 15.2	254	63.5 × 66.0 × 94.0	94
FDM	Objet Dimension series	Stratasys	40,9C0	25.4 × 25.4 × 30.5	178	83.8 × 73.7 × 114.3	148
FDM	Fortus series	Stratasys	184,C00	91.4 × 61.0 × 91.4	127	277.2 × 168.3 × 202.7	2869

Where a 3D printer series is characterized, the lowest cost, largest print area, lowest print resolution, largest printer size, and greater printer weight are selected for comparison. *BJT*, binder jet technique; *cm*, centimeter; *FDM*, fused deposition modeling; *kg*, kilograms; *MJM*, multijet modeling; *nm*, nanometers; *N/A*, not available; *SLA*, stereolithography; *SLS*, selective laser sintering.

Reprint with permission from Chae et al.[72].

TABLE 10.3
A Summary of Average Raw Material Cost of Each 3D Printing Technique.

Type of 3D Printing	Average Cost of Print Material (USD)
SLA	200 per L
MJM	300 per kg
SLS	500 per kg
BJT	100 per kg
FDM	50 per kg

BJT, binder jet technique; *FDM*, fused deposition modeling; *L*, liter; *MJM*, multijet modeling; *SLA*, stereolithography; *SLS*, selective laser sintering. Reprint with permission from Chae et al.[72]

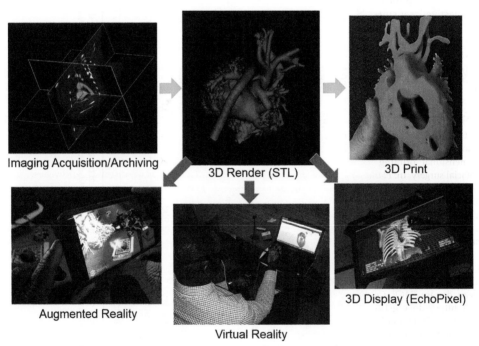

FIG. 10.5 Maturation of digital technology. Starting with imaging acquisition, 3D rendered heart models are no longer just available for 3D printing. Virtual reality, augmented reality, and interactive 3D displays are now available options for advanced visualization and virtual surgical planning. (Reprint with permission from Moore et al.[74].)

CONCLUSION

Clinicians and biomedical researchers often question the value of subjective measure of health because they are perceived as unreliable.[77] We are often uncomfortable with results based on survey questionnaires and would rather prefer data derived from objective meta-analysis. However, subjective measures based on individual awareness and personal experience are certainly an important characteristic of the variables related to health and clinical practice which should not be disregarded. Structural and CHD are such complex and multifaceted specialties that multiple indicators to assess different aspects of outcomes and health are required, in which measures exist on a continuum of biological, social, phycological, and clinical complexity.

Future work should definitively include large randomized studies and evaluate the impact on surgical morbidity, mortality, and cost-effectiveness of 3D printing in CHD.

ABBREVIATIONS

AR	Augmented reality
BJT	Binder jet technique
CHD	Congenital heart defect
CT	Computed tomography
FDM	Fused deposition modeling
MJM	Multijet modeling
MRI	Magnetic resonance imaging
SLA	Stereolithography
SLS	Selective laser sintering
TGA	Transposition of the great arteries
UVH	Univentricular heart
VR	Virtual reality
VSD	Ventricular septal defect

REFERENCES

1. Jacobs CA, Lin AY. A new classification of three-dimensional printing technologies: systematic review of three-dimensional printing for patient-specific cranio-maxillofacial surgery. In: *Plastic and Reconstructive Surgery.* Vol. 139. 2017:1211−1220. https://doi.org/10.1097/PRS.0000000000003232.
2. Zweifel DF, Simon C, Hoarau R, Pasche P, Broome M. Are virtual planning and guided surgery for head and neck reconstruction economically viable? *J Oral Maxillofac Surg.* 2015;73(1):170−175. https://doi.org/10.1016/j.joms.2014.07.038.
3. Mathur M, Patil P, Bove A. The role of 3D printing in structural heart disease. *JACC Cardiovasc Imaging.* 2015;8(8):987−988. https://doi.org/10.1016/j.jcmg.2015.03.009.
4. Bhatla P, Tretter JT, Ludomirsky A, et al. Utility and scope of rapid prototyping in patients with complex muscular ventricular septal defects or double-outlet right ventricle: does it alter management decisions? *Pediatr Cardiol.* 2017;38(1):103−114. https://doi.org/10.1007/s00246-016-1489-1.
5. Bhatla P, Tretter JT, Chikkabyrappa S, Chakravarti S, Mosca RS. Surgical planning for a complex double-outlet right ventricle using 3D printing. *Echocardiography.* 2017; 34(5):802−804. https://doi.org/10.1111/echo.13512.
6. Biglino G, Capelli C, Wray J, et al. 3D-manufactured patient-specific models of congenital heart defects for communication in clinical practice: feasibility and acceptability. *BMJ Open.* 2015;5(4):e007165. https://doi.org/10.1136/bmjopen-2014-007165.
7. Biglino G, Capelli C, Leaver L-K, Schievano S, Taylor AM, Wray J. Involving patients, families and medical staff in the evaluation of 3D printing models of congenital heart disease. *Commun Med.* 2016;12(2−3):157−169. https://doi.org/10.1558/cam.28455.
8. Biglino G, Capelli C, Koniordou D, et al. Use of 3D models of congenital heart disease as an education tool for cardiac nurses. *Congenit Heart Dis.* 2017;12(1):113−118. https://doi.org/10.1111/chd.12414.
9. Biglino G, Koniordou D, Gasparini M, et al. Piloting the use of patient-specific cardiac models as a novel tool to facilitate communication during cinical consultations. *Pediatr Cardiol.* 2017;38(4):813−818. https://doi.org/10.1007/s00246-017-1586-9.
10. Costello JP, Olivieri LJ, Krieger A, et al. Utilizing three-dimensional printing technology to assess the feasibility of high-fidelity synthetic ventricular septal defect models for simulation in medical education. *World J Pediatr Congenit Hear Surg.* 2014;5(3):421−426. https://doi.org/10.1177/2150135114528721.
11. Costello JP, Olivieri LJ, Su L, et al. Incorporating three-dimensional printing into a simulation-based congenital heart disease and critical care training curriculum for resident physicians. *Congenit Heart Dis.* 2015;10(2):185−190. https://doi.org/10.1111/chd.12238.
12. Farooqi KM, Lengua CG, Weinberg AD, Nielsen JC, Sanz J. Blood pool segmentation results in superior virtual cardiac models than myocardial segmentation for 3D printing. *Pediatr Cardiol.* 2016;37(6):1028−1036. https://doi.org/10.1007/s00246-016-1385-8.
13. Farooqi KM, Gonzalez-Lengua C, Shenoy R, Sanz J, Nguyen K. Use of a three dimensional printed cardiac model to assess suitability for biventricular repair. *World J Pediatr Congenit Hear Surg.* 2016;7(3):414−416. https://doi.org/10.1177/2150135115610285.
14. Garekar S, Bharati A, Chokhandre M, et al. Clinical application and multidisciplinary assessment of three dimensional printing in double outlet right ventricle with remote ventricular septal defect. *World J Pediatr Congenit Hear Surg.* 2016;7(3):344−350. https://doi.org/10.1177/2150135116645604.
15. Greil GF, Wolf I, Kuettner A, et al. Stereolithographic reproduction of complex cardiac morphology based on high spatial resolution imaging. *Clin Res Cardiol.* 2007; 96(3):176−185. https://doi.org/10.1007/s00392-007-0482-3.
16. Hadeed K, Dulac Y, Acar P. Three-dimensional printing of a complex CHD to plan surgical repair. *Cardiol Young.* 2016;26(7):1432−1434. https://doi.org/10.1017/S104795 1116000755.
17. Jones TW, Seckeler MD. Use of 3D models of vascular rings and slings to improve resident education. *Congenit Heart Dis.* 2017;12(5):578−582. https://doi.org/10.1111/chd.12486.
18. Kappanayil M, Koneti N, Kannan R, Kottayil B, Kumar K. Three-dimensional-printed cardiac prototypes aid surgical decision-making and preoperative planning in selected cases of complex congenital heart diseases: early

experience and proof of concept in a resource-limited environment. *Ann Pediatr Cardiol.* 2017;10(2):117. https://doi.org/10.4103/apc.APC_149_16.

19. Kiraly L, Tofeig M, Jha NK, Talo H. Three-dimensional printed prototypes refine the anatomy of post-modified Norwood-1 complex aortic arch obstruction and allow presurgical simulation of the repair. *Interact Cardiovasc Thorac Surg.* 2016;22(2):238–240. https://doi.org/10.1093/icvts/ivv320.

20. Loke Y-H, Harahsheh AS, Krieger A, Olivieri LJ. Usage of 3D models of tetralogy of Fallot for medical education: impact on learning congenital heart disease. *BMC Med Educ.* 2017;17(1):54. https://doi.org/10.1186/s12909-017-0889-0.

21. Ma XJ, Tao L, Chen X, et al. Clinical application of three-dimensional reconstruction and rapid prototyping technology of multislice spiral computed tomography angiography for the repair of ventricular septal defect of tetralogy of Fallot. *Genet Mol Res.* 2015;14(1): 1301–1309. https://doi.org/10.4238/2015.February.13.9.

22. Mottl-Link S, Hübler M, Kühne T, et al. Physical models aiding in complex congenital heart surgery. *Ann Thorac Surg.* 2008;86(1):273–277. https://doi.org/10.1016/j.athoracsur.2007.06.001.

23. Olejník P, Nosal M, Havran T, et al. Utilisation of three-dimensional printed heart models for operative planning of complex congenital heart defects. *Kardiol Pol.* 2017; 75(5):495–501. https://doi.org/10.5603/KP.a2017.0033.

24. Olivieri LJ, Krieger A, Loke YH, Nath DS, Kim PCW, Sable CA. Three-dimensional printing of intracardiac defects from three-dimensional echocardiographic images: feasibility and relative accuracy. *J Am Soc Echocardiogr.* 2015;28(4):392–397. https://doi.org/10.1016/j.echo.2014.12.016.

25. Olivieri LJ, Su L, Hynes CF, et al. "Just-In-Time" simulation training using 3-D printed cardiac models after congenital cardiac surgery. *World J Pediatr Congenit Hear Surg.* 2016; 7(2):164–168. https://doi.org/10.1177/2150135115623961.

26. Riesenkampff E, Rietdorf U, Wolf I, et al. The practical clinical value of three-dimensional models of complex congenitally malformed hearts. *J Thorac Cardiovasc Surg.* 2009;138(3):571–580. https://doi.org/10.1016/j.jtcvs.2009.03.011.

27. Shiraishi I, Yamagishi M, Hamaoka K, Fukuzawa M, Yagihara T. Simulative operation on congenital heart disease using rubber-like urethane stereolithographic biomodels based on 3D datasets of multislice computed tomography. *Eur J Cardio-thoracic Surg.* 2010;37(2): 302–306. https://doi.org/10.1016/j.ejcts.2009.07.046.

28. Sodian R, Weber S, Markert M, et al. Stereolithographic models for surgical planning in congenital heart surgery. *Ann Thorac Surg.* 2007;83(5):1854–1857. https://doi.org/10.1016/j.athoracsur.2006.12.004.

29. Valverde I, Gomez G, Gonzalez A, et al. Three-dimensional patient-specific cardiac model for surgical planning in Nikaidoh procedure. *Cardiol Young.* 2015;25(4): 698–704. https://doi.org/10.1017/S1047951114000742.

30. Valverde I, Gomez G, Coserria JF, et al. 3D printed models for planning endovascular stenting in transverse aortic arch hypoplasia. *Cathet Cardiovasc Interv.* 2015;85(6): 1006–1012. https://doi.org/10.1002/ccd.25810.

31. Valverde I, Sarnago F, Prieto R, Zunzunegui JL. Three-dimensional printing in vitro simulation of percutaneous pulmonary valve implantation in large right ventricular outflow tract. *Eur Heart J.* 2017;38(16):1262–1263. https://doi.org/10.1093/eurheartj/ehw546.

32. Valverde I, Gomez-Ciriza G, Hussain T, et al. Three-dimensional printed models for surgical planning of complex congenital heart defects: an international multicentre study. *Eur J Cardio-thoracic Surg.* 2017;52(6):1139–1148. https://doi.org/10.1093/EJCTS/EZX208.

33. Mendez A, Gomez-Ciriza G, Raboisson M-J, et al. Apical muscular ventricular septal defects: surgical strategy using three-dimensional printed model. *Semin Thorac Cardiovasc Surg.* 2018;0(0). https://doi.org/10.1053/j.semtcvs.2018.07.002.

34. Forte MNV, Byrne N, Perez IV, et al. 3D printed models in patients with coronary artery fistulae: anatomical assessment and interventional planning. *EuroIntervention.* 2017;13(9):e1080–e1083. https://doi.org/10.4244/EIJ-D-16_00897.

35. Velasco Forte MN, Byrne N, Valverde I, et al. Interventional correction of sinus venosus atrial septal defect and partial anomalous pulmonary venous drainage. Procedural planning using 3D printed models. *JACC Cardiovasc Imaging.* 2017;11(2 Pt 1):2372. https://doi.org/10.1016/j.jcmg.2017.07.010.

36. Lau I, Sun Z. Three-dimensional printing in congenital heart disease: a systematic review. *J Med Radiat Sci.* 2018. https://doi.org/10.1002/jmrs.268.

37. McDonald PJ, Kulkarni AV, Farrokhyar F, Bhandari M. Ethical issues in surgical research. *Can J Surg.* 2010; 53(2):133–136. http://www.ncbi.nlm.nih.gov/pubmed/20334746.

38. Valent F, Brusaferro S, Barbone F. A case-crossover study of sleep and childhood injury. *Pediatrics.* 2001;107(2). https://doi.org/10.1542/peds.107.2.e23. e23-e23.

39. Hernández-Díaz S, Hernán MA, Meyer K, Werler MM, Mitchell AA. Case-crossover and case-time-control designs in birth defects epidemiology. *Am J Epidemiol.* 2003; 158(4):385–391. https://doi.org/10.1093/aje/kwg144.

40. Lashkarinia SS, Piskin S, Bozkaya TA, Salihoglu E, Yerebakan C, Pekkan K. Computational pre-surgical planning of arterial patch reconstruction: parametric limits and in vitro validation. *Ann Biomed Eng.* 2018;46(9):1–17. https://doi.org/10.1007/s10439-018-2043-5.

41. Sun X, Zhang H, Zhu K, Wang C. Patient-specific three-dimensional printing for Kommerell's diverticulum. *Int J Cardiol.* 2018;255(C):184–187. https://doi.org/10.1016/j.ijcard.2017.12.065.

42. Scanlan AB, Nguyen AV, Ilina A, et al. Comparison of 3D echocardiogram-derived 3D printed valve models to molded models for simulated repair of pediatric atrioventricular valves. *Pediatr Cardiol.* 2018;39(3):538–547. https://doi.org/10.1007/s00246-017-1785-4.

43. Zhao L, Zhou S, Fan T, Li B, Liang W, Dong H. Three-dimensional printing enhances preparation for repair of double outlet right ventricular surgery. *J Card Surg.* 2018; 33(1):24−27. https://doi.org/10.1111/jocs.13523.

44. Farooqi KM, Nielsen JC, Uppu SC, et al. Use of 3-dimensional printing to demonstrate complex intracardiac relationships in double-outlet right ventricle for surgical planning. *Circ Cardiovasc Imaging.* 2015;8(5). https://doi.org/10.1161/CIRCIMAGING.114.003043. e003043-e003043.

45. Biglino G, Moharem-Elgamal S, Lee M, Tulloh R, Caputo M. The perception of a three-dimensional-printed heart model from the perspective of different stakeholders: a complex case of truncus arteriosus. *Front Pediatr.* 2017;5: 171−175. https://doi.org/10.3389/fped.2017.00209.

46. Smith ML, McGuinness J, O'Reilly MK, Nolke L, Murray JG, Jones JFX. The role of 3D printing in preoperative planning for heart transplantation in complex congenital heart disease. *Ir J Med Sci.* 2017;186(3): 753−756. https://doi.org/10.1007/s11845-017-1564-5.

47. Sodian R, Weber S, Markert M, et al. Pediatric cardiac transplantation: three-dimensional printing of anatomic models for surgical planning of heart transplantation in patients with univentricular heart. *J Thorac Cardiovasc Surg.* 2008;136(4):1098−1099. https://doi.org/10.1016/j.jtcvs.2008.03.055.

48. Schmauss D, Juchem G, Weber S, Gerber N, Hagl C, Sodian R. Three-dimensional printing for perioperative planning of complex aortic arch surgery. *Ann Thorac Surg.* 2014;97(6):2160−2163. https://doi.org/10.1016/j.athoracsur.2014.02.011.

49. Sodian R, Schmauss D, Markert M, et al. Three-dimensional printing creates models for surgical planning of aortic valve replacement after previous coronary bypass grafting. *Ann Thorac Surg.* 2008;85(6):2105−2108. https://doi.org/10.1016/j.athoracsur.2007.12.033.

50. Yang DH, Kang JW, Kim N, Song JK, Lee JW, Lim TH. Myocardial 3-dimensional printing for septal myectomy guidance in a patient with obstructive hypertrophic cardiomyopathy. *Circulation.* 2015;132(4):300−301. https://doi.org/10.1161/CIRCULATIONAHA.115.015842.

51. Manso B, García-Díaz L, Valverde I. TGA+VSD and subpulmonary Conus: from fetus to a 3-dimensional model. *Rev Esp Cardiol.* 2017;70(11):1007. https://doi.org/10.1016/j.recesp.2017.01.020.

52. Lau IWW, Liu D, Xu L, Fan Z, Sun Z. Clinical value of patient-specific three-dimensional printing of congenital heart disease: quantitative and qualitative assessments. *PLoS One.* 2018;13(3). https://doi.org/10.1371/journal.pone.0194333. e0194333-15.

53. Jacobs S, Grunert R, Mohr FW, Falk V. 3D-Imaging of cardiac structures using 3D heart models for planning in heart surgery: a preliminary study. *Interact Cardiovasc Thorac Surg.* 2008;7(1):6−9. https://doi.org/10.1510/icvts.2007.156588.

54. Yuan D, Luo H, Yang H, Huang B, Zhu J, Zhao J. Precise treatment of aortic aneurysm by three-dimensional printing and simulation before endovascular intervention. *Sci Rep.* 2017;7(1):795. https://doi.org/10.1038/s41598-017-00644-4.

55. Mafeld S, Nesbitt C, McCaslin J, et al. Three-dimensional (3D) printed endovascular simulation models: a feasibility study. *Ann Transl Med.* 2017;5(3). https://doi.org/10.21037/atm.2017.01.16, 42-42.

56. Hernández-Enríquez M, Brugaletta S, Andreu D, et al. Three-dimensional printing of an aortic model for transcatheter aortic valve implantation: possible clinical applications. *Int J Cardiovasc Imaging.* 2017;33(2): 283−285. https://doi.org/10.1007/s10554-016-0983-0.

57. Wang Z, Liu Y, Xu Y, Gao C, Chen Y, Luo H. Three-dimensional printing-guided percutaneous transcatheter closure of secundum atrial septal defect with rim deficiency: first-in-human series. *Cardiol J.* 2016;23(6): 599−603. https://doi.org/10.5603/CJ.a2016.0094.

58. Chaowu Y, Hua L, Xin S. Three-dimensional printing as an aid in transcatheter closure of secundum atrial septal defect with rim deficiency: in vitro trial occlusion based on a personalized heart model. *Circulation.* 2016;133(17):e608−e610. https://doi.org/10.1161/CIRCULATIONAHA.115.020735.

59. Olivieri L, Krieger A, Chen MY, Kim P, Kanter JP. 3D heart model guides complex stent angioplasty of pulmonary venous baffle obstruction in a Mustard repair of D-TGA. *Int J Cardiol.* 2014;172(2):e297−e298. https://doi.org/10.1016/j.ijcard.2013.12.192.

60. Phillips ABM, Nevin P, Shah A, Olshove V, Garg R, Zahn EM. Development of a novel hybrid strategy for transcatheter pulmonary valve placement in patients following transannular patch repair of tetralogy of fallot. *Cathet Cardiovasc Interv.* 2016;87(3):403−410. https://doi.org/10.1002/ccd.26315.

61. Schievano S, Migliavacca F, Coats L, et al. Percutaneous pulmonary valve implantation based on rapid prototyping of right ventricular outflow tract and pulmonary trunk from MR data. *Radiology.* 2007;242(2):490−497. https://doi.org/10.1148/radiol.2422051994.

62. Macario A. What does one minute of operating room time cost? *J Clin Anesth.* 2010;22(4):233−236. https://doi.org/10.1016/j.jclinane.2010.02.003.

63. Tack P, Victor J, Gemmel P, Annemans L. 3D-printing techniques in a medical setting: a systematic literature review. *Biomed Eng Online.* 2016;15(1):115. https://doi.org/10.1186/s12938-016-0236-4.

64. Kim JYS, Khavanin N, Rambachan A, et al. Surgical duration and risk of venous thromboembolism. *JAMA Surg.* 2015;150(2):110. https://doi.org/10.1001/jamasurg.2014.1841.

65. Rebollo MH, Bernal JM, Llorca J, Rabasa JM, Revuelta JM. Nosocomial infections in patients having cardiovascular operations: a multivariate analysis of risk factors. *J Thorac Cardiovasc Surg.* 1996;112(4):908−913. https://doi.org/10.1016/S0022-5223(96)70090-9.

66. López-Sendón J, González-Juanatey JR, Pinto F, et al. Quality markers in cardiology. Main markers to measure quality of results (Outcomes) and quality measures related to better results in clinical practice (Performance Metrics).

INCARDIO (Indicadores de Calidad en Unidades Asistenciales del Área del Corazón. *Rev Esp Cardiol.* 2015;68(11):976–995. https://doi.org/10.1016/j.rec.2015.07.003.

67. Birkhäuer J, Gaab J, Kossowsky J, et al. Trust in the health care professional and health outcome: a meta-analysis. *PLoS One.* 2017;12(2):e0170988. https://doi.org/10.1371/journal.pone.0170988.

68. McMurray R, Kendall L, Parsons JM, et al. A life less ordinary: growing up and coping with congenital heart disease. *Coron Health Care.* 2001;5(1):51–57. https://doi.org/10.1054/chec.2001.0112.

69. Martelli N, Serrano C, Van Den Brink H, et al. Advantages and disadvantages of 3-dimensional printing in surgery: a systematic review. *Surgeon.* 2016;159(6):1485–1500. https://doi.org/10.1016/j.surg.2015.12.017.

70. Giannopoulos AA, Mitsouras D, Yoo S-J, Liu PP, Chatzizisis YS, Rybicki FJ. Applications of 3D printing in cardiovascular diseases. *Nat Rev Cardiol.* 2016;13(12):701–718. https://doi.org/10.1038/nrcardio.2016.170.

71. Byrne N, Velasco Forte M, Tandon A, Valverde I, Hussain T. A systematic review of image segmentation methodology, used in the additive manufacture of patient-specific 3D printed models of the cardiovascular system. *JRSM Cardiovasc Dis.* 2016;5(0). https://doi.org/10.1177/2048004016645467, 204800401664546.

72. Chae MP, Rozen WM, McMenamin PG, Findlay MW, Spychal RT, Hunter-Smith DJ. Emerging applications of bedside 3D printing in plastic surgery. *Front Surg.* 2015;2:25. https://doi.org/10.3389/fsurg.2015.00025.

73. Valverde I, Gomez G, Suarez-Mejias C, et al. 3D printed cardiovascular models for surgical planning in complex congenital heart diseases. *J Cardiovasc Magn Reson.* 2015;17(Suppl 1):P196. https://doi.org/10.1186/1532-429X-17-S1-P196.

74. Moore RA, Riggs KW, Kourtidou S, et al. Three-dimensional printing and virtual surgery for congenital heart procedural planning. *Birth Defects Res.* 2018;110(13):1082–1090. https://doi.org/10.1002/bdr2.1370.

75. Riener R, Harders M. Virtual reality in medicine. *Virtual Real Med.* 2012;9781447140(1):1–294. https://doi.org/10.1007/978-1-4471-4011-5.

76. Ong CS, Krishnan A, Huang CY, et al. Role of virtual reality in congenital heart disease. *Congenit Heart Dis.* 2018;13(3):357–361. https://doi.org/10.1111/chd.12587.

77. Ferlie E. Increasing top management turnover: is it true and does it matter? *J Health Serv Res Policy.* 1997;2(1):1–2. http://journals.sagepub.com/doi/pdf/10.1177/135581969700200102%0Ahttp://www.ncbi.nlm.nih.gov/entrez/query.fcgi?cmd=Retrieve&db=PubMed&dopt=Citation&list_uids=10180647.

CHAPTER 11

3D Modeling as a Medical Education Resource, Simulation, and Communication Tool

LAURA OLIVIERI, MD

INTRODUCTION

3D modeling of human anatomy offers an invaluable tool for a deeper and more precise understanding of the human body. Possibilities are nearly endless when applying 3D modeling to biomedical uses. This chapter will cover the specific evidence for use of 3D modeling as a medical education resource, a simulation tool, and a communication tool. Arguably, these three uses are actually a single, shared concept, resting on the foundation of creation of a shared mental model of an extremely complex disease. Once a group of viewers can all convincingly see the same thing at the same time, education, communication, and simulation can take place. Over the last 10 years, significant advances in 3D printing technology have made it possible to create lifelike, printed models of any part of the human anatomy, including congenital heart defects. These printed models have considerable educational value wherein defects can be examined from every angle, and complex 3D relationships of cardiac structures no longer need to be inferred from 2D imaging, they can be displayed in three dimensions and held in the hand.

3D models have long been used to enhance learners' understanding of the human anatomy. Plastic, 3D models of the most complex organs, including the heart, have been in production for decades, and can illustrate general features of normal human anatomy. However, when learners set out to understand pathology beyond what is considered normal, more complex, detailed 3D guides are required. For example, when learning about congenital heart disease (CHD), postmortem specimens are frequently employed for this purpose, requiring guided sessions with experts in the field who handle the specimens and teach small groups of learners the most important, and often the most subtle, features that define CHD.

These sessions form the basis for the framework that many of us use to understand all of human CHD, day in and day out. We go back in our memories to recapture important details as we go forward to care for the next patient. This is an immersive educational experience; however, access to these specimens is limited, and over time becomes more and more limited as specimens are subject to degradation and loss of integrity of these very important features. They cannot be labeled, they cannot be "resliced," and their utility is time-limited.

Enter 3D cardiovascular modeling and additive manufacturing.[1,2] With the advent of 3D printing, complex shapes are able to be manufactured relatively quickly and cheaply, without constraining the 3D print. A variety of methods are available now which help to build 3D shapes from various types of polymers,[3] as discussed in detail in Chapter 2. These tools can be used to create both digital and printed models of cardiovascular pathology at any scale and sliced and resliced in multiple planes to demonstrate characteristics of the heart from various angles. 3D printed and digital heart models are unconstrained and incredibly useful, as the following chapter will show.

The utility of a 3D anatomic model is easy to understand and difficult to measure as noted in the previous chapter. Some have compared it to the backup cameras that are now standard on vehicles sold in the United States.[4] For generations, people have backed into and out of parking spaces. One does not require a backup camera to back a car out of a parking space on a Saturday at a busy neighborhood grocery store. However, the confidence with which one can back a car out increases dramatically with use of the camera, and thus the value is measured in driver confidence and satisfaction. The same can be true for management of CHD; surgeons

3-Dimensional Modeling in Cardiovascular Disease. https://doi.org/10.1016/B978-0-323-65391-6.00011-9

and cardiologists do not need 3D heart models to manage patients and perform surgery. Likewise, trainees do not need 3D heart models to learn cardiac pathology. However, holding an accurate, detailed 3D heart model in your hand, or viewing one in virtual reality, improves the confidence with which these groups move forward in their knowledge and with their management plans.

The drivers are more confident; the pedestrians are also safer. Likewise can be said for providers and patients.

3D MODELS AS A COMMUNICATION TOOL

A picture is worth a 1000 words, and a 3D lifelike model is probably worth more than this when communicating complex information. A prime example of this can be seen in the care of patients with CHD, due to the importance of subtle anatomic features that are open to interpretation in different ways by different people. Cardiologists, cardiovascular surgeons, cardiac intensivists, cardiac anesthesiologists, nurses, therapists, and most importantly, parents and caregivers, need to have a shared mental model of a patient's congenital heart defect. Creating cohesion in understanding of these various groups of people is complicated by the presence of anatomic variation within types of CHD and nonspecific and, at times, imprecise language used to describe CHD.

Patient-specific 3D models created from patient data may also be beneficial during consultations with family members regarding a patient's diagnosis of CHD. The models make the details of a particular congenital heart defect more readily understandable, regardless of educational background.

Biglino et al. report on their experience with 3D printed, patient-specific heart models and their impact on communication. In a well-designed study, 103 parents of children with known CHD were randomized to either a 3D model group or a control group for cardiac consultation. Based on pre- and postintervention questionnaires, there were no statistically significant differences in knowledge of their child's heart defect between the two groups; however, a large (>70%) portion of the parents found the model to be "very useful" in the cardiac consultation. Clinicians involved were also polled and gave high marks to utility and quality of the model. From objective data gathered from the study, the 3D model increased the duration of the visit by an average of only 5 min; interestingly, clinicians reported that they did not feel that the visit was prolonged when models were used. Parent freeform feedback was grouped into three main themes; first, 3D models are much easier to understand than standard medical images and in some cases offered families their first true understanding of their child's disease. Second, models can be shocking at first, when families realize that it is a lifelike reproduction of their child's heart, but quickly become a centerpiece of engagement in the conversation and in the care of their child. Finally, 3D models can be particularly helpful during the initial encounter when a diagnosis is first being discussed with a family.[5,6]

These precious insights gained from the Biglino study should inform our approach to discussion of CHD as we look to how we will utilize these valuable adjuncts in the future for communication and team building.

3D MODELS AS AN EDUCATIONAL RESOURCE

3D cardiovascular models are well suited to providing education about cardiac anatomy to learners of various levels. Whether it is a group of postdoctoral students, parents, or cardiac intensive care unit (CICU) practitioners, 3D printed heart models depicting CHD can summarize large amounts of complex spatial data and make it easily digestible for these learners.

Examples of the value added by 3D models in the medical education literature abound, including orthopedic, ophthalmologic, urologic examples. For example, in a randomized trial assessing the understanding of spinal fracture types among a group of medical students in China, the group with access to 3D printed models of the various spinal fracture types had faster recall and more confidence in the subject matter when compared to peers who had been randomized to standard imaging (CT) and 3D imaging for their learning session.[7] Trainees in ophthalmology and optometry gain improved visualization of all portions of the human eye through reproduction of an orbital dissection.[8] Yammine et al. performed a meta-analysis of educational programs using 3D models, including on 2226 participants including 2128 from studies with comparison groups. 3D visualization technologies (1) resulted in higher (d = 0.30, 95% CI: 0.02−0.62) factual knowledge, (2) yielded significantly better results (d = 0.50, 95% CI: 0.20−0.80) in spatial knowledge acquisition, and (3) produced significant increases in user satisfaction (d = 0.28, 95% CI = 0.12−0.44) and in learners' perception of the effectiveness of the learning tool (d = 0.28, 95% CI = 0.14−0.43).[9] The authors conclude that, in an era where anatomy knowledge is diminishing among students, 3D visualization technology may be a potential solution to the problem of inadequate anatomy pedagogy.

Impact on Cardiovascular Disease Education

3D printed models of the human anatomy have long been shown to be excellent teaching aids for all of human anatomy; however, this is particularly the case in CHD, a heterogeneous collection of lesions with a wide spectrum of severity within each type of cardiac defect. This wide spectrum of severity creates complexity for learning, thus it is encouraging that several studies show efficacy in learning about CHD with use of 3D models. Complex anatomical pathologies, including malalignment-type ventricular septal defects, double outlet right ventricle, and the heterotaxy syndromes can be more easily demonstrated with a 3D model that offers hands-on education. Trainees can have a tactile experience with any type of heart defect. More recently, time and attention have been paid to fine-tuning the material in which 3D heart models are printed, with development of lifelike materials that can hold sutures, which provide a realistic "practice" model that can be used to perform simulated procedures in anticipation of a complex surgical procedure.[10]

In an effort to understand the value that 3D models add to education, multiple groups have designed experiments specifically to assess the value of 3D printed teaching tools in the field of cardiology and CHD. Loke et al.[11] report on the value of 3D printed models of various types of tetralogy of Fallot (TOF) at various stages of growth and development, including a preoperative model from an unrepaired infant, a postoperative model of repaired TOF with pulmonary atresia that was repaired with a right ventricle to pulmonary artery conduit, and a postoperative model of repaired TOF by a transannular patch. Forty pediatric residents were randomized to receive an educational session on TOF with either standard, 2D depictions of TOF or 3D printed models. The session content, pace, and style were otherwise identical between the two groups. Pediatric residents showed no difference in understanding of the content, which is an expected result (Fig. 11.1). Learning of content can occur without 3D models. What 3D models provide is an enhanced understanding of the content, which is typically measured by ratings that correlate with confidence, recall, and learner satisfaction. In adult learners, satisfaction and engagement have been shown to directly affect subject matter retention,[12,13] making these important outcome variables to describe quality of education.

A 3D model–based approach to enhancing content surrounding ventricular septal defect education for large groups of postdoctoral and medical students was reported on by Costello et al. These investigators demonstrated that all students reported significant improvement in knowledge acquisition, knowledge reporting, and structural conceptualization of ventricular septal defects following their educational session.[14] Similar results were reported by Su et al., who undertook a similar experiment with the addition of a control arm, in which medical students were taught with standard teaching aids. Scores here indicated superior knowledge acquisition and learner satisfaction in the 3D print group compared with standard teaching aids.[15]

Finally, 3D printed models were pitted head to head against cadaveric cardiac specimens in a double-blind randomized controlled trial of 52 undergraduate medical students where postintervention test scores were significantly higher in the 3D prints group (60.8% vs. 44.8%, $P = .01$), suggesting at least noninferiority, and possibly superior demonstration of external cardiovascular anatomy with the 3D printed heart models.[16]

Impact on Collaboration Between Academic Institutions

3D cardiovascular models have the potential to align educational content between academic institutions, so that resources may be shared and teaching curricula may be enhanced by being developed with a wider spectrum of human anatomy. An example of this is the codevelopment of pathology educational session between institutions in Ireland and California in which unique specimens from each location were shared at both locations thanks to 3D segmentation tools and 3D printing.[17] Each site imaged, segmented, and created virtual 3D models of some of their specimens, and then shared with the other site, in effect doubling their collections, and exposing learners to specimens beyond their local environment. Medical education dedicated toward presentation of rare diseases and congenital defects, about which there are fewer educational resources available, benefits from institutions sharing their local case-specific and patient-specific variations to curate an improved educational collection for all contributors. Resources such as the 3D Print Exchange,[18] hosted by the National Institute of Immunology, Allergy and Infectious Diseases, have created a publicly accessible location to share such resources, and they have dedicated ongoing resources toward developing a 3D Cardiovascular Library.[18]

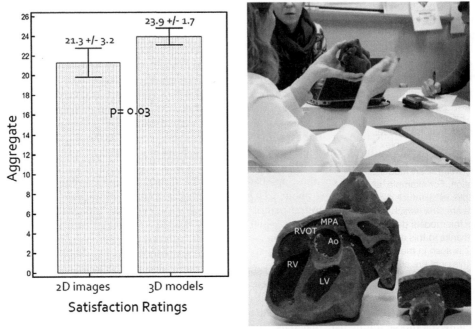

FIG. 11.1 Figure shows the main results from the Loke et al. study, where an important and statistically significant impact on learner satisfaction scores (out of 26), $P = .03$, was observed in a randomized controlled trial of 2D versus 3D models used during a trainee educational session. The right panels demonstrate a model used in the study of repaired tetralogy of Fallot (TOF) by placement of a right ventricle to pulmonary artery conduit, and a session where an instructor is utilizing the model to teach a group of trainees. (Photo courtesy Dr. Yue-Hin Loke.)

Increase Access to Pathology Specimens

Access to human pathologic specimens is limited, and financial, legal, and ethical concerns surrounding such specimens have contributed to use of alternative teaching techniques for human anatomy, including cardiovascular anatomy. Advances in both 3D cardiac modeling and web-based access to this information have broken significant barriers in anatomic and pathologic education and information dissemination.[19] Traditionally, each institution largely relied on its own local library of pathology specimens to create a curriculum for local learners. The result is highly variable quality of specimens as well as gaps in the educational curriculum that centers around the availability of specific types of specimens. Each institution's medical imaging archives likely contain thousands more 3D representations of CHD than the pathology specimens that may be used to develop a robust 3D-based educational curriculum. 3D printing and 3D modeling can allow for easier sharing of 3D replicas of pathology specimens, as files containing the 3D spatial information are easily transmitted, and these files can be printed using a local printer, obviating the need for expensive packing, shipping, and storing.

Improved Visualization of Critical Features

An important attribute of 3D cardiac models, particularly digital models, is that they are free of constraints for visualizing internal anatomic details. One can virtually "slice" the 3D object with 360 degrees of freedom. In addition, there is incredible value in addition of various colors to the 3D model to create layers of embedded information indicating specific parts of the heart, including atria, ventricles, outflows, and veins, all within one print[18,20,21] (Fig. 11.2).

3D MODELS FOR SIMULATION

Again, we see trends where 3D models have allowed for simulation of correction of various anatomic defects prior to performing the surgery or procedure on a patient. For example, researchers 3D printed abdominal models of choledochal cysts, as well as surrounding structures including the liver capsule and

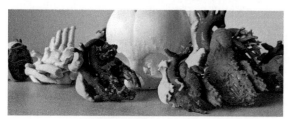

FIG. 11.2 Figure demonstrates the impact of adding color to a 3D printed anatomic model. In the foreground, multiple colorful 3D models of complex congenital heart defects are seen with a standard application of colors to various parts of the heart between heart models, to enhance visual communication. For example, all of the right ventricles are colored purple, left ventricles are peach, right atria are teal, and left atria are pink, which allow the congenital heart disease that the models depict to be more easily accessible to learners thanks to this embedded information. In contrast, a white skull is seen in the background, where various portions of this print are all the same color, and the observer is left to make decisions about the boundaries of the various portions of the skull. (Photo courtesy Dr. Justin Ryan.)

pancreatic ducts. Trainees performed a simulated surgery, with feedback showing that the 3D printed trainer was useful and easily reproducible in other centers. In addition, 100% of trainees would recommend the simulation to their colleagues for professional development.[22]

Procedural Simulation

Regarding cardiovascular simulation, there has been a sharp increase in reported uses of 3D cardiac models in simulation over the last 10 years. The concept of simulation of surgical procedure prior to surgery will be covered in Chapters 3 and 8, and so will only be briefly touched on here. A recent example from Ong et al. describes selection of the proper right ventricle to pulmonary artery conduit size and type through use of a "virtual surgery" in which the entire chest and right ventricular outflow tract were modeled with various types of conduits.[23] Similar assessments have been made for the Norwood arch reconstruction.[24] Beyond surgical simulation, there are numerous examples of how 3D printed, patient-specific heart models have assisted in simulation of catheter-based interventions in patients with structural and CHD. For example, our group reported on an early use of 3D printing to help guide a complex stent angioplasty of an obstructed pulmonary venous baffle in a patient with D-transposition of the great arteries who previously underwent a Mustard atrial switch operation. Important

elements of the case, including stent sizing and selection as well as camera angle selection, were informed by preprocedural simulation with the 3D heart model.[25]

Care Delivery Simulation

An emerging and innovative area of use of 3D cardiac models is for use in simulating care delivery by bedside providers, including anesthesiologists, intensivists, and cardiologists. Understanding patient-specific anatomy is critical to effective delivery of care in highly specialized inpatient units, particularly the Pediatric CICU. 3D printed heart models were used during a "just-in-time," patient-specific simulation in the CICU with the bedside team who were about to accept a patient from the operating room after a congenital heart surgery. Seventy clinicians participated in 10 patient-specific group simulations on common postoperative care scenarios relevant to the anatomy. Authors found that 3D models enhanced anatomic understanding and were generally more helpful than a standard hand-off, with a higher effect noted with higher case complexity by STAT mortality score.[26]

A similar experiment was conducted at the same institution, but instead of using printed 3D heart models, virtual 3D heart models were used for asynchronous, "just-in-time" patient-specific simulation and care handoff, in the pediatric CICU. Again, both nurses and physicians reported significant improvement in handoff and confidence with the use of the patient-specific 3D virtual heart models (Table 11.1).

When a subanalysis was conducted comparing the printed versus digital 3D models, printed models scored higher than digital models as adjuncts to handoffs. Otherwise there were no significant differences between the two types of models, with both types being very highly rated by all types of CICU providers (score greater than 7 out of 10). Interestingly, despite similar satisfaction and confidences scores, cost analysis for 3D patient-specific model construction for "just-in-time" patient simulation showed that the digital 3D model strategy was roughly 1/15th the cost of the printed 3D model strategy[27] (Fig. 11.3).

Finally, the Society for Cardiovascular Angiography and Interventions (SCAI) assessed the current use of medical simulators in interventional cardiology and concluded that simulation will take on a larger role in cardiovascular training and maintenance of certification in the future.[28] These simulators may include 3D virtual and printed patient-specific models as part of the training materials.[29]

TABLE 11.1

Questionnaire and Response Scores [Median (IQR)] for Virtual 3D Model Simulation From the Olivieri et al. Study Which Demonstrates That Both Physicans and Nurses Report a Significant and Positive Impact on Their Ability to do Their Job With the Use of a 3D Heart Model in a "Just-In-Time" Simulation Session in the Cardiac Intensive Care Unit.

Question	Physicians n = 19 Providers	Nurses/Trainees, n = 34 Providers	All Combined, n = 53 Providers[a]	P Value[b]
1. Previously familiar with surgery	8 (5–10)	9 (7–10)	8 (7–10)	.64
2. Ability to describe anatomy	9 (8–10)	9 (8–10)	9 (8–10)	.83
3. Ability to describe surgery	8 (6–9)	8 (7–9)	8 (7–9)	.99
4. Ability to manage clinically	8 (7–9)	8 (7–9)	8 (7–9)	.78
5. Enhanced anatomy understanding	9 (7–10)	10 (8–10)	10 (8–10)	.09
6. Enhanced surgical understanding	9 (7–10)	9 (7–10)	9 (7–10)	.56
7. Enhanced management clinically	9 (7–10)	8 (7–10)	8 (7–10)	.50
8. More helpful than handoffs	7 (4–9)	6 (5–10)	7 (5–9)	.78

3D, three dimensional.
[a] Data are median score (interquartile range). Two groups were compared by the nonparametric Mann-Whitney U-test.
[b] No significant differences between physicians and nurses/trainees.

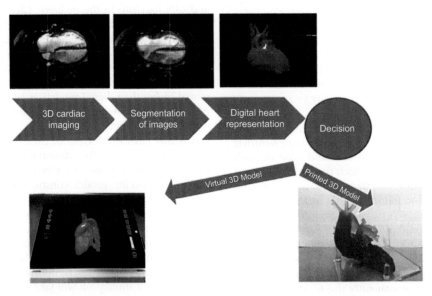

$1300 - $3500 over 100 cases $16,000 to $55,960 over 100 cases

FIG. 11.3 Figure depicts the process for creation of both 3D virtual and 3D printed models; both models begin with a standardized process using 3D cardiac imaging as a roadmap for creation of a 3D heart reconstruction as a digital file. From there, a decision is made to further render the file to display as a 3D virtual model (bottom left) or as a 3D printed model (bottom right). Cost differential between the two methods was approximately $5000–$10,000 for the 20 cases described in this publication. (Reprinted with permission.)

CONCLUSION

Evidence exists which supports the use of 3D models of the heart to enhance trainee education, care simulation (both procedural and bedside care), and particularly communication. As 3D visualization and segmentation technology continues to advance, inclusion of a 3D heart model into almost any area of cardiovascular medicine should become easier, and should simplify even the most complex task at hand, whether that is explaining a complex, life-sustaining procedure to worried parents of a newborn, or performing that procedure. 3D printed hearts can be a tool that will enhance our abilities and improve our already high standards of care.

REFERENCES

1. Greil GF, Wolf I, Kuettner A, et al. Stereolithographic reproduction of complex cardiac morphology based on high spatial resolution imaging. *Clin Res Cardiol.* 2007; 96:176–185. Available from: http://link.springer.com. proxygw.wrlc.org/article/10.1007/s00392-007-0482-3.
2. Kim MS, Hansgen AR, Wink O, Quaife RA, Carroll JD. Rapid prototyping a new tool in understanding and treating structural heart disease. *Circulation.* 2008;117: 2388–2394. Available from: http://circ.ahajournals.org/content/117/18/2388.
3. Bramlet M, Olivieri L, Farooqi K, Ripley B, Coakley M. Impact of three-dimensional printing on the study and treatment of congenital heart disease. *Circ Res.* 2017;120: 904–907.
4. News ABC. All new cars in US now required to have backup cameras. *ABC News*; 2018. Available from: https://abcnews.go.com/US/cars-us-now-required-backup-cameras/story?id=54854404.
5. Biglino G, Capelli C, Wray J, et al. 3D-manufactured patient-specific models of congenital heart defects for communication in clinical practice: feasibility and acceptability. *BMJ Open.* 2015;5. Available from: https://www.ncbi.nlm.nih.gov/pmc/articles/PMC4420970/.
6. Biglino G, Capelli C, Leaver L-K, Schievano S, Taylor AM, Wray J. Involving patients, families and medical staff in the evaluation of 3D printing models of congenital heart disease. *Commun Med.* 2015;12:157–169.
7. Li Z, Li Z, Xu R, et al. Three-dimensional printing models improve understanding of spinal fracture—a randomized controlled study in China. *Sci Rep.* 2015;5. Available from: https://www.ncbi.nlm.nih.gov/pmc/articles/PMC4477328/.
8. 3D printed reproductions of orbital dissections: a novel mode of visualising anatomy for trainees in ophthalmology or optometry. *Br J Ophthalmol;* 2015. Available from: https://bjo.bmj.com/content/99/9/1162.long.
9. Yammine K, Violato C. A meta-analysis of the educational effectiveness of three-dimensional visualization technologies in teaching anatomy. *Anat Sci Educ.* 2015;8:525–538.
10. Shiraishi I, Yamagishi M, Hamaoka K, Fukuzawa M, Yagihara T. Simulative operation on congenital heart disease using rubber-like urethane stereolithographic biomodels based on 3D datasets of multislice computed tomography. *Eur J Cardiothorac Surg.* 2010;37:302–306.
11. Loke Y-H, Harahsheh AS, Krieger A, Olivieri LJ. Usage of 3D models of tetralogy of Fallot for medical education: impact on learning congenital heart disease. *BMC Med Educ.* 2017;17. Available from: https://www.ncbi.nlm.nih.gov/pmc/articles/PMC5346255/.
12. Anderson KT. *Linking Adult Learner Satisfaction With Retention: The Role of Background Characteristics, Academic Characteristics, and Satisfaction Upon Retention.* 2011:98.
13. Kang M. *Increasing Student Engagement and Knowledge Retention in an Entry-Level General Nutrition Course with Technology and Innovative Use of a Graduate-Level Teaching Assistant.* 2017:118.
14. Costello JP, Olivieri LJ, Krieger A, et al. Utilizing three-dimensional printing technology to assess the feasibility of high-fidelity synthetic ventricular septal defect models for simulation in medical education. *World J Pediatr Congenit Heart Surg.* 2014;5:421–426.
15. Su W, Xiao Y, He S, Huang P, Deng X. Three-dimensional printing models in congenital heart disease education for medical students: a controlled comparative study. *BMC Med Educ.* 2018;18. Available from: https://www.ncbi.nlm.nih.gov/pmc/articles/PMC6090870/.
16. Lim KHA, Loo ZY, Goldie SJ, Adams JW, McMenamin PG. Use of 3D printed models in medical education: a randomized control trial comparing 3D prints versus cadaveric materials for learning external cardiac anatomy. *Anat Sci Educ.* 2016;9:213–221.
17. Mahmoud A, Bennett M. Introducing 3-dimensional printing of a human anatomic pathology specimen: potential benefits for undergraduate and postgraduate education and anatomic pathology practice. *Arch Pathol Lab Med.* 2015;139, 1048–51. Available from: http://www.archivesofpathology.org/doi/10.5858/arpa.2014-0408-OA.
18. Coakley MF, Hurt DE, Weber N, et al. The NIH 3D print Exchange: a public resource for bioscientific and biomedical 3D prints. *3D Print Addit Manuf.* 2014;1, 137–40. Available from: http://online.liebertpub.com/doi/10.1089/3Dp.2014.1503.
19. Ghazanfar H, Rashid S, Hussain A, Ghazanfar M, Ghazanfar A, Javaid A. Cadaveric dissection a thing of the past? The insight of consultants, fellows, and residents. *Cureus.* 2018;10. Available from: https://www.ncbi.nlm.nih.gov/pmc/articles/PMC5991920/.
20. Ryan JR, Moe TG, Richardson R, Frakes DH, Nigro JJ, Pophal S. A novel approach to neonatal management of tetralogy of Fallot, with pulmonary atresia, and multiple aortopulmonary collaterals. *JACC Cardiovasc Imaging.* 2015;8:103–104.
21. How multi-colour 3D printing helps communicate ideas. *3D Print;* 2016. Available from: https://3Dprinting.com/3D-printing-use-cases/how-multi-colour-3D-printing-helps-communicate-ideas/.

22. Burdall OC, Makin E, Davenport M, Ade-Ajayi N. 3D printing to simulate laparoscopic choledochal surgery. *J Pediatr Surg.* 2016;51:828−831.

23. Ong CS, Loke Y-H, Opfermann J, et al. Virtual surgery for conduit reconstruction of the right ventricular outflow tract. *World J Pediatr Congenit Heart Surg.* 2017;8:391−393.

24. Kiraly L, Tofeig M, Jha NK, Talo H. Three-dimensional printed prototypes refine the anatomy of post-modified Norwood-1 complex aortic arch obstruction and allow presurgical simulation of the repair. *Interact Cardiovasc Thorac Surg.* 2016;22:238−240.

25. Olivieri L, Krieger A, Chen MY, Kim P, Kanter JP. 3D heart model guides complex stent angioplasty of pulmonary venous baffle obstruction in a Mustard repair of D-TGA. *Int J Cardiol.* 2014.

26. O'Brien SM, Jacobs JP, Pasquali SK, et al. The society of thoracic surgeons congenital heart surgery database mortality risk model: Part 1—statistical methodology. *Ann Thorac Surg.* 2015;100, 1054−62. Available from: https://www.ncbi.nlm.nih.gov/pmc/articles/PMC4728716/.

27. Olivieri LJ, Zurakowski D, Ramakrishnan K, et al. Novel, 3D display of heart models in the postoperative care setting improves CICU caregiver confidence. *World J Pediatr Congenit Heart Surg.* 2018;9, 206−13. Available from: https://doi.org/10.1177/2150135117745005.

28. Green SM, Klein AJ, Pancholy S, et al. The current state of medical simulation in interventional cardiology: a clinical document from the Society for Cardiovascular Angiography and Intervention's (SCAI) Simulation Committee. *Catheter Cardiovasc Interv.* 2014;83:37−46. Available from: https://onlinelibrary.wiley.com/doi/abs/10.1002/ccd.25048.

29. Valverde I, Gomez G, Coserria JF, et al. 3D printed models for planning endovascular stenting in transverse aortic arch hypoplasia. *Catheter Cardiovasc Interv.* 2015;85:1006−1012.

CHAPTER 12

Computational Modeling and Personalized Surgery

WEIGUANG YANG, PHD • JEFFREY A. FEINSTEIN, MD, MPH •
ALISON L. MARSDEN, PHD

INTRODUCTION

Hemodynamics plays an important role in the initiation, progression, and treatment of cardiovascular diseases in adults and children. There is increasing evidence that treatments for cardiovascular disease can be improved by quantification and prediction of changing hemodynamics and its interaction with the physiology and biology of the cardiovascular system. Computational blood flow simulation uses computer modeling to simulate blood flow by numerically solving the governing equations of flow and tissue mechanics that characterize the cardiovascular system, producing blood pressure, velocity, and additional variables of clinical and biological interest. Complementing in vivo imaging techniques such as magnetic resonance imaging (MRI), a unique advantage of computational modeling is the capability to predict the response of the flow field to physiologic changes or surgical interventions. Thus, computational modeling is a promising tool to supplement current imaging techniques for surgical planning.

Modeling pulsatile flow in rigid and elastic vessel dates back to the 1950s. Womersley derived analytical solutions for pulsatile Newtonian fluid in an axisymmetric one-dimensional (1D) circular tube by linearizing the Navier—Stokes equations.[1,2] Later, analogy to electrical circuits (also called the 0D model) was used to model the circulatory system.[3,4] In contrast to many methods that were applied to cardiovascular modeling from other areas, immersed boundary methods (IBMs) were originally developed by Peskin[5] in the 1970s for modeling blood flow in the heart with moving boundaries. Starting from the late 1980s, three dimensional (3D) blood flow simulations have been used with increasing anatomic detail.[6-9] Since the late 1990s, MRI and computed tomography (CT) data with other in vivo clinical data have become essential to patient-specific 3D blood

flow simulations, and regions of interest have been expanded from the carotid artery to other arteries.[10-15]

The remainder of this chapter is organized as follows: we first outline the fundamentals needed to model cardiovascular flow, including the equations and principles governing 0D, 1D, and 3D blood flow modeling. Then, procedures for patient-specific 3D simulations, choices of boundary conditions (BCs), 0D—3D coupling to multiscale physiologic models, and fluid—structure interactions (FSIs) for 3D modeling are introduced, followed by representative case studies from adult and congenital heart diseases. Finally, we discuss current challenges and future perspectives.

ELECTRIC ANALOGY OF BLOOD FLOW

It is simple and surprisingly effective to model the circulatory system by making an analogy between blood flow and electrical current, in which pressure drop is analogous to voltage and flow rate is analogous to current. Starting in the 1960s, lumped parameter models (LPMs) comprised of electrical circuit components have been used to model the circulatory system. The resistive, elastic, and inertial properties of blood flow through a vessel can be modeled by basic circuit components: resistors, capacitors, and inductors, respectively. These elements can be mathematically described as follows:

$$R = \frac{\Delta P}{Q}, \tag{12.1}$$

$$Q = C\frac{dP}{dt}, \tag{12.2}$$

$$\Delta P = L\frac{dQ}{dt}, \tag{12.3}$$

where R, P, Q, C, L, t are resistance, pressure, flow rate, capacitance, inductance, and time, respectively. Additional components can be added to simulate active

3-Dimensional Modeling in Cardiovascular Disease. https://doi.org/10.1016/B978-0-323-65391-6.00012-0

(A)   **(B)**

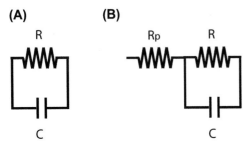

FIG. 12.1 Diagrams for **(A)** a resistor–capacitor (RC) model and **(B)** a three-element Windkessel (RCR) model.

contraction of the ventricles, intramyocardial pressure, and variable and nonlinear resistances.

Since the electric analogy does not have any spatial dimension, it is also called 0D modeling. An LPM is created by lumping these circuit components into a resulting model. The simplest LPM is to use a single resistor to represent blood vessels. Based on Ohm's law, the pressure drop down the length of the vessel is proportional to the inflow. In the resistor model, the vessel compliance is ignored. A resistor–capacitor (RC) model (Fig. 12.1A) connects a resistor and a capacitor in parallel to account for the resistive and compliant properties. By applying Kirchhoff's current law to the RC circuit, the flow rate is related to pressure as follows.

$$Q = C\frac{dP}{dt} + \frac{P}{R},\qquad(12.4)$$

and if $Q(t)$ is known, Eq. (12.4) can be solved for $P(t)$. The RC model is also called a two-element Windkessel (German for air chamber) model. Similarly, a three-element Windkessel (RCR) model is formed by adding an additional resistor (R_p) to the RC circuit (Fig. 12.1B). The equation for the RCR model is given as follows:

$$\frac{dP}{dt} + \frac{P}{CR} = Q\left(\frac{1}{C} + \frac{R_p}{CR}\right) + R_p\frac{dQ}{dt}.\qquad(12.5)$$

By solving Eq. (12.5), the pressure for the RCR model is given by

$$P(t) = e^{-\frac{t}{RC}}[P(0) - R_pQ(0)] + R_pQ + \int_0^t \frac{e^{-(t-s)/(RC)}}{C}Q(s)ds.\qquad(12.6)$$

Pulsatile blood flow is generated by the contraction and relaxation of heart chambers. Ventricular pressure elevates rapidly during systole while the atrial pressure pulse remains small. In an LPM for the left heart

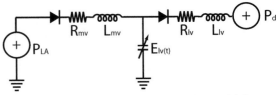

FIG. 12.2 A lumped parameter model for the left heart.

(Fig. 12.2), the left atrium is modeled by a constant pressure head and the left ventricle is modeled by a time-varying capacitor $C(t)$. Ventricular pressure $P_v(t)$ is usually related to ventricular volume $V(t)$ by

$$P_v(t) = \frac{1}{C(t)}(V(t) - V_0),\qquad(12.7)$$

where V_0 is the volume of the ventricular chamber at zero pressure. We define an elastance function E as the inverse of capacitance so that $P_v(t) = E(t)(V(t) - V_0)$ Heart valves are modeled by a diode, through which flow goes only in one direction. In Fig. 12.2, a resistor and an inductor are added for each valve to model viscous and inertial effects. Thus, the equations for the heart model are given as follows:

$$P_{la} = Q_{la}R_{mv} + \frac{dQ_{la}}{dt}L_{la} + P_{lv},\qquad(12.8)$$

$$P_{lv} = E(t)(V(t) - V_0),\qquad(12.9)$$

$$\frac{dV}{dt} = Q_{la} - Q_{ao},\qquad(12.10)$$

$$P_d = P_{lv} - Q_{ao}R_{av} - \frac{dQ_{ao}}{dt}L_{av},\qquad(12.11)$$

where L is inductance and subscripts la, mv, lv, av, ao and d represent the left atrium, mitral valve, left ventricle, aortic valve, aorta, and distal vasculature, respectively. Q_{la} is set to 0 when $P_{la} < P_{lv}$. Similarly, Q_{ao} is set to 0 when $P_{lv} < P_d$. If parameters $R_{mv}, L_{mv}E(t), V_0, R_{av}$ and P_d are known, Eqs. (12.8)–(12.11) can be solved numerically for unknowns Q_{la}, P_{lv} and Q_{ao}. In practice, these parameters need to be tuned iteratively to match target clinical values such as end diastolic volume, end systolic volume, systolic and diastolic ventricular pressures. Generally, $E(t)$ is a patient-specific function. A standard normalized elastance function E_N can be scaled to achieve desired ventricular pressures and volumes for each patient.[16]

$$E(t) = E_N \times E_{max},\qquad(12.12)$$

$$t = t_N \times E_{max},\qquad(12.13)$$

where E_{max} is the maximum elastance value and t_{max} is the time difference between the onset of systole and the time at the maximum elastance. While the above LPM examples can be solved analytically, with increasing complexity of LPMs, analytical solutions become unavailable and the governing ordinary differential equations (ODEs) need to be solved numerically. Standard time integration schemes such as Runge–Kutta methods are effective and easily implemented. To model diseased or pathological heart valve behavior, a valve model with parameters designed for valvar stenosis and insufficiency can be used.[17] Theoretical analysis of the 0D model showed that 0D models for vessel network are a first-order approximation of the 1D flow model (see Milisic et al.[18]).

Applications

LPMs are useful to study global hemodynamics when LPMs for different organs are connected to form a lumped parameter network (LPN). Some early LPM studies for congenital heart defects include Peskin et al.[19] in which an LPM was used to model patients with patent ductus arteriosus and ventricular septal defect or atrial septal defect, and Pennati et al.[20] in which the impact of the bidirectional Glenn procedure for single ventricle defects has been studied. Applications to modeling tetralogy of Fallot and pulmonary arterial hypertension can be found in Refs.[21,22] Because LPMs offer a computationally cheap method to model a large-scale circulatory system with no local hemodynamic information, LPMs are usually coupled to a higher order model (1D and 3D) that describes the region of interest. The coupling between LPMs and 3D models is reviewed in Marsden et al.[23] Examples of 0D–3D coupling will be shown in the case studies for 3D flow modeling in Section 4.3.

ONE-DIMENSIONAL BLOOD FLOW MODELING

Because spatial variables are absent in LPMs, wave propagation or reflection in blood vessels cannot be captured. To characterize these phenomena, 1D flow modeling is needed. A generalized 1D blood flow theory without an assumption of axisymmetry was developed by Hughes and Lubliner[24] in the 1970s. The 1D equations for Newtonian flow in a deformable domain are given as follows:

$$\frac{\partial S}{\partial t} + \frac{\partial Q}{\partial z} = -\Psi \qquad (12.14)$$

$$\frac{\partial Q}{\partial t} + \frac{\partial}{\partial t}\left[(1+\delta)\frac{Q^2}{S}\right] + \frac{S}{\rho}\frac{\partial p}{\partial z} = Sf + N\frac{Q}{S} + \nu\frac{\partial^2 Q}{\partial z^2}, \qquad (12.15)$$

where S and Q are cross-sectional area and volumetric flow rate, respectively, Ψ is an outflow function with $\Psi = 0$ for impermeable walls, f is the external force, ν is kinematic viscosity, and δ and N are parameters for velocity profile. For a Poiseuille profile $\delta = \frac{1}{3}$ and $N = -8\pi\nu$. In addition, N can be modified to account for additional viscous loss due to stenosis.

Eqs. (12.14) and (12.15) are the continuity and momentum equations, respectively. A constitutive equation is needed to close the system, and a popular constitutive relationship is suggested by Olufsen[25] using linear elasticity:

$$p(z,t) = p_0(z) + \frac{4}{3}\frac{Eh}{r_0(z)}\left(1 - \sqrt{\frac{S_0(z)}{S(z,t)}}\right), \qquad (12.16)$$

where $p_0(z) = p(z,0), r_0(z) = \sqrt{S_0(z)/\pi}$ and $S_0(z)$ is the stress-free cross-sectional area. Eh/r_0 can be further approximated by an empirical exponential function:

$$\frac{Eh}{r_0} = k_1 \exp(k_2 r_0) + k_3, \qquad (12.17)$$

where parameters k_1, k_2 and k_3 can be obtained by fitting to experimental data.

A common choice for the inlet BC is to prescribe the flow rate. Pressure, flow rate, resistance, impedance, and RCR BCs can be prescribed at the outlets. Eqs. (12.14)–(12.16) are highly nonlinear and coupled, making analytical solutions unavailable. To solve the 1D blood flow equations, finite difference, finite volume, and finite element methods have been used.[26] Further details of the relevant formulations and numerical methods can be found in Refs. 25, 27–29. A review of 1D cardiovascular flow solution methods and applications is given by Shi et al.[26]

Applications

Because 1D flow models are computationally less expensive than 2D or 3D models, they are suitable for characterizing large-scale cardiovascular flow and pressure propagation. In Refs. 25,30, large arteries were modeled by the 1D flow equations and smaller arteries were represented by a parameterized structured tree whose root impedance is used to provide outflow BCs for the 1D model. This approach was used to compute the flow and pressure waveforms along the pulmonary arterial tree with and without pulmonary hypertension. Mynard et al.[31] incorporated a ventricular model, aortic valve, and coronary flow to the 1D flow model. Steele et al.[32] validated 1D model–derived flow distribution in the aorta of porcine aortic bypass models against with PCMRI measurements. Recently the use of 1D

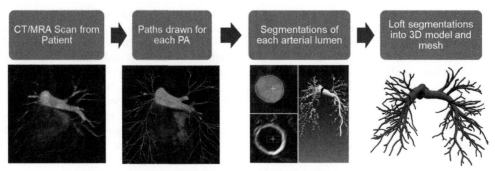

FIG. 12.3 Steps for patient-specific model construction using SimVascular.

models for fractional flow reserve (FFR) was explored following studies on noninvasive 3D modeling for FFR.[33] 1D models can also be used as BCs for 3D simulations, with appropriate coupling methods, allowing for wave propagation across the 3D—1D domain.

THREE-DIMENSIONAL FLOW MODELING

In the 1D flow equations, only the axial component of the velocity is considered and pressure is assumed uniform over the vessel cross-section. However, in large arteries, flow separation and nonlinear affects are often encountered. More detailed flow fields are needed when the interaction between blood flow and tissue is studied locally (e.g., wall shear stress [WSS] on a coronary artery with a stenosis). Therefore, 3D flow modeling is particularly suitable for large arteries. Three-dimensional modeling requires a pipeline progressing from medical imaging to anatomical model construction, flow simulation, and analysis. Below, we describe each step in this pipeline, with references provided for additional detail.

Patient-Specific Model Construction

In contrast to many conventional engineering systems, the geometry of the cardiovascular system is highly complex and irregular with considerable heterogeneity among patients. Although idealized models with a parameterized description provide useful insights, it is usually necessary to perform patient-specific modeling to obtain sufficiently realistic results. Typical patient-specific model construction for the arterial and venous systems derives from CT or MRI data. Invasive intravascular ultrasound (IVUS)[34] and optical coherence tomography (OCT)[35] can also be used for coronary model construction when a higher resolution is needed. Fig. 12.3 illustrates the three major steps for patient-

specific model construction. First, a center line path is created by the user along each vessel of interest. Second, the lumen boundary is identified manually or automatically using algorithms such as level set methods to create 2D segmentation for cross-sections sampled along the vessel. Third, the 2D segmentations are lofted to form a 3D solid model. This "path planning" model construction method is suitable for cylindrical vessels with treelike branch structure. Alternative methods, such as 3D segmentation, are typically better suited to model construction in vessels with aneurysms or in ventricular or cardiac mechanics. Center lines for the coronary artery tree can be automatically extracted from CT images.[36,37] Lumen boundary segmentation can be carried out in a semiautomatic way while manual correction is still required.[38] In our experience, automatic segmentation often underperforms when image quality is reduced and branching patterns become complex such as in the pulmonary arteries (PAs), and manual intervention is needed in these cases. A number of software packages can be used for model construction including open source packages SimVascular (www.simvascular.org),[39—41] ITK-SNAP[42] and VMTK (www.vmtk.org), freely available CRIMSON (www.crimson.software) package, and the commercial package MIMICS (Materialise NV, Leuven, Belgium).

Governing Equations and Boundary Conditions

Three-dimensional blood flow can be described by the 3D Navier—Stokes equations of incompressible flow that may be written as follows:

$$\rho\left(\frac{\partial \mathbf{u}}{\partial t} + \mathbf{u} \cdot \nabla \mathbf{u} - \mathbf{f}\right) - \nabla \cdot \sigma = 0, \qquad (12.18)$$

$$\nabla \cdot \mathbf{u} = 0, \qquad (12.19)$$

where $\mathbf{u} = (u, v, w), \rho, p$ and $\mathbf{f}$ are the velocity vectors, flow density, pressure, and external force, respectively, and the stress tensor σ is defined as follows:

$$\sigma = -p\mathbf{I} + 2\mu\varepsilon(\mathbf{u}), \qquad (12.20)$$

$$\varepsilon(\mathbf{u}) = \frac{1}{2}\left(\nabla\mathbf{u} + \nabla\mathbf{u}^{\mathrm{T}}\right), \qquad (12.21)$$

where $\mathbf{I}, \mu$, and ε are the identity tensor, dynamic viscosity, and strain-rate tensor, respectively. Here a Newtonian assumption is employed. In large arteries, shear rates are usually high $(> 100s^{-1})$ and blood flow can be approximated as a Newtonian fluid with a constant viscosity. When shear rates decrease $(< 10s^{-1})$, red blood cells aggregate and non-Newtonian effects may become prominent. The shear-rate-dependent viscosity can be modeled by a class of generalized Newtonian fluids (e.g., power-law fluids) in which the viscosity is related to the shear rate.[43] In addition, blood also shows viscoelastic properties at low shear rates due to the elasticity of red blood cells.[44] Typical BCs for 3D blood flow in a vessel are given as follows:

$$\mathbf{u} = 0, \text{ on } \Gamma_{\text{wall}}, \qquad (12.22)$$

$$\mathbf{u} = \mathbf{g(t)} \text{ on } \Gamma_{\text{inlets}}, \qquad (12.23)$$

$$\sigma \cdot \mathbf{n} = -p\mathbf{n} \text{ on } \Gamma_{\text{outlets}}, \qquad (12.24)$$

where Γ denotes the boundary faces of the model and $\mathbf{g}(t)$ and P are velocity and pressure values prescribed at the inlets and outlets, respectively. When solution values or their derivatives are imposed on the boundary, BCs are referred to as Dirichlet or Neumann BCs. Dirichlet BCs are usually employed on vessel walls with a rigid wall assumption and on inlet faces. In rigid wall simulations, velocity on vessel wall is set to 0. At the inlets, flow rates with a predefined velocity profile such as parabolic or Womersley are prescribed. At the outlets, Neumann BCs are often employed. Because of attractive advantages in handling complex geometry, finite element methods[8,11,14,45] are widely used in 3D blood flow modeling, though finite volume[46,47] and finite difference schemes[48-50] are also employed. An alternative approach to modeling fluid flow is the lattice Boltzmann method (LBM) that simulates the process of microscopic particle streaming and collision to obtain macroscopic behaviors of fluids.[51] Examples of modeling 3D cardiovascular flow by LBM can be found in Refs. [52-54]

Limited by computational cost and medical imaging resolution, 3D flow modeling is typically performed in a region of interest which is a subset of the entire vasculature. However, the flow field in the 3D model is influenced by the upstream and downstream domains. For example, the changes in cardiac output can significantly alter the pressure gradient in coarctation of the aorta and pulmonary vascular resistance in each lung has a great impact on the flow distribution in the PAs. Therefore, BCs play a crucial role in blood flow simulations. For 3D computational modeling for large vessels, the inflow data can be measured relatively easily by phase contrast MRI (PCMRI) or by echocardiography. Prescribing inflow rates with an analytical profile such as parabolic is commonly used. Using nonidealized velocity profiles from PCMRI data has also been reported.[55-57] Simulation results with parabolic profiles are shown to have good agreement with those with patient-specific profiles though aortic abnormalities could alter the inlet profile resulting in a substantial change in flow patterns.[56,57]

For outflow BCs, a traction-free BC,

$$\sigma\mathbf{n} = 0 \qquad (12.25)$$

is the simplest; however, this often results in a nonphysiologic flow distribution to the outlets in models with branching vessels. It is also not possible to achieve a physiologic value of mean pressure when using a traction-free BC. The desired flow distribution may not be achieved when a 3D model contains branches. In addition, it is not uncommon to be lacking measurements for distal branches. Therefore, LPMs are useful to represent the downstream vasculature and supply the outflow BCs for 3D models. With the resistance BC, the outlet mean pressure is given by,

$$P = QR \qquad (12.26)$$

where Q and R are outflow rate and resistance value, respectively. Similarly, an RCR BC prescribes the outlet mean pressure by Eq. (12.6). Compared to the resistance BC, the RCR BC damps the pressure pulse due to the capacitor, and allows for parameter tuning to match the pressure waveform amplitude. Details of numerical implementation in a finite element formulation can be found in the classic paper of Vignon-Clementel et al.[58]

Fig. 12.4 is an example in which flow in an aortic bifurcation model is simulated with steady inflow and two different outflow BCs, traction-free and resistance, in a stenotic model (55% stenosis) versus a normal model. In Fig. 12.4A and B, for the stenotic model, there are significant differences in the flow split and local velocity fields between traction-free and resistance BCs. With a stenosis and traction-free BCs, flow to the left

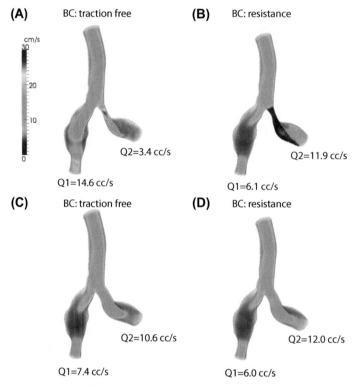

FIG. 12.4 Examples of influence of outflow boundary conditions (BCs) on the flow field. Constant inflow of 18 *cc/s* with a parabolic profile is prescribed at the inlet. Traction-free and resistance BCs are applied to an aortic bifurcation model with **(A−B)** and without (C-D)a narrowing in the left common iliac artery. Resistance value for outlets 1 (the right common iliac artery) and 2 (the left common iliac artery) is 16,662 and 8331 *dyn ·s· cm^{-5}*, respectively.

common iliac is substantially diminished (Fig.12.4A). However, with resistance BCs, outflow to the left common iliac artery (outlet 2) remains greater than that to the right common iliac artery (outlet 1) due to a higher resistance value prescribed at outlet 1 (Fig.12.4B). When the stenosis is relieved, the flow split change from 81/19 to 41/59 under the traction-free BC (Fig. 12.4A to C) while the value hardly changes under the resistance BC (Fig. 12.4B to D) because the downstream resistance dominates the resistance created by the stenosis in this example. This example demonstrates both local geometry and distal vascular resistance should be carefully considered in simulations. These considerations are also crucially important for predicting other derived quantities such as WSS and residence times.

0D−3D Coupling

In addition to resistance and RCR models, more complex LPMs can be coupled to provide BCs for 3D simulations. For example, a heart model described in Fig. 12.2 can be coupled to a 3D aorta or a PA model to provide inlet conditions. LPMs for the inlets and outlets can be connected forming a closed-loop LPN with the advantage that the each part is coupled together allowing one to examine the influence of local hemodynamic changes on global physiology.

For simple 0D LPMs coupled to a 3D model, analytical solutions are available and can be directly hard-coded into the 3D flow solver to get robust and efficient performance. When complex LPMs are coupled to a 3D model, no analytical solution exists and pressure and flow information is exchanged iteratively between 3D and 0D domains. Numerical instabilities may arise, necessitating time-step restrictions. Moghadam et al.[59] compared explicit, semi-implicit, and implicit coupling strategies (Adding contributions from the 0D−3D coupling to the tangent matrix at each Newton−Raphson iteration is referred to as implicit coupling.) and found a semi-implicit implementation for 0D−3D coupling to be robust and versatile in cardiovascular finite element simulations. Coupling a 3D model to 0D physiology models can be done in an open loop or closed loop configuration, depending on the application.

Data Assimilation and Uncertainty Quantification

In 3D cardiovascular simulations, BCs are tuned such that quantities derived from simulation results match clinical measurements such as pressures and cardiac output. In 0D−3D coupled simulations, the number of input parameters is greatly increased with increasing complexity of LPMs, making manual tuning inefficient. Systematic tuning methods in which optimization algorithms were utilized to minimize the difference between computed results and targets have been used in cardiovascular modeling[22,60−62]. Furthermore, clinical measurements for patients are discrete observations with uncertainties and errors. Methods to identify proper parameters for cardiovascular modeling while accounting for uncertain inputs are receiving increased attention. Data assimilation is widely used in geophysical fluid dynamics as a process to combine observations data, which are often sparse and heterogeneous in space and time with errors, and numerical models to optimally represent the state of a system.

Next, we use a simple example to illustrate the process of parameter estimation using a Markov chain Monte Carlo (MCMC) method (Metropolis−Hastings sampling). In the context of cardiovascular modeling, MCMC methods can be used to estimate input parameters such that simulation results match the distribution of clinical data.[63] Suppose outlet resistance is needed for modeling blood flow in a bifurcation model with two outlets and the flow split measured by MRI has a normal distribution $P(f_s)$ centered at 60/40 with a standard deviation = 0.05. We aim to find a set of resistance ratios, θ, such that the simulation results denoted by $y = \mathbf{G}(\theta)$ match the target clinical distribution $P(f_s) = N(0.6, 0.05)$. We perform Metropolis−Hastings sampling as follows:

1. Choose an arbitrary starting point θ_0.
2. For iteration i, compute the flow split $y_i = \mathbf{G}(\theta_i)$ and evaluate the probability density function $P(y_i)$. A user-defined symmetric probability density function Q is used to draw the next candidate point. For example, we can randomly draw a point θ_{i+1} with a normal distribution $N(\theta_i, \sigma)$ centered at θ_i.
3. Calculate the acceptance ratio $\alpha = P(y_{i+1})/P(y_i)$. A uniform random number u is generated between 0 and 1. If $\alpha \geq u$, the candidate is accepted. If $\alpha < u$, the candidate is rejected and set $\theta_{i+1} = \theta_i$. In other

words, we always accept candidate when $\alpha \geq 1$ and accept candidates with probability of α if $\alpha < 1$.
4. Repeat steps 2−3 until stopping criteria are met.

Fig. 12.5A shows that the MCMC sampling performs random walks and move to a region that matches target clinical distribution (high posterior probability). Fig. 12.5B shows good agreement between the computed flow splits using MCMC-sampled resistance ratios and the target flow split distribution. Starting from these sample points, optimization algorithms can be used to further minimize the difference between simulation results and target values.[63] The method outlined above has been employed to identify input parameters in 3D hemodynamic simulations for single ventricle defects and the coronary arteries.[63,64] In addition to MCMC, other techniques including Kalman filtering[65,66] and variational data assimilation[67,68] were also used in cardiovascular modeling.

In cardiovascular modeling, uncertainties refer to a potential deviation from true values due to the lack of knowledge and inevitably exist as follows:

- Model construction: Patient-specific models are created from image data with uncertainties due to image noise and segmentation methods.
- Boundary conditions: Clinical data are often incorporated into BCs resulting in significant uncertainties due to physiologic conditions, measurement methods, and data unavailability.
- Choice of physical models: Physical models represent a system with assumptions in which certain properties or phenomena are ignored.

Uncertainty quantification (UQ) allows one to provide simulation outputs with error bars or confidence intervals and may improve modeling efficiency and enhance error tolerance for surgical planning. Recently several UQ techniques used in engineering have been applied to cardiovascular modeling problems. The Monte Carlo simulation quantifies the impacts of parameters of interest on model outputs by running hundreds or thousands of simulations randomly sampled from the probability distribution of uncertain parameters. Statistical quantities such as mean and variance can be extracted directly from simulation results. To obtain converged results, a large number of simulations is required, making it unaffordable for expensive modeling such as 3D Navier−Stokes simulations, though several techniques, for example Latin hypercube sampling, have been introduced to reduce computational cost. The Monte Carlo simulation is considered the reference for other UQ techniques. Similar to Monte Carlo sampling, stochastic collocation methods strategically sample grid points in the space of stochastic

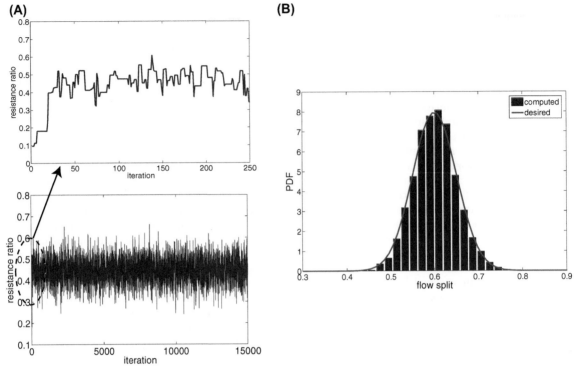

FIG. 12.5 A Markov chain Monte Carlo (MCMC) sampling for parameter estimation. **(A)** The trace plot shows MCMC takes random walks to identify resistance ratios for target flow splits. Starting from an initial value of 0.1, candidate points jump to regions near 0.45. **(B)** Probability density functions for computed flow splits using samples given by MCMC and the clinical target.

variables. For each grid point, a deterministic simulation is performed. Values between grid points are interpolated by orthogonal polynomials:

$$g(\mathbf{x}, t, \theta) = \sum_{i=1}^{m} \mathbf{u}(\mathbf{x}, t, \theta_i) L_i(\theta), \qquad (12.27)$$

where $\mathbf{x}$ is the coordinates, t is the time, g is the approximated solution, $\mathbf{u}$ is the solution, θ_i are uncertain parameters on collocation points, m is the number of collocation points, and L_i are Lagrange polynomials. Sparse grids such as Smolyak algorithms can be used with increasing dimensions.[69,70] Since stochastic collocation methods are nonintrusive, existing solvers can be used directly to perform UQ.

If solutions with random variables are expanded by polynomial chaos expansions to $p + 1$ terms,

$$g(\mathbf{x}, t, \theta) = \sum_{i=0}^{p} \widehat{\mathbf{u}}_i(x, t) \mathbf{\Phi}_i(\theta), \qquad (12.28)$$

where $\mathbf{\Phi}_i$ are orthogonal polynomials, and substituted into the governing equations, one can obtain $p + 1$ coupled equations using the Galerkin projection. The polynomial chaos expansion can also be considered as a spectral expansion in the random space with random modes $i = 0 \ldots p$. For each mode i, $\widehat{\mathbf{u}}_i$ is deterministic and conventional numerical methods can be used to solve the equations.[71,72] This method is shown to achieve fast converge;[72] however, the implementation may be more challenging. Nonintrusive pseudo-spectral methods approximate $\widehat{\mathbf{u}}_i$ by summing deterministic simulation solutions on collocation points with polynomial chaos and weights.[73,74] Both stochastic collocation methods and pseudo-spectral methods perform deterministic simulations on grid points in stochastic space. A major difference is that grid values are used to estimate coefficients for known basis functions in pseudo-spectral methods while each grid value is used as a known coefficient for Lagrange interpolations in stochastic collocation methods.[75]

Conventional polynomial chaos methods may become unstable due to the use of global polynomial expansions when quantities of interest exhibit nonlinear behaviors such as discontinuities and steep gradients.[76] Multiresolution expansions have been proposed to address these limitations for intrusive[77] and nonintrusive[78] uncertainty propagation.

The propagation of uncertainty from clinical data/BCs to simulation results has been studied for coronary flow[64,79,80], abdominal aortic aneurysms,[70,81] carotid arteries,[82] bypass graft models,[83] Fontan circulation,[70] and 1D arterial networks.[84–86]

Fluid—Structure Interaction

Blood flow with moving boundaries is ubiquitous in the cardiovascular system from the heart valves to blood vessels. Although a rigid wall assumption is justified in many 3D cardiovascular flow simulations, the influence of structural deformation on hemodynamics is important in many cases necessitating FSI models. When the forces on boundaries exerted by the blood flow are negligible compared to the forces exerted on blood flow by moving boundaries, hemodynamic modeling with deformable walls can be performed by prescribing the boundary motions.[87,88] Wall motion can be prescribed analytically or extracted from in vivo MRI data, often using image registration methods. However, the application is limited by the availability of data and the desire for the wall motion to be emergent from the simulations. With advances in computing power, there has been an increased tendency to study cardiovascular FSI problems by solving the structural and flow equations simultaneously. Despite increased complexity and cost, fully coupled FSI is capable of characterizing both hemodynamics and wall tissue mechanics in cardiovascular modeling.

Cardiovascular FSI can be simulated on a body-fitted mesh or a fixed mesh using different numerical approaches. In the arbitrary Lagrangian—Eulerian (ALE) formulations, meshes for structure and fluid are separated and conformal to the structure.[89] The solid mesh moves with the structure in a Lagrangian way and fluid mesh is deformed to conform to the moving boundary by solving an additional elastic problem. The fluid momentum equations are related to the structure momentum equations by the fluid—solid interface condition which ensures continuity in velocity and traction on the boundary. The advantage of conformal mesh—based method is that the mesh near the fluid—solid boundary can be refined to better resolve near-wall flow. However, additional computational cost is required for deforming the fluid mesh and remeshing

when the fluid mesh becomes severely distorted. It is particularly challenging to handle biological tissues with large deformation and complex contact conditions such as valves. Alternatively, IBMs originally developed by Peskin[5] for modeling heart valves allow one to simulate FSI using a fixed mesh. In IMBs, solids are immersed in a stationary background mesh. Navier—Stokes equations are modified by adding a forcing function that exerts forces to fluids in the vicinity of the boundary to simulate the presence of solids.[90] A major advantage for IBMs is the ease of mesh generation because structured Cartesian grids can be used. However, challenges lie in reduced resolution near the fluid-solid interface and the geometric representation for IBMs. In addition, it is noteworthy that the coupled momentum method proposed by Figueroa, Taylor and colleagues[91] provides an efficient alternative to model arteries with small deformations. Under the assumption of thin walls and small deformations, a linear membrane model is coupled to the Navier—Stokes equations by replacing the Dirichlet BC (prescribing no slip velocity) with a Neumann BC (prescribing a traction) for vessel walls. Since the wall displacement is given by a linear model and the mesh is fixed, it is computationally efficient to model FSI in 3D artery models with small displacements. Mathematical formulations and numerical methods for solving FSI problems are involved and technical. We therefore refer the interested readers to Bazilevs et al.,[89] Quarteroni et al.,[45] and Formaggia et al.[92] for relevant details.

Applications

Case study: coronary bypass graft surgery

Coronary artery disease is a leading cause of death in the United States (1 in 7 deaths) and worldwide.[93] In 2011, more than 200,000 coronary bypass graft (CABG) procedures were performed in the United States.[94] Approximately 70% of patients receive a saphenous vein graft (SVG).[95] The failure rate of SVG is approximately 50% within 10 years postsurgery[96] while internal mammary artery (IMA) grafts can maintain patency in 90% over 10–15 years postoperatively.[97] Given this drastic difference between two common types of grafts, there is a pressing clinical need to understand the biomechanical mechanisms of these failures.

In this case study, patient-specific modeling of CABG patients is employed to elucidate mechanical conditions in grafts. Following previous studies, patient-specific models are created based on CT images and discretized by linear tetrahedral elements. Due to the size of the coronary arteries, it is difficult to directly measure coronary flow. Therefore LPMs were coupled

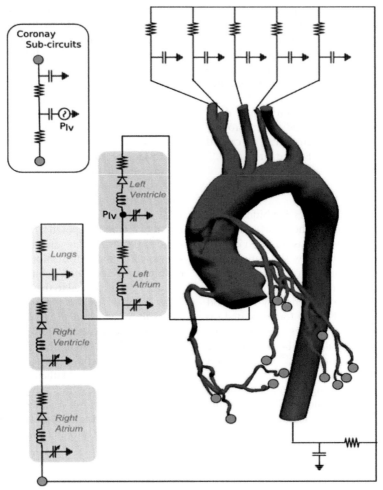

FIG. 12.6 Schematic view of a closed loop 0D–3D coupling for a patient-specific coronary model.[64]

to the 3D models of the aorta and coronary arteries. Fig. 12.6 shows a schematic view of a closed-loop 0D–3D model. A heart LPM is used to provide BCs for the aortic inlet. Conventional RCR BCs are used for the outlets of the 3D model except the coronary outlets. A striking difference between the coronary arteries and other arteries is that coronary artery flow drops during systole due to ventricular contraction and peaks during diastole. As shown in Fig. 12.6, a coronary LPM consists of RC circuits with an intramyocardial pressure added to a capacitor to regulate coronary flow in synchrony with cardiac contraction.[98] The intramyocardial pressures for the right and left coronary arteries were approximated by the right and left ventricular pressures given by the heart LPMs. Due to a large difference

between RV and LV pressures, the out-of-phase flow is more pronounced in the left coronary artery.

In Fig. 12.7, WSS and strains were shown to have significant differences in five patients with venous and arterial coronary grafts.[99] These results may shed light on the higher failure rate of vein grafts for coronary artery bypass surgery. This computational modeling framework was also used to study the anastomosis angle for the bypass graft in a patient-specific setting.[100]

Tran et al.[64] applied an automatic parameter estimation framework based on adaptive MCMC sampling to coronary flow simulations. Fig. 12.8 shows the WSS and oscillatory shear index (OSI) values with standard deviation in the coronary arteries when uncertainties for clinical input data were taken into account.

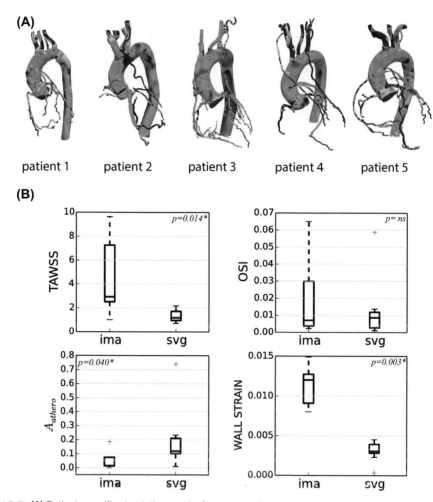

FIG. 12.7 **(A)** Patient-specific simulation results for coronary bypass graft models. Time-averaged wall shear stress for five patients with venous and arterial coronary grafts. (B) Significant differences are found in shear stress and wall strains for the five patients.[99]

Case study: surgerical design for the Fontan procedure

Single ventricle defects, among the most severe congenital heart defects in newborns, are uniformly fatal without intervention. Typically, a three-stage palliative surgical approach is performed. In the first week after birth, the Norwood procedure reconstructs the aorta and an aortopulmonary shunt is inserted to provide blood flow to the lungs. In the second stage, the Glenn procedure, the superior vena cava (SVC) is connected to the PA and the aortopulmonary shunt is taken down, typically within 6 months of birth. At the age of 3–4 years, the Fontan procedure connects the inferior vena cava (IVC) to the PA such that all venous return is redirected to the lungs, bypassing the heart, and the functional ventricle is used to drive the systemic circulation only. In the extracardiac Fontan procedure, a Gore-tex graft is used to connect the IVC to the PA forming a T-junction.

Three-dimensional hemodynamics modeling for the Fontan procedure dates back to the 1990s when Dubini et al.[101] used CFD to show that an offset design reduces energy loss compared to the T-junction, in which the IVC flow aligns with SVC flow in an idealized Fontan model. Their computational studies led to a clinical adoption of the offset design by surgeons and are perhaps the earliest example of CFD impacting clinical practice. Since then, CFD has gained increased popularity for hemodynamic

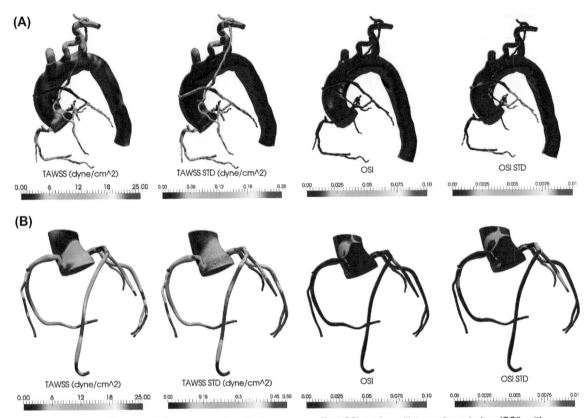

FIG. 12.8 Computed time averaged wall shear stress (TAWSS) and oscillatory shear index (OSI) with standard deviation (STD) for **(A)** a vein graft model and **(B)** a normal coronary model with uncertainties in clinical measurements taken into account.[64]

evaluations in the Fontan circulation.[102−107] Later, a Y-shaped design was proposed to replace the conventional tube-shaped Gore-Tex graft.[103,108] Three-dimensional blood flow simulations were performed to evaluate the energy loss, SVC pressure, and hepatic flow distribution at rest and exercise conditions between conventional and Y-graft designs. Clinically, a lower SVC pressure is correlated with favorable outcomes, and the lack of hepatic flow to the lungs leads to pulmonary arteriovenous malformations (PAVMs).[109,110] In Fig. 12.9, three patient-specific Glenn models were virtually converted to a Fontan circuit comparing three surgical modifications: T-junction, offset, and Y-graft. Pulsatile inflow waveforms and RCR BCs were applied to the inlets and outlets, respectively. Lagrangian particle tracking[111] was used to quantify the hepatic flow distribution, defined as the percentage of IVC flow streaming to the right PA. Simulation results showed that the anastomosis location relative to the SVC for the Fontan graft and the overall pulmonary flow split play an important role in

distributing the hepatic flow evenly to the lungs. Due to a large variety of anatomy, flow conditions in Fontan patients, 3D flow simulations demonstrate that customized surgical planning is needed for each subject.

Shape optimization has been the norm in engineering design, while trial and error and surgeon experience is still the method of choice in routine surgical planning. Recently, shape optimization was applied to the Fontan and shunt designs for single ventricle defects to identify optimal geometry.[107,112,113,114] Fig. 12.10 shows idealized Y-graft models optimized for even hepatic flow distribution under a wide range of pulmonary flow splits.

Case study: modeling surgical repair for peripheral pulmonary stenosis

In this case study, we demonstrate how 3D flow modeling is used to predict postoperative pulmonary flow distribution in children with peripheral pulmonary artery stenosis (PPS). PPS is characterized by multiple

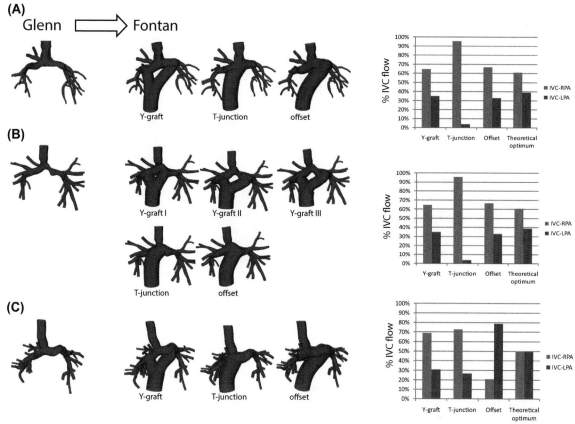

FIG. 12.9 Three patient-specific Glenn models (A, B and C) virtually converted into extracardiac Fontan models with Y-graft, T-junction, and offset designs. Hepatic flow distribution was quantified by Lagrangian particle tracking seeding from the IVC inlet. The theoretical optimum for HFD is defined as a value that is closest to 50/50 for given inflow conditions and an overall pulmonary flow split.[106]

and often diffusely distributed narrowed ostia of the branch PAs, resulting in pulmonary flow disparity and right ventricular (RV) hypertension.

PPS is frequently associated with Alagille syndrome, a rare genetic disorder affecting multiple organs.[115–117] Alagille patients may develop liver failure requiring liver transplantation. Treatment of significant PA stenoses and the resulting reduction in the RV pressures improve both the long-term cardiac performance and liver transplant outcomes. In addition, restoring pulmonary perfusion in the affected PAs is beneficial to lung development. Staged surgical repair is occasionally employed in order to achieve even pulmonary flow distribution in some complex cases.

Three-dimensional CT-based preoperative PA models (Fig. 12.1) were constructed using SimVascular (simvascular.org).[39–41] Creation of virtual postoperative models were constructed in consultation with the surgeon. Blood flow was modeled using three-dimensional Navier–Stokes equations under incompressibility and Newtonian assumptions with density and viscosity values set at 1.06 g/cm^3 and 0.04 g/(cm·s), respectively. We employed the coupled momentum method to account for arterial compliance.[91] Initial values for the Young's modulus and wall thickness were 2.6 –4.2 × 10^6 dyn/cm^2 and 0.05 cm, respectively. Young's modulus and wall thickness were tuned to match cath-derived pressures. Pulmonary mean flow rates were based on the catheterization-derived values. Inflow waveforms were taken from Tang et al.[118] and scaled iteratively with Young's modulus for the wall and outflow BCs to match preoperative PA systolic, diastolic, and mean pressures obtained by catheterization. For outflow BCs,

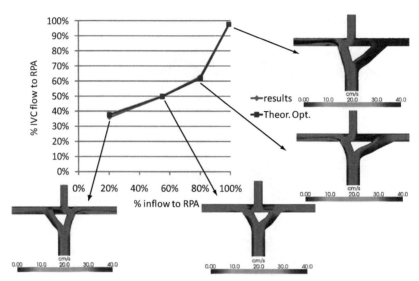

FIG. 12.10 Idealized Y-graft models optimized for even hepatic flow distribution under a wide range of pulmonary flow splits using surrogate management framework with adaptive mesh direct search (SMF-MADS).[107]

three-element Windkessel models were employed to model the distal PAs.[119] In contrast to previous surgical designs, outflow BCs were adapted in addition to the geometric modification in order to account for distal vascular adaptation (vasodilation) in response to increased blood flow.[120–122] A structured tree model representing the distal vascular bed in conjunction with the constant WSS assumption was used to estimate the postoperative resistance.[30] For each outlet, a baseline structured tree was generated such that the total resistance is equal to the resistance of the Windkessel model used for the preoperative simulations. A simulation is then performed on the virtual postoperative model using the same preoperative BCs. By comparing flow changes, the segments in the baseline structured trees will be dilated or constricted to restore WSS level in the preoperative stage. A new set of outlet resistances is given by the adapted structured trees. Then we obtain the predicted postoperative flow distribution by applying the adapted resistance to the postoperative model.

Fig. 12.11 shows the mean pressure distribution and velocity magnitude between pre- and postoperative stages. Table 12.1 compares the predicted postoperative flow distribution using adaptive and constant outflow BCs to in vivo lung perfusion scans, suggesting that satisfactory agreement with in vivo data could be achieved by

incorporating the downstream vascular adaptation in response to the surgical repair into the simulation.

Previous simulations for surgical planning usually assumed that the outflow BCs do not change significantly for postoperative simulations. The discrepancies between the in vivo measurements and results predicted by the use of constant outflow BCs indicate that the distal PAs, which are not included in the 3D model, also play a role in redistributing pulmonary flow as they can adapt to the changes from the upstream. Previous animal experiments showed that surgically induced flow perturbations lead to changes in vessel size to maintain shear stress.[120,123] In patients with PPS, surgical reconstruction created an initial change in pulmonary flow distribution; then, mechanobiological responses were triggered by the altered pulmonary perfusion making the downstream resistance different from the baseline. Thus, the resulting postoperative pulmonary flow distribution was determined by the obstruction relief in the proximal PAs combined with the vasoactive responses in the distal PAs. In summary, this study demonstrates the importance of downstream vascular adaptation in surgical planning for complex PPS repair.

Challenges and Future Perspective

In the past 2 decades, the capability of computational cardiovascular modeling has been greatly increased

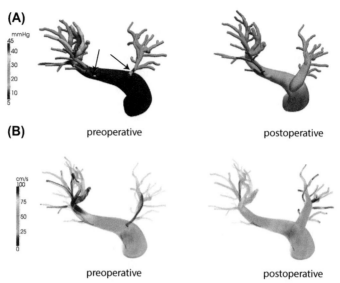

FIG. 12.11 Pre and postoperative time-average pressure (A) and velocity magnitude (B) for representative Alagille patients with pulmonary artery stenosis (PPS). The preoperative baseline BCs are tuned to match the clinical measurements. Postoperative results are obtained with adaptive outflow BCs. PPS is marked by arrows.[124]

TABLE 12.1

Immediate Post-operative Lung Perfusion Scans (LPSs) and Simulation-Derived Pulmonary Flow Distribution (RPA/LPA). Simulations are Performed on Virtual Postoperative models With Constant and Adaptive Outflow Boundary Conditions (BCs). Prediction Errors are Relative to the measured Flow Distribution to the RPA.

Patient	Postop LPS	Constant BCs	Adaptive BCs	Errors
A	53%/47%	65%/35%	52%/48%	23% → 2%
B	63%/37%	74%/26%	67%/33%	17% → 6%
C	49%/51%	59%/41%	54%/46%	20% → 10%

due to advances in computing power and the development of sophisticated software packages for image-based modeling. Computational modeling not only is a research tool for cardiovascular fluid mechanics but has also started making clinical impacts.[125,126] Of note, the recent FDA approval and clinical adoption of HeartFlow's FFRCT technology is a striking example of the potential of computational modeling to impact clinical decision-making.[125–127]

However, there remain many challenges ahead. Algorithms for automated segmentation have been developed for specific problems. However, performance of these methods in complex model construction tasks with multiple branching vessels is often lacking.

Congenital heart diseases are noted for complex and diverse abnormalities with relatively low incidence creating difficulties for data-driven segmentation algorithms. In addition, small vessel size and constraints in scan time and imaging modality decrease the quality of image data for pediatric patients. Laborious manual segmentation is often required to create accurate 3D models in patients with congenital abnormalities such as PA models with segmental/subsegmental vessels. Therefore, large cohort studies with complex anatomic features or poor image resolution are often hindered by the lack of robust automated segmentation algorithms for model construction. Machine learning and deep learning methods offer potential avenues to overcome these barriers in large cohort studies with complex anatomic models.[128,129]

Validation and UQ of computational modeling are not fully addressed despite some important recent efforts on these topics. Recent benchmark tests showed considerable variations in simulations produced by multiple solvers and research groups.[130,131] Comprehensive validations against in vivo measurements remain lacking due to ethical considerations and imaging limitations. With the increasing use of 0D−3D coupled simulations, input data (clinical data and parameters for BCs) increase significantly. It is of importance to quantify how those uncertainties in input parameter and numerical methods influence simulation outputs before a wider adoption of CFD-based design and modeling techniques in clinical research and practice.

Although FSI has been employed in a number of cardiovascular problems, the majority of 3D cardiovascular flow simulations still employ the rigid wall assumption. The computational cost, numerical stability, and software availability for FSI should be improved in the future to facilitate the use of FSI. Of note, the SimVascular project provides ALE FSI capabilities through its newly released svFSI solver. Biological soft tissues are known to be nearly incompressible, anisotropic, and viscoelastic with large deformations and pose a particular challenge to FSI modeling. Currently, most if not all FSI simulations compromise on the incompressibility. A recent study by Liu et al.[132] shows a promising formulation for cardiovascular FSI to handle incompressible biomaterials. In addition, predicting vessel growth and remodeling (G&R) in realistic geometry may benefit from coupling G&R models[133,134] to FSI to create a fluid-solid-growth framework. Integrating cardiac and valvar FSI with electrophysiologic modeling is another emerging topic in cardiovascular FSI.

For simulation-based surgical planning, there are several important issues to be improved to enhance postoperative predictions and foster clinical adoption. First, changing the geometry only without modifications to BCs may not fully characterize postoperative hemodynamics. In the example of modeling PPS, we showed that the use of constant outflow BCs can lead to inaccurate predictions even for the immediate postoperative stage. There is a need to incorporate adaptive models into surgical planning to account remodeling and autoregulatory responses to surgical interventions. This could be particularly challenging for pediatric cardiovascular surgeries because the patients not only respond adaptively to surgical repair but also experience

somatic growth. Second, there is a lack of physical models for modeling the process of surgical repair. In most surgical planning studies, vascular modifications such as graft anastomosis and stenosis relief were made under the guidance of surgeons and implemented manually. There is a growing need for interactive tools to allow for seamless and smooth model manipulations, particularly to place simulations tools directly in the hands of clinicians. Postoperative pressure and flow patterns are also influenced by the geometry, such as changes in patch sizes and anastomosis angles. Future studies should reduce the discrepancies between virtually reconstructed models and the actual postoperative geometry.

Apart from improving accuracy and increasing complexity of the computational framework, there are several practical barriers that currently hinder the impact of computational modeling in clinical practice. Current methods often require laborious model construction, access to high-performance computing resources, and substantial engineering expertise. HeartFlow provides a great example of overcoming these barriers to achieve initial success. Three-dimensional flow simulations generate dozens of gigabytes of hemodynamics data. From these massive data, what information and how much information should we extract to make a clinical decision or understand the progression of cardiovascular diseases? There are only a few endpoints derived from computational modeling proved to be clinically beneficial and accepted by clinicians. Large cohort studies and multidisciplinary collaborations with experimentalists are needed to catalyze computational modeling as a routine clinical tool.

REFERENCES

1. Womersley JR. Method for the calculation of velocity, rate of flow and viscous drag in arteries when the pressure gradient is known. *J Physiol.* 1955;127(3):553−563.
2. Womersley J. *An Elastic Tube Theory of Pulse Transmission and Oscillatory Flow in Mammalian Arteries, Air Research and Development Command, united states Air Force.* Ohio: Wright Air Development Center, Wright-Patterson Air Force Base; 1957.
3. Westerhof N, Bosman F, De Vries CJ, Noordergraaf A. Analog studies of the human systemic arterial tree. *J Biomech.* 1969;2:121−143.
4. Thiry PS, Roberge FA. Analogs and models of systemic arterial circulation. *Rev Canad Biol.* 1976;35(4):217−238.
5. Peskin C. Flow patterns around heart valves: a numerical method. *J. comp. Phys.* 1972;10(2):252−271.
6. Perktold K, Resch M, Peter RO. Three-dimensional numerical analysis of pulsatile flow and wall shear stress

in the carotid artery bifurcation. *J Biomech.* 1991;24(6): 409–420.

7. Perktold K, Resch M, Florian H. Pulsatile non-Newtonian flow characteristics in a three-dimensional human carotid bifurcation model. *J Biomech Eng.* 1991;113(4): 464–475.

8. Perktold K, Rappitsch G. Computer simulation of local blood flow and vessel mechanics in a compliant carotid artery bifurcation model. *J Biomech.* 1995;28:845–856.

9. Taylor CA, Hughes TJR, Zarins CK. Computational investigations in vascular disease. *Comput Phys.* 1996;10(3): 224–232.

10. Milner J, Moore J, Rutt B, Steinman D. Hemodynamics of human carotid artery bifurcations: computational studies with models reconstructed from magnetic resonance imaging of normal subjects. *J Vasc Surg.* 1998;28(1): 143–156.

11. Taylor CA, Hughes TJR, Zarins CK. Finite element modeling of blood flow in arteries. *Comput Methods Appl Mech Eng.* 1998;158(1–2):155–196.

12. Hsia T, Migliavacca F, Pittaccio S, et al. Computational fluid dynamic study of flow optimization in realistic models of the total cavopulmonary connections. *J Surg Res.* 2004;116(2):305–313.

13. Taylor CA, Draney MT, Ku JP, et al. Predictive medicine: computational techniques in therapeutic decision-making. *Comput Aided Surg.* 1999;4(5):231–247.

14. Taylor CA, Figueroa CA. Patient-specific modeling of cardiovascular mechanics. *Annu Rev Biomed Eng.* 2009;11: 109–134.

15. Taylor CA, Steinman DA. Image-based modeling of blood flow and vessel wall dynamics: applications, methods and future directions. *Ann Biomed Eng.* 2010; 38(3):1188–1203.

16. Senzaki H, Chen CH, Kass DA. Single-beat estimation of end-systolic pressure-volume relation in humans, a new method with the potential for noninvasive application. *Circulation.* 1996;15(94):2497–2506.

17. Mynard JP, Davidson MR, Penny DJ, Smolich JJ. A simple, versatile valve model for use in lumped parameter and one-dimensional cardiovascular models. *Int J Numer Meth Biomed Eng.* 2012;28(6–7):626–641.

18. Milisic V, Quarteroni A. Analysis of lumped parameter models for blood flow simulations and their relation with 1D models. *ESAIM M2AN.* 2004;38(4):613–632.

19. Peskin C, Tu C. Hemodynamics in congenital heart disease. *Comput Biol Med.* 1986;16(5):331–359.

20. Pennati G, Migliavacca F, Dubini G, Pietrabissa R, de Leval MR. A mathematical model of circulation in the presence of the bidirectional cavopulmonary anastomosis in children with a univentricular heart. *Med Eng Phys.* 1997;19(3):223–234.

21. Kilner PJ, Balossino R, Dubini G, et al. Pulmonary regurgitation: the effects of varying pulmonary artery compliance, and of increased resistance proximal or distal to the compliance. *Int J Cardiol.* 2009;133(2):157–166.

22. Yang W, Marsden AL, Ogawa MT, et al. Right ventricular stroke work correlates with outcomes in pediatric

pulmonary arterial hypertension. *Pulm Circ.* 2018;8(3), 2045894018780534.

23. Marsden AL, Esmaily-Moghadam M. Multiscale modeling of cardiovascular flows for clinical decision support. *Appl Mech Rev.* 2015;67(3), 030804–030804–11.

24. Hughes T, Lubliner J. On the one-dimensional theory of blood flow in the larger vessels. *Math Biosci.* 1973; 18(1–2):161–170.

25. Olufsen MS, Peskin C, Kim WY, Pedersen EM, Nadim A, Larsen J. Numerical simulation and experimental validation of blood flow in arteries with structured-tree outflow conditions. *Ann Biomed Eng.* 2000;28(11):1281–1299.

26. Shi Y, Lawford P, Hose R. Review of zero-D and 1-D models of blood flow in the cardiovascular system. *Biomed Eng Online.* 2011;10(33).

27. Wan J, Steele B, Spicer SA, et al. A one-dimensional finite element method for simulation-based medical planning for cardiovascular disease. *Comput Methods Biomech Biomed Eng.* 2002;5(3):195–206.

28. Sherwin SJ, Formaggia L, Peiró J, Franke V. Computational modelling of 1D blood flow with variable mechanical properties and its application to the simulation of wave propagation in the human arterial system. *Int J Numer Methods Fluids.* 2003;43(6–7):673–700.

29. Formaggia L, Lamponi D, Quarteroni A. One-dimensional models for blood flow in arteries. *J Eng Math.* 2003;47(3–4):251–276.

30. Olufsen MS. Structured tree outflow condition for blood flow in larger systemic arteries. *Am J Physiol.* 1999;276(1 Pt 2). H257–268.

31. Mynard JP, Nithiarasu P. A 1D arterial blood flow model incorporating ventricular pressure, aortic valve and regional coronary flow using the locally conservative galerkin (LCG) method. *Commun Numer Methods Eng.* 2008;24(5):367–417.

32. Steele B, Wan J, Ku J, Hughes T, Taylor C. In vivo validation of a one-dimensional finite-element method for predicting blood flow in cardiovascular bypass grafts. *IEEE Trans Biomed Eng.* 2003;50(6):649–656.

33. Boileau E, Pant S, Roobottom C, et al. Estimating the accuracy of a reduced-order model for the calculation of fractional flow reserve (FFR). *Int J Numer Method Biomed Eng.* 2018;34(1):e2908.

34. Krams R, Wentzel JJ, Oomen JA, et al. Evaluation of endothelial shear stress and 3D geometry as factors determining the development of atherosclerosis and remodeling in human coronary arteries in vivo combining 3D reconstruction from angiography and ivus (angus) with computational fluid dynamics. *Arterioscler Thromb Vasc Biol.* 1997;7(10):2061–2065.

35. Chiastra C, Montin E, Bologna M, et al. Reconstruction of stented coronary arteries from optical coherence tomography images: feasibility, validation, and repeatability of a segmentation method. *PLoS One.* 2017;12(6): e0177495.

36. Gülsün MA, Tek H. Robust vessel tree modeling. In: Metaxas D, Axel L, Fichtinger G, Székely G, eds. *Medical*

Image Computing and Computer-Assisted Intervention — MICCAI 2008. Berlin, Heidelberg: Springer Berlin Heidelberg; 2008:602−611.

37. Zheng Y, Tek H, Funka-Lea G. Robust and accurate coronary artery centerline extraction in CTA by combining model-driven and data-driven approaches. *Med Image Comput Comput Assist Interv.* 2013;16(Pt3):74−81.

38. Slomka PJ, Dey D, Sitek A, Motwani M, Berman DS, Germano G. Cardiac imaging: working towards fully-automated machine analysis and interpretation. *Expert Rev Med Devices.* 2017;14(3):197−212.

39. Schmidt JP, Delp SL, Sherman MA, Taylor CA, Pande VS, Altman RB. The simbios national center: systems biology in motion. *Proc IEEE Inst Electr Electron Eng.* 2008;96(8):1266−1280. special issue on Computational System Biology.

40. Updegrove A, Wilson NM, Merkow J, Lan H, Marsden AL, Shadden SC. SimVascular: an open source pipeline for cardiovascular simulation. *Ann Biomed Eng.* 2017;45(3):525−541.

41. Lan H, Updegrove A, Wilson NM, Maher GD, Shadden SC, Marsden AL. A Re-engineered software interface and work-flow for the open- source SimVascular cardiovascular modeling package. *J Biomech Eng.* 2018;140(2).

42. Yushkevich PA, Piven J, Hazlett HC, et al. User-guided 3d active contour segmentation of anatomical structures: significantly improved efficiency and reliability. *Neuroimage.* 2006;31(3):1116−1128.

43. Cho YI, Kensey KR. Effects of the non-Newtonian viscosity of blood on flows in a diseased arterial vessel. part 1: steady flows. *Biorheology.* 1991;28(3−4):241−262.

44. Thurston GB. Viscoelasticity of human blood. *Biophys J.* 1972;12(9):1205−1217.

45. Quarteroni A, Manzoni A, Vergara C. The cardiovascular system: mathematical modelling, numerical algorithms and clinical applications. *Acta Numer.* 1998;26, 365−590.

46. Bove EL, Migliavacca F, de Leval MR, et al. Use of mathematic modeling to compare and predict hemodynamic effects of the modified blalock−taussig and right ventricle−pulmonary artery shunts for hypoplastic left heart syndrome. *J Thorac Cardiovasc Surg.* 2008;136(2), 312−320.e2.

47. Kheyfets V, Thirugnanasambandam M, Rios L, et al. The role of wall shear stress in the assessment of right ventricle hydraulic workload. *Pulm Circ.* 2015;5(1):90−100.

48. Le TB, Sotiropoulosa F. On the three-dimensional vortical structure of early diastolic flow in a patient-specific left ventricle. *Eur J Mech B Fluid.* 2012;35:20−24.

49. Seo JH, Mittal R. Effect of diastolic flow patterns on the function of the left ventricle. *Phys Fluids.* 2013;25(11):110801.

50. Anupindi K, Delorme Y, Shetty DA, Frankel SH. A novel multiblock immersed boundary method for large eddy simulation of complex arterial hemodynamics. *J Comput Phys.* 2013;254(1):200−218.

51. Chen S, Doolen GD. Lattice Boltzmann method for fluid flows. *Annu Rev Fluid Mech.* 1998;30(1):329−364.

52. Krafczyk M, Cerrolaza M, Schulz M, Rank E. Analysis of 3d transient blood flow passing through an artificial aortic valve by lattice−Boltzmann methods. *J Biomech.* 1998;31(5):453−462.

53. Artoli A, Hoekstra A, Sloot P. Mesoscopic simulations of systolic flow in the human abdominal aorta. *J Biomech.* 2006;39(5):873−884.

54. Yu H, Chen X, Wang Z, et al. Mass-conserved volumetric lattice Boltzmann method for complex flows with willfully moving boundaries. *Phys Rev E.* 2014;89:063304.

55. Ku JP, Elkins CJ, Taylor CA. Comparison of CFD and MRI flow and velocities in an *in vitro* large artery bypass graft model. *Ann Biomed Eng.* 2005;33(3):257−269.

56. Campbell IC, Ries J, Dhawan SS, Quyyumi AA, Taylor WR, Oshinski JN. Effect of inlet velocity profiles on patient-specific computational fluid dynamics simulations of the carotid bifurcation. *J Biomech Eng.* 2012;134(5):051001.

57. Youssefi P, Gomez A, Arthurs C, Sharma R, Jahangiri M, Figueroa CA. Impact of patient-specific inflow velocity profile on hemodynamics of the thoracic aorta. *J Biomech Eng.* 2017;140(1):011002.

58. Vignon-Clementel IE, Figueroa CA, Jansen KE, Taylor CA. Outflow boundary conditions for three-dimensional finite element modeling of blood flow and pressure in arteries. *Comput Methods Appl Mech Eng.* 2006; 195(29−32):3776−3796.

59. Esmaily Moghadam M, Vignon-Clementel IE, Figliola R, Marsden AL. A modular numerical method for implicit 0D/3D coupling in cardiovascular finite element simulations. *J Comput Phys.* 2013;244:63−79.

60. Spilker RL, Feinstein JA, Parker DW, Reddy VM, Taylor CA. Morphometry-based impedance boundary conditions for patient-specific modeling of blood flow in pulmonary arteries. *Ann Biomed Eng.* 2007;35(4):546−549.

61. Spilker RL, Taylor CA. Tuning multidomain hemodynamic simulations to match physiological measurements. *Ann Biomed Eng.* 2010;38(8):2635−2648.

62. Xiao N, Alastruey J, Alberto Figueroa C. A systematic comparison between 1-D and 3-D hemodynamics in compliant arterial models. *Int J Numer Method Biomed Eng.* 2014;30(2):204−231.

63. Schiavazzi DE, Arbia G, Baker C, et al. Uncertainty quantification in virtual surgery hemodynamics predictions for single ventricle palliation. *Int J Numer Method Biomed Eng.* 2016;32(3):e02737.

64. Tran JS, Schiavazzi DE, Ramachandra AB, Kahn AM, Marsden AL. Automated tuning for parameter identification and uncertainty quantification in multi-scale coronary simulations. *Comput Fluids.* 2017;142:128−138.

65. Moireau P, Bertoglio C, Xiao N, et al. Sequential identification of boundary support parameters in a fluid-structure vascular model using patient image data. *Biomechanics Model Mechanobiol.* 2013;12(3):475−496.

66. Pant S, Corsini C, Baker C, Hsia T-Y, Pennati G, Vignon-Clementel IE. Data assimilation and modelling of patient-specific singleventricle physiology with and without valve regurgitation. *J Biomech.* 2016;49(11): 2162–2173.

67. D'Elia M, Perego M, Veneziani A. A variational data assimilation procedure for the incompressible Navier-Stokes equations in hemodynamics. *J Sci Comput.* 2012; 52(2):340–359.

68. Veneziani A, Vergara C. Inverse problems in cardiovascular mathematics: toward patient-specific data assimilation and optimization. *Int J Numer Method Biomed Eng.* 2013;29(7):723–725.

69. Smolyak SA. Quadrature and interpolation formulas for tensor products of certain classes of functions. *Dokl Akad Nauk SSSR.* 1963;148(5):1042–1045.

70. Sankaran S, Marsden A. A stochastic collocation method for uncertainty quantification and propagation in cardiovascular simulations. *ASME J Biomech Eng.* 2011;133(3), 031001–031001–12.

71. Xiu D, Karniadakis G. The wiener–askey polynomial chaos for Stochastic differential equations. *SIAM J Sci Comput.* 2002;24(2):619–644.

72. Xiu D, Karniadakis GE. Modeling uncertainty in flow simulations via generalized polynomial chaos. *J Comput Phys.* 2003;187(1):137–167.

73. Xiu D. *Stochastic Collocation Methods: A Survey.* Cham: Springer International Publishing; 2016:1–18.

74. Xiu D. Fast numerical methods for stochastic computations: a review. *Commun Comput Phys.* 2009;5(2–4): 242–272.

75. Eldred MS, Burkardt J. *Comparison of non-intrusive polynomial chaos and stochastic collocation methods for uncertainty quantification*, 47th AIAA Aerospace Sciences Meeting Including The New Horizons Forum and Aerospace Exposition 5–8 January 2009, Orlando, Florida. 2009.

76. Maitre OL, Knio O, Najm H, Ghanem R. Uncertainty propagation using wiener–haar expansions. *J Comput Phys.* 2004;197(1):28–57.

77. Le Maitre O, Najm H, Pébay P, Ghanem R, Knio O. Multiresolution analysis scheme for uncertainty quantification in chemical systems. *SIAM J Sci Comput.* 2007;29(2): 864–889.

78. Schiavazzi D, Doostan A, Iaccarino G, Marsden A. A generalized multiresolution expansion for uncertainty propagation with application to cardiovascular modeling. *Comput Methods Appl Mech Eng.* 2017;314: 196–221.

79. Sankaran S, Kim HJ, Choi G, Taylor CA. Uncertainty quantification in coronary blood flow simulations: impact of geometry, boundary conditions and blood viscosity. *J Biomech.* 2016;49(12):2540–2547.

80. Eck VG, Donders WP, Sturdy J, et al. A guide to uncertainty quantification and sensitivity analysis for cardiovascular applications. *Int J Numer Method Biomed Eng.* 2015;32(8):e02755. e02755 cnm.2755.

81. Biehler J, Gee MW, Wall WA. Towards efficient uncertainty quantification in complex and large-scale biomechanical problems based on a bayesian multi-fidelity scheme. *Biomechanics Model Mechanobiol.* 2015; 14(3):489–513.

82. D'Elia M, Veneziani A. Uncertainty quantification for data assimilation in a steady incompressible Navier-Stokes problem. *ESAIM M2AN.* 2013;47(4):1037–1057.

83. Sankaran S, Marsden AL. The impact of uncertainty on shape optimization of idealized bypass graft models in unsteady flow. *Phys Fluids.* 2010;22(12):121902.

84. Xiu D, Sherwin SJ. Parametric uncertainty analysis of pulse wave propagation in a model of a human arterial network. *J Comput Phys.* 2007;226(2):1385–1407.

85. Chen P, Quarteroni A, Rozza G. Simulation-based uncertainty quantification of human arterial network hemodynamics. *Int J Numer Method Biomed Eng.* 2013; 29(6):698–721.

86. Brault A, Dumas L, Lucor D. Uncertainty quantification of inflow boundary condition and proximal arterial stiffness–coupled effect on pulse wave propagation in a vascular network. *Int J Numer Method Biomed Eng.* 2017; 33(10):e2859.

87. Schenkel T, Malve M, Reik M, Markl M, Jung B, Oertel H. Mri-based CFD analysis of flow in a human left ventricle: methodology and application to a healthy heart. *Ann Biomed Eng.* 2009;37(3):503–515.

88. Lantz J, Dyverfeldt P, Ebbers T. Improving blood flow simulations by incorporating measured subject-specific wall motion. *Cardiovasc Eng Technol.* 2014;5(3): 261–269.

89. Bazilevs Y, Takizawa K, Tezduyar TE. *Computational Fluid-Structure Interaction: Methods and Applications.* Wiley; 2013.

90. Mittal R, Iaccarino G. A review of the numerical analysis of blood flow in arterial bifurcations. *Annu Rev Fluid Mech.* 2005;37:239–261.

91. Figueroa CA, Vignon-Clementel IE, Jansen KF, Hughes TJ, Taylor CA. A coupled momentum method for modeling blood flow in three-dimensional deformable arteries. *Comput Methods Appl Mech Eng.* 2006;195(41–43): 5685–5706.

92. Formaggia L, Quarteroni A, Veneziani A. *Cardiovascular Mathematics: Modeling and Simulation of the Circulatory System.* Springer Science & Business Media; 2010.

93. Benjamin EJ, Virani SS, Callaway CW, et al. *Heart disease and stroke statistics—2018 update.* Circulation: A report from the American Heart Association; 2018.

94. Weiss AJ, Elixhauser A. *Trends in Operating Room Procedures in u.S. Hospitals, 2001–2011, STATISTICAL BRIEF 171, Healthcare Cost and Utilization Project.* 2014.

95. Goldman S, Zadina K, Moritz T, et al. Long-term patency of saphenous vein and left internal mammary artery grafts after coronary artery bypass surgery: results from a department of veterans affairs cooperative study. *J Am Coll Cardiol.* 2004;44(11):2149–2156.

96. Harskamp RE, Lopes R, Baisden CE, de Winter RJ, Alexander JH. Saphenous vein graft failure after coronary artery bypass surgery: pathophysiology, management, and future directions. *Ann Surg.* 2013;257(5):824–833.

97. Taggar DP. Current status of arterial grafts for coronary artery bypass grafting. *Ann Cardiothorac Surg.* 2013;2(4): 427−430.

98. Kim H, Vignon-Clementel I, Coogan J, Figueroa CA, Jansen KE, Taylor CA. Patient-specific modeling of blood flow and pressure in human coronary arteries. *Ann Biomed Eng.* 2010;38(10):3195−3209.

99. Ramachandra AB, Kahn AM, Marsden AL. Patient-specific simulations reveal significant differences in mechanical stimuli in venous and arterial coronary grafts. *J Cardiovasc Transl Res.* 2016;9(4):279−290.

100. Sankaran S, Esmaily Moghadam M, Kahn A, Guccione J, Tseng E, Marsden A. Patient-specific multiscale modeling of blood flow for coronary artery bypass graft surgery. *Ann Biomed Eng.* 2012;40(1):2228−2242.

101. Dubini G, de Leval MR, Pietrabissa R, Montevecchi FM, Fumero R. A numerical fluid mechanical study of repaired congenital heart defects: application to the total cavopulmonary connection. *J Biomech.* 1996;29(1): 111−121.

102. Bove EL, de Leval MR, Migliavacca F, Guadagni G, Dubini G. Computational fluid dynamics in the evaluation of hemodynamic performance of cavopulmonary connections after the Norwood procedure for hypoplastic left heart syndrome. *J Thorac Cardiovasc Surg.* 2003;126: 1040−1047.

103. Marsden AL, Reddy VM, Shadden SC, Chan FP, Taylor CA, Feinstein JA. A new multi-parameter approach to computational simulation for Fontan assessment and redesign. *Congenit Heart Dis.* 2010;5(2):104−117.

104. Whitehead KK, Pekkan K, Kitahima HD, Paridon SM, Yoganathan AP, Fogel MA. Nonlinear power loss during exercise in singleventricle patients after the Fontan: insights from computational fluid dynamics. *Circulation.* 2007;116. I−165 − I−171.

105. Itatani K, Miyaji K, Nakahata Y, Ohara K, Takamoto S, Ishii M. The lower limit of the pulmonary artery index for the extracardiac fontan circulation. *J Thorac Cardiovasc Surg.* 2011;142(1):127−135.

106. Yang W, Vignon-Clementel IE, Troianowski G, Reddy VM, Feinstein JA, Marsden AL. Hepatic blood flow distribution and performance in traditional and Y-graft Fontan geometries: a case series computational fluid dynamics study. *J Thorac Cardiovasc Surg.* 2012;143: 1086−1097.

107. Yang W, Feinstein JA, Shadden SC, Vignon-Clementel IE, Marsden AL. Optimization of a Y-graft design for improved hepatic flow distribution in the Fontan circulation. *J Biomech Eng.* 2013;135(1):011002.

108. Soerensen DD, Pekkan K, de Zelicourt D, et al. Introduction of a new optimized total cavopulmonary connection. *Ann Thorac Surg.* 2007;83(6):2182−2190.

109. Duncan BW, Desai S. Pulmonary arteriovenous malformations after cavopulmonary anastomosis. *Ann Thorac Surg.* 2003;76:1759−1766.

110. Pike NA, Vricella LA, Feinstein JA, Black MD, Reitz BA. Regression of severe pulmonary arteriovenous malformations after Fontan revision and hepatic factor rerouting. *Ann Thorac Surg.* 2004;78:697−699.

111. Shadden SC, Taylor CA. Characterization of coherent structures in the cardiovascular system. *Ann Biomed Eng.* 2008;36(7):1152−1162.

112. Yang W, Feinstein JA, Marsden AL. Constrained optimization of an idealized Y-shaped baffle for the Fontan surgery at rest and exercise. *Comput Methods Appl Mech Eng.* 2010;199(33−36):2135−2149.

113. Moghadam ME, Migliavacca F, Vignon-Clementel IE, Hsia TY, Marsden AL. M. of Congenital Hearts Alliance (MOCHA) Investigators, Optimization of shunt placement for the Norwood surgery using multidomain modeling. *J Biomech Eng.* 2012;134(5):051002.

114. Verma A, Esmaily M, Shang J, et al. Optimization of the assisted bidirectional glenn procedure for first stage single ventricle repair. *World J Pediatr Congenit Heart Surg.* 2018;134(5):157−170.

115. Krantz ID, Piccoli DA, Spinner NB. Alagille syndrome. *J Med Genet.* 1997;34(2):152−157.

116. Turnpenny PD, Ellard S. Alagille syndrome: pathogenesis, diagnosis and management. *Eur J Hum Genet.* 2012;20(3): 251−257. https://doi.org/10.1038/ejhg.2011.181.

117. Cunningham JW, McElhinney DB, Gauvreau K, et al. Outcomes after primary transcatheter therapy in infants and young children with severe bilateral peripheral pulmonary artery stenosis. *Circ Cardiovasc Interv.* 2013; 6(4):460−467.   https://doi.org/10.1161/ CIRCINTERVENTIONS.112.000061.

118. Tang BT, Fonte TA, Chan FP, Tsao PS, Feinstein JA, Taylor CA. Three-dimensional hemodynamics in the human pulmonary arteries under resting and exercise conditions. *Ann Biomed Eng.* 2011;39(1):347−358.

119. Vignon-Clementel IE, Figueroa CA, Jansen KE, Taylor CA. Outflow boundary conditions for 3D simulations of non-periodic blood flow and pressure fields in deformable arteries. *Comput Methods Biomech Biomed Eng.* 2010; 13(5):625−640.

120. Kamiya A, Togawa T. Adaptive regulation of wall shear stress to flow change in the canine carotid artery. *Am J Physiol.* 1980;239(1). H14−21.

121. Langille BL, O'Donnell F. Reductions in arterial diameter produced by chronic decreases in blood flow are endothelium-dependent. *Science.* 1986;231(4736): 405−407.

122. Yang W, Feinstein JA, Vignon-Clementel IE. Adaptive outflow boundary conditions improve post-operative predictions after repair of peripheral pulmonary artery stenosis. *Biomechanics Model Mechanobiol.* 2016. https:// doi.org/10.1007/s10237-016-0766-5.

123. Razavi H, Stewart SE, Xu C, et al. Chronic effects of pulmonary artery stenosis on hemodynamic and structural development of the lungs. *Am J Physiol Lung Cell Mol Physiol.* 2013;304(1):L17−L28. https://doi.org/10.1152/ ajplung.00412.2011.

124. Yang FP, Chan W, Reddy VM, Marsden AL, Feinstein JA. Flow simulations and validation for the first cohort of

patients undergoing the Y-graft fontan procedure. *J Thorac Cardiovasc Surg.* 2015;149(1):247–255.

125. Douglas PS, Pontone G, Hlatky MA, et al. Clinical outcomes of fractional flow reserve by computed tomographic angiography-guided diagnostic strategies vs. usual care in patients with suspected coronary artery disease the prospective longitudinal trial of FFRCT: outcome and resource impacts study. *Eur Heart J.* 2015;36(47): 3359–3367.

126. Benton Jr SM, Tesche C, De Cecco CN, Duguay TM, Schoepf UJ, Bayer RR. Noninvasive derivation of fractional flow reserve from coronary computed tomographic angiography: a review. *J Thorac Imaging.* 2018; 33(2):88–96.

127. Taylor CA, Fonte TA, Min JK. Computational fluid dynamics applied to cardiac computed tomography for noninvasive quantification of fractional flow reserve: scientific basis. *J Am Coll Cardiol.* 2013;61(22): 2233–2241.

128. Merkow J, Tu Z, Kriegman D, Marsden A. Structural edge detection for cardiovascular modeling. In: Navab N, Hornegger J, Wells WM, Frangi AF, eds. *Medical Image Computing and Computer-Assisted Intervention – MICCAI 2015.* Cham: Springer International Publishing; 2015: 735–742.

129. Litjens G, Kooi T, Bejnordi BE, et al. A survey on deep learning in medical image analysis. *Med Image Anal.* 2017;42:60–88.

130. Stewart SFC, Paterson EG, Burgreen GW, et al. Assessment of CFD performance in simulations of an idealized medical device: results of FDA's first computational interlaboratory study. *Cardiovasc Eng Technol.* 2012;3(2): 139–160.

131. Steinman DA, Hoi Y, Fahy P, et al. Variability of computational fluid dynamics solutions for pressure and flow in a giant aneurysm: the ASME 2012 summer bioengineering conference cfd challenge. *ASME J Biomech Eng.* 2013;135(2), 021016–021016–13.

132. Liu J, Marsden AL. A unified continuum and variational multiscale formulation for fluids, solids, and fluid–structure interaction. *Comput Methods Appl Mech Eng.* 2018;337:549–597.

133. Gleason RL, Humphrey JD. A mixture model of arterial growth and remodeling in hypertension: altered muscle tone and tissue turnover. *J Vasc Res.* 2004;41(4): 352–363. https://doi.org/10.1159/000080699.

134. Valentín A, Cardamone L, Baek S, Humphrey J. Complementary vasoactivity and matrix remodelling in arterial adaptations to altered flow and pressure. *J R Soc Interface.* 2009;6(32):293–306.

CHAPTER 13

3D Bioprinting: What Does the Future Hold?

LUCY L. NAM, BA • NARUTOSHI HIBINO, MD, PHD

INTRODUCTION

For the general public, 3D bioprinting of the heart often refers to biofabrication of the entire human heart. However, with current technologies, this is infeasible, and remains a long-term goal in the field of cardiac tissue engineering. What are less commonly discussed and more tangible are the current advances in printing vascular networks for the delivery of nutrients and immune cells and in printing the myocardium to repair tissue injury from cardiovascular disease (CVD).[1] Using 3D bioprinting to repair injured cardiac tissue in the case of CVD has been of great interest in the field of tissue engineering. This is especially important as CVD accounts for approximately 30% of deaths globally, of which coronary heart disease is the single largest cause of death in developed countries.[2] If blood flow is interrupted to the coronary arteries, blood supply to the cardiomyocytes occurs, resulting in myocardial infarction (heart attack).[3] After inflammatory cells respond to the site of injury, fibroblasts migrate and form noncontracting tissue. Scar formation with minimal cardiomyocytes results. With limited cardiomyocytes that rarely divide in the human body, a heart transplant is often the last option for individuals suffering from end-stage CVD.[4] However, given the shortage of organ heart donors, especially given that hearts can only be transplanted from deceased donors (which is different from the kidney for example), attempting to provide heart transplants for all who suffer from advanced CVD is impossible. Current 3D bioprinting technologies offer the ability to create tissue patches that heal scarred myocardial tissue.

Researchers working on 3D bioprinting of cardiac tissues advanced techniques in the last decade by improving their physiological mimicry of human cardiovascular tissue, expanding therapeutic avenues such as drug screening and partial tissue replacement.[5] What seemed like a long-term, often-unreachable goal

of printing the whole human heart now seems more attainable and in the less-distant future. This is because researchers have taken advantage of unique features of 3D bioprinters to create cardiac tissues that resemble native tissue. 3D printers present unique advantages in the field of cardiac tissue engineering—they offer a method for automating the process of biofabricating tissue by using biocompatible materials. They also provide a technique for introducing the complexity needed for successful creation of heart tissue: diffusion, integration, vascularization, high cell density, and spatial organization.[6,7]

To generate viable bioprinted cardiac tissue, several key characteristics must be addressed. First, the cells used for 3D bioprinting must allow for cardiac tissue regeneration. There has been active research with cardiac stem cells that has the potential for use in future treatment.[8] Second, the cells must self-organize and demonstrate spontaneous and synchronous contractions seen in functional tissues. Third, the printed tissue must survive in an environment suitable for in vivo integration.[9] Fourth, the tissue must allow for the introduction of microvascular networks to provide oxygen and nutrients for growth and proliferation. This network must also promote vessel anastomosis with the host vasculature.[10] Lastly, the construct must show and maintain proper cell phenotypes without eliciting an adverse reaction.[9] Over the past several years, through experimentation with bioinks, cell types, printing techniques and mouse models, researchers have worked toward addressing and improving these key features, and are continuously developing new, unique methods to create cardiac tissue models using 3D bioprinting.[9] The current techniques in 3D bioprinting of heart tissue exciting prospects for the field of cardiac engineering.

In this review, we will (1) discuss the development of 3D bioprinting in cardiac tissue regeneration to

3-Dimensional Modeling in Cardiovascular Disease. https://doi.org/10.1016/B978-0-323-65391-6.00013-2

underscore the advancements in tissue printing and highlight the uniqueness of biofabrication using printing, (2) compare the current methods of 3D bioprinting to one another, and (3) discuss the future of 3D bioprinting of cardiac tissue.

DEVELOPMENT OF 3D BIOPRINTING OF CARDIAC TISSUE: CURRENT APPROACHES

What can be accomplished now with 3D bioprinting is due to both biological and technological advances that have been occurring over many decades. Since the development of cell theory in 1839[11] and the creation of the first 3D printer by Charles Hull in 1986,[12] there have been substantial advances in the capacity to 3D bioprint organs. Biofabrication of cardiac tissue using 3D bioprinting allows researchers to accomplish feats that cannot be addressed by other methods of tissue engineering. In particular, these are the bioprinter's ability to simultaneously print various cell types in predefined locations, and its ability to reproducibly create constructs with high accuracy.[13,14] Here, we will discuss the development of 3D printing of cardiac tissue by discussing the myriad ways in which the technology has addressed key features required for developing a functional cardiac tissue. This will provide insight to the history of the techniques currently possible with 3D cardiac bioprinting and will elucidate potential paths for improving the technology in the future.

Early Studies with Cardiac Progenitor Cells

One of the most primitive 3D-bioprinted cardiac tissues involved printed cardiac progenitor cells (CPCs) within an alginate scaffold,[15] as seen in Fig. 13.1A. Researchers used alginate as bioink material to mimic an extracellular matrix environment that supports the cells during and after printing.[16] Many researchers investigated the potential of stem cell therapy as a promising method to restore cardiac function in patients with heart failure.[17] Because of their cardiac developmental origins, CPCs are a more promising cell source for heart regeneration than stem cells from other organs such as bone marrow and adipose tissue. Gaetani et al. isolated human cardiac-derived cardiomyocytes progenitor cells (hCMPCs) from both fetal and adult human heart biopsies. These cells are committed to the cardiac lineage, can be differentiated into cardiomyocytes, and can also secrete a variety of factors that can activate stem cell pools, making them an ideal cell population for cardiac regeneration. Researchers demonstrated the ability to create a homogeneous distribution of cells in the scaffold when printed. Furthermore, they demonstrated

that 3D bioprinting could retain functional properties of cardiac cells. In particular, these cells showed high viability (89% at 7 days), demonstrated cardiogenic potential, and retained their commitment to cardiac lineage through the expression of early cardiac transcription factors. In addition, the printed cells seemed to migrate within the low-adherent alginate scaffold to a matrigel layer, forming a positive CD31 (vascular marker) tube on the matrigel matrix, suggesting possible in vivo applications where the cells can migrate from the scaffold to the infarcted region.

Three years later, the same research group progressed the work by studying the function of these cells in mice models of myocardial infarction (MI),[18] as seen in Fig. 13.1B. They attempted to demonstrate the therapeutic potential of a 3D-printed patch that similarly consisted of hCMPCs but this time with a hyaluronic acid/gelatin (HA/gel) matrix. This new biomaterial enhanced cell attachment and survival compared to the alginate from their previous experiment.[15] They created a cardiac tissue patch that measured 2 × 2 cm with 400 µm thickness and demonstrated that these cells maintained their cardiogenic phenotype for up to 1 month and were able to proliferate. After applying their patch into a mouse model of MI, the patch preserved heart function by reducing LV remodeling and improving myocardial viability. Although this study only followed this patch for a short period of time and did not evaluate the progression of hCMPC differentiation in the mouse model, this demonstrated the initial therapeutic effect of incorporating cells into biomaterials for the regenerative application of stem cells.[18]

These early studies with cardiac progenitor cells demonstrated a translational approach to enhancing hCMPC delivery to the heart using 3D bioprinting methods. Cardiac stem cell therapy using CMPCs suffered from inefficient delivery and engraftment and the extracellular matrix (ECM) being replaced with scar tissue, and thus researchers used 3D bioprinting to print stem cells to regenerate myocardial tissue while also using the bioink to replace the ECM.[15,18,19] They focused on the possibility of replenishing the heart with new myocytes after CVD using a hybrid combination of bioink and stem cells developed by printing. This advancement of stem-cell therapy using tissue printing is pivotal to the advancement of cardiac printing in tissues.

Over the years, researchers have also explored using other cell types, including induced pluripotent stem cells (iPSCs). Because of the ability of iPSCs to differentiate into multiple cell lineages, including

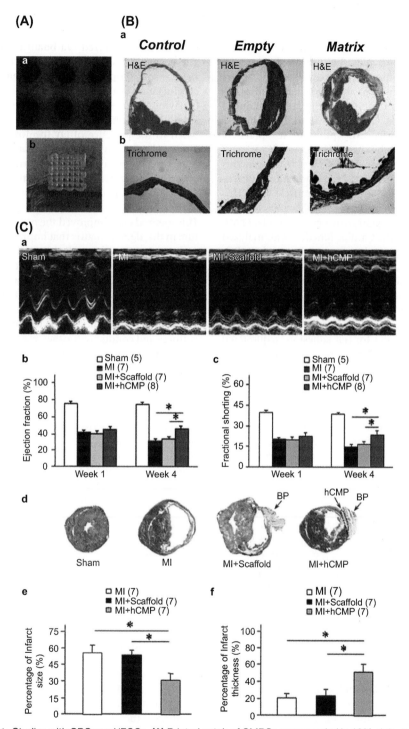

FIG. 13.1 Studies with CPCs and iPSCs. **(A)** Printed patch of CMPCs resuspended in 10% alginate scaffold: (a) confocal image, (b) aerial view; **(B)** Effect of patch implantation on myocardium: (a) matrix + CMPCs increased wall thickness, (b) matrix + CMPCs decreased infarct fibrosis. **(C)** CMPC transplantation improves cardiac function and reduces infarct size after myocardial infarction: (a) echocardiograph assessment (b) left ventricular ejection fraction (c) fractional shortening (d) Masson trichome stain showing reduction in infarct size and thickness with hCMPs derived from iPSCs (e) infarct size (f) infarct wall thickness. BP indicates bovine pericardium. (Credit: Reproduced with permission from Refs. 15, 18, and 21.)

cardiomyocytes, they hold great promise in tissue regeneration, and thus have been studied intensely. Zhang et al.[20] advanced personalized medicine by showing a proof-of-concept ability to create cardiac tissue from cardiomyocytes induced from human-induced pluripotent stem cells. Gao et al.[21] used multiphoton-excited photochemistry 3D printing to precisely generate a scaffold with native-like cardiac ECM architecture and seeded the scaffold with a heterogeneous mix of cells derived from iPSCs, including cardiomyocytes, endothelial cells, and smooth muscle cells. This resulted in a robust hiPSC-derived cardiac muscle patch that was capable of integration in a mouse model of MI, as shown in Fig. 13.1C. Cardiac function was analyzed 28 days after injury, and the transplanted hCMPCs improved recovery of MI by reducing apoptosis, promoting angiogenesis and increasing cell proliferation, compared to the mouse model without cell implantation. Multiphoton 3D printing created a high-resolution ECM that was structurally native-like, and thus provided substrates for cell adhesion, sequestered soluble factors and served as a structure for mechanical signaling.[21]

By exploring new ways of 3D printing, researchers developed techniques to generate an ECM scaffold with unprecedented resolution, and then seeded it with hiPSC-derived cardiac-derived cells, which showed high levels of cell engraftment and improvements in cardiac function, infarct size, apoptosis, and vascularity.

Experimentation with Bioinks

After the demonstration of the potential therapeutic effects of a cardiac patch inside a mouse model that consisted of both bioink and cells, researchers began to alter the bioink, which is the printable material used while printing the cells to prevent cell damage. Many individual ECM components such as hydrogels like collagen, fibrin, gelatin, and alginate have been used as bioinks, which mimic an ECM that supports the adhesion and proliferation of the cells in the ink.[22,23]

However, achieving a hydrogel that is electrically conductive, mechanically robust, and biologically functional remains a challenge. Alginate and collagen are common natural bioinks used in 3D bioprinting. Alginate is a highly biocompatible hydrogel, generally nondegradable, and has wide pore sizes that facilitate the diffusion of large molecules, which is beneficial for drug testing.[24] However, alginate lacks the nanofibrous structural features found in native ECM, and collagen is mechanically weak, and both alginate and collagen have poor electrical conductance. To address these limitations, Mohammad et al.[22] explored using

surface functionalized carbon nanotubes (CNTs). These have shown the potential to improve hydrogel mechanical properties because their high electrical conductance can improve the matrix electrical behavior.[22] Furthermore, methacrylated type-I collagen (MeCol) is a photolabile derivative of collagen that, when in the presence of UV, can induce cross-linking and enhance hydrogel stiffness. By using UV-integrated bioprinting of CNT-incorporated hybrid implants with alginate and MeCol, the researchers were able to create a patch that demonstrated higher electrical conductivity and compressive modulus in vitro. This method even improved the nanofilamentous structure in the alginate matrix that improved cell elongation and attachment. Although this study was not assessed in MI animal models, it demonstrates important techniques to develop conductive, robust, and hybrid cardiac patches, which offer opportunities for myocardial regeneration.

Although researchers have worked to improve the stiffness and conductivity of hydrogel patches, synthetic and natural bioinks such as collagen and alginate still present limitations as they are only partial components of the ECM. Natural ECM, on the other hand, includes fibrous proteins, glycosaminoglycans, and growth factors that mimic the environmental factors found in vivo.[25] Organ-derived decellularized ECM (dECM) bioinks are arguably the most biomimetic bioinks, but dECM derived from the heart has a very low stiffness compared to that found in normal cardiac muscle tissue.[23] It is important to tailor the dECM bioink to match that found in a native cardiac tissue environment by combining it with either natural or synthetic materials.[23,26]

To do this, researchers have combined dECM with vitamin B2 and Ultraviolet A irradiation (to induce cross-linking) to create the appropriate viscosity and stiffness necessary for printing and creating tissue,[27] as seen in Fig. 13.2A. With this technique, they are able to create a construct that matches the biomechanical properties of native cardiac tissue, supports high cell viability, and allows for the proliferation of cardiac progenitor cells.[27] This two-step solidification of dECM bioink enables the tailoring of the mechanical properties of the dECM to create tissue that is similar in stiffness to native tissue. The techniques developed for the printing of the dECM will have a variety of applications in the future of cardiac tissue engineering.

To avoid the limitations of both natural and synthetic polymers as well as dECM, researchers have begun to bioprint cardiac patches free of biomaterials. The use of biomaterials is advantageous during

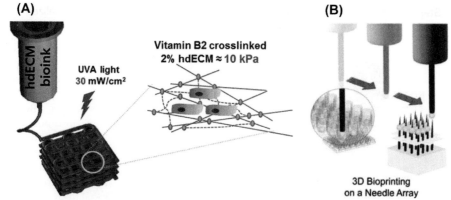

FIG. 13.2 Experimentation with bioinks: **(A)** schematic illustration of cross-linking process of dECM using vitamin B2 and UVA irradiation; **(B)** schematic of biomaterial-free 3D bioprinting process. (Credit: Reproduced with permission from Refs 27 and 29.)

extrusion printing to prevent cell damage as the cells exit the nozzle, but using biomaterials presents many challenges including immunogenicity, host inflammatory responses, fibrous tissue formation, and toxicity of degradation products.[28] Ong et al.[29] demonstrated a method to create cardiac patches that consisted of cells derived from human iPSCs using a 3D bioprinter that picks up individual cardiospheres using vacuum suction and loads them onto a needle array, as seen in Fig. 13.2B. These spheres fused and were taken off the needle by day 3, and were allowed to grow over time. The patch spontaneously beated after printing and exhibited ventricular-like action potential waveforms and electrical conduction. The researchers also demonstrated functional capabilities through immunohisto chemistry and through implantation into a native rat myocardium.[29]

The ability to manipulate the bioink for 3D bioprinting is powerful because it presents a way to tailor the tissue construct to match native tissue. It allows for the optimization of a variety of features of the tissue, including the ability of the bioink to support cells, reorganize the tissue, or allow for the production of the cell's own extracellular matrix.[30]

Introduction of Vasculature

Other researchers tackled another important challenge when trying to engineer cardiac tissue: the tissues must be laden with a microvascular network. A vascular network within a cardiac tissue construct is important for several reasons: (1) it provides oxygen and nutrients and removes waste products, (2) it allows for the expansion and proliferation of tissue growth without cell death, (3) it allows for vessel anastomosis with the host vasculature for in vivo considerations.[31] Zhang et al.[20] proposed a novel hybrid strategy to fabricate endothelialized myocardium, as shown in Fig. 13.3. The researchers printed endothelial cells with a composite bioink that included GelMA + alginate that then migrated toward the periphery to form a layer of endothelium. By seeding cardiomyocytes around this endothelial scaffold, they were able to induce the formation of vascularized endothelialized myocardium that they were able to use to screen pharmaceutical compounds for cardiovascular toxicity by using a microfluidic perfusion bioreactor.[32] This novel technique utilizing endothelialized myocardium in a microfluidic perfusion bioreactor introduces not only ways to engineer human organ models, but also ways to screen drugs to elucidate cardiovascular toxicity and treatment efficacy.[20] Others, on the other hand, have introduced vasculature by creating a heterogenous structure that includes endothelial cells.[21] The ability to create vasculature using 3D printing techniques in cardiac tissue is very important, as coronary artery disease results from deficient blood supply in cardiac tissue.[9]

Spatially Patterning Tissues

So far, researchers have demonstrated the ability of the 3D bioprinter to successfully print spontaneously contracted patches with different cell lines, bioinks, and vasculature, and have demonstrated their function in vitro and in vivo. However, organs are complex systems composed of different cells and molecules that are arranged in a highly ordered structure to create function. Therefore, one of the unique characteristics of 3D

Step 1. Bioprinting of microfibrous scaffold encapsulating endothelial cells.   **Step 2.** Formation of the endothelialized structure and the vascular bed.

Step 3. Seeding with cardiomyocytes.   **Step 4.** Formation of endothelialized myocardium.

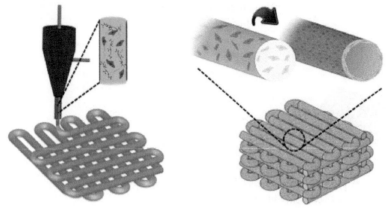

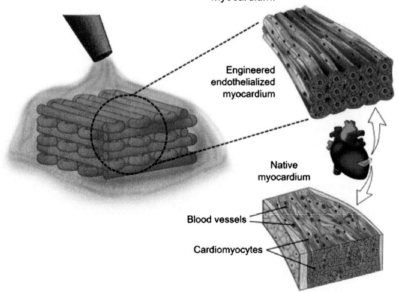

Engineered endothelialized myocardium

Native myocardium

Blood vessels

Cardiomyocytes

FIG. 13.3 Introduction of vasculature. Schematic of biofabricating endothelialized myocardium. (Credit: Reproduced with permission from Ref. 20.)

bioprinting is its ability to create predefined spatial organization through precise deposition and assembly of materials and cells.[33] Although multiphoton 3D printing can manufacture micron-level ECM resolutions and made a significant contribution to developing a native-like environment of the resulting construct, it introduced a conglomeration of cells within the scaffold, which does not allow for the cellular organization that is normally seen in heart tissue.

Early work in 2011 used laser printing techniques to successfully pattern human mesenchymal stem cells and endothelial cells on a cardiac patch, as seen in Fig. 13.4A, which enhanced angiogenesis at the site of infarction and preserved cardiac infarction.[34] However, more recent work created a printed structure that had a patterned patch which was composed of a spatial pattern of dual stem cells to provide cell-to-cell interaction and differentiation capabilities, as seen in

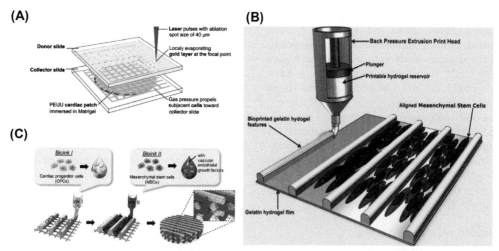

FIG. 13.4 Spatial patterning of cells: **(A)** schematic bioprinting setup of laser printing technique; **(B)** illustration of stem cell patch with multiple bioinks; **(C)** schematic representation of process of aligning cells. (Credit: Reproduced with permission from Refs. 34, 36 and 37.)

Fig. 13.4B. This patterned patch, when implanted in vivo, increased the migration from the patch to the infarcted area and improved cardiac function as well as reduced cardiac hypertrophy and fibrosis.[35]

Utilizing 3D bioprinting to create a spatially organized construct introduces many unique advances to the field of cardiac tissue engineering, as it enhances the function and maturity of cardiomyocytes (CMs). This is because spatially organizing the cells allows for a controlled alignment of beating cardiomyocytes that matches in the same direction as the functional myocardium. Tijore et al.[36] generated a cell guidance scaffold using gelatin to align human mesenchymal stem cells, as seen in Fig. 13.4C. This printed microchannel scaffold seeded with CMs showed rhythmic beating while also supporting CM growth and stem cell differentiation.

The ability for 3D bioprinting to create spatially organized cardiac tissue advances the field because it means we can create complex, heterogeneous tissue constructs that can be immediately implanted into the body. Researchers have continued to demonstrate the potential to create highly organizeds structure with unique physiological and biomechanical properties that are similar to native myocardium.[37] Wang et al.[37] isolated primary cardiomyocytes from infant rat hearts, and suspended them in a fibrin-based bioink to create a highly organized structure with physiologic, mechanical, and electrical properties found in vivo. Their resulting bioprinted tissue stained for factors demonstrating that the cardiac cells were uniformly aligned, dense, and electromechanically coupled.

The development of 3D bioprinting of the cardiac tissue has involved many pivotal advances that have greatly impacted the field. As an alternative technique for traditional ways to engineer cardiac tissue, 3D bioprinting is capable of introducing functionality and producing heterogenous constructs. Over the past several years, 3D bioprinting has introduced the potential for vasculature, synchronous electric coupling, spatial and heterogenous organization, personalized patches, seamless integration in mice, reduction in cardiotoxicity, and therapeutic potential in diseased mice.

A discussion and comparison of the methods that have been used for cardiac tissue engineering will elucidate the benefits of certain techniques that can pave the path for the future of bioprinting in 3D cardiac tissue engineering.

METHODS OF 3D BIOPRINTING CARDIAC TISSUE: A COMPARISON

There are myriad ways to create cardiac tissues using 3D bioprinting. Most individuals are generally familiar with the method that extrudes material out of a nozzle. However, there are many other ways to bioprint including the inkjet bioprinting, laser-based printing, omnidirectional printing using sacrificial ink, and vacuum-suction printing. Of these, only a few have been explored for printing cardiac tissues: microextrusion-based printing, laser-based printing, and vacuum-suction printing. Although many cells can survive in carefully controlled culture conditions for up to 3 months, high pressure, speeds, sheer force, and heat created by extrusion- or droplet-based printing cannot not tolerated. In fact, extrusion-based printing causes significant cell death, while inkjet and other methods have reported higher cell viability.[38] Of these techniques, the one most commonly used in 3D bioprinting has been microextrusion-based printing.

Here, we will solely focus on the various methods used in cardiac 3D printing and will compare the results obtained from these methods to discuss their advantages and disadvantages. We will also introduce a negative printing method that has not yet been used in cardiac printing but provides a promising direction for the future of the field.

Microextrusion-Based Printing

The most commonly used method for 3D printing cardiac tissue is pneumatic or mechanical pressure (piston) microextrusion printing. This technique involves a robotic system that is under the control of a computer, allowing for the consistent and reliable deposition of cells.[39,40] It easily incorporates software such as computer-aided design to enable users to load files for printing. Furthermore, it allows for customization through adjusting the size and type of nozzle, the dispensing rate, and the velocity of the dispensing head.[5] Through this method, cells are directly encapsulated in the ECM-like bioink.[5,41]

However, determining the bioink ideal for printing cardiac tissue is not trivial.[41,42] The selection of the bioink depends on the target tissue, type of cell, and the bioprinter, which is further complicated by the need to allow for cell growth while possessing the proper mechanical, rheological, and biological properties of the target tissue.[30] Both natural and synthetic biomaterials have been used as bioinks, and each have their own advantages and disadvantages. Natural biomaterials are isolated from natural sources and improve biological features, but experience less mechanical stability and higher variation in molecular weight from batch to batch, relative to synthetic biomaterials.[43]

There have been several bioinks suitable for the printing and survival of cardiac tissue. The most primitive tissue printing experiment used alginate, a protein-based bioink, which did not alter the viability or proliferation of hCMPs when printed with the scaffold. Specifically, there was a significant increase in gene expression of early cardiac transcription factors (Nkx2.5, GATA-A, and Mef-2C) and a substantial upregulation of sarcomeric protein TnT for up to 1 week.[15] hCMPCs have also been printed in HA/gel bioink, and have similarly demonstrated enhanced cell

attachment and survival. The tissue provided therapeutic potential by reducing LV remodeling in mouse heart infarction models but has not yet been studied for a period exceeding 1 month. Because printed hydrogels are often mechanically weak, researchers have explored cross-linking the bioinks using UVA light postprinting as a method of mimicking the stiffness and conductivity found in native cardiac tissue.[22] Researchers have also been experimenting with cross-linking dECM bioink, a bioink that mimics a native microenvironment. This construct also showed high cell viability and active proliferation and increased cardiomyogenic differentiation.[27]

Microextrusion printing has also been used to construct endothelialized-myocardial tissues by printing endothelial cells and then seeding them with cardiomyocytes to generate aligned myocardium from hiPSCs. The endothelial cells migrate to resemble a blood vessel structure but were not shown to allow perfusion through the vessels. This structure, after connecting to a bioreactor, was demonstrated as a possible platform for cardiovascular drug screening.[20] Microextrusion-based bioprinting allows for continuous deposition of biomaterial and has been shown to be a convenient and rapid technique for the continuous deposition of cells, which explains its ubiquitous use in cardiac tissue bioprinting. Bioprinters can be equipped with multiple extruders, allowing for the printing of multiple cell types and bioinks, enabling heterogeneous tissue patches and allowing for organization within a patch.[5]

Despite the successes shown with microextrusion printing, the limitations of this technique must be kept in mind especially when considering it for large-scale tissue printing, including the shear stress induced by the nozzle tip that could affect cell viability when the cell density is high.[44] Microextrusion printing has been the most studied method of printing cardiac tissues and researchers will continue to experiment with various bioinks to provide the sufficiently high viscosity necessary for printing and stiffness needed for in vitro modeling. Given the ease of microextrusion printing in depositing a high volume of cells, microextrusion printing will likely continue to be a popular technique in 3D cardiac printing.

Laser Printing

Another 3D bioprinting method that researchers have used for cardiac tissue printing is laser-based. Laser direct writing (LDW or laser-induced forward transfer) uses high-energy laser beams to propel bioink from one surface to another.[14,34,45] This method requires three parts: the laser source, a film with cell-containing bioink (called a ribbon), and a receiving substrate that contains biopolymer or cell culture medium. The laser irradiates the film, evaporating the liquid material and producing droplets onto the receiving substrate.[14] This technique avoids the limitations imposed by nozzle clogging and permits high-resolution printing.[34,45] It also has proven useful for cardiac regeneration and has many unique advantages, including a nozzle-free process, with high resolution and precision of delivery.[34] Finally, it is able to sustain high-viscosity bioinks, allowing for robust 3D structures,[5] but has not been demonstrated in creating cardiac tissue.

Vacuum-Suction Printing

In every variant of 3D bioprinting described earlier, a scaffold is needed for a successful print. Another way to approach layer-by-layer printing is without the use of biomaterials, eliminating the concern for the presence of cytotoxic materials during printing via the polymers or other bioink.[46] This method utilizes "spheroids," which are dense aggregates of cells.[29,47] A Kenzan 3D bioprinter suctions up individual spheroids and lays them down to form a predesigned contiguous structure. Stainless steel microneedles are used as temporary support to align the spheroids together, allowing them to fuse into aggregates and to synthesize their own extracellular matrix.[48] Research has shown this method to be compatible with in vivo structures and to exhibit comparable contractile and mechanical strength, making it a highly promising technology for cardiac tissue regeneration and disease modeling.[49]

Omnidirectional Printing

The printing techniques described so far have addressed ways to print a range of materials that can incorporate and sustain live cells. However, the layer-by-layer printing method limits the print to always be mechanically supported as it prints, and thus the printer is unable to create complex hollow structures. As a solution, omnidirectional printing utilizes extrusion printing in a free-form method, instead of layer by layer.[50,51] Although this method has not yet been introduced with cardiac tissues, the technique presents many advantages that can be applied to cardiac tissue engineering. This method uses a sacrificial material to allow temporary suspension and support of the printed material during the printing process. The sacrificial material is dissolved postprinting after heating the result to body temperature.[52] Not only can this method anisotropically deposit material, but it also has a greater capacity to print soft hydrogels that are

currently limited in other 3D bioprinting methods by supporting soft structures as they are printed. It can also keep the cells alive because of the aqueous printing environment.[51,52]

The method described produces a "positive" print: the postprocessed product is that which was printed. Another method that researchers have investigated uses sacrificial ink to create hollow structures by printing sacrificial ink and encapsulating it within living cells. This form of "negative" printing is used to create microchannels within the finished product.[53-55] This method of anisotropic printing introduces 3D bioprinting techniques that can form complex 3D structures. However, the sacrificial material must be compatible with the biomaterial and cells, so that when the breakdown and diffusion of sacrificial material occurs, the cells are still in an environment that promotes survival. Although these techniques have not yet been applied to cardiac tissues, they may have a significant impact on methods to improve vasculature and printing of large-scaled cardiac tissue. Researchers have already used this technique to fabricate a 3D construct replete with vasculature.[53]

Researchers have used a variety of techniques for cardiac tissue printing, but by far the most commonly used has been microextrusion-based printing. However, many of the other techniques present advantages that may influence the further development that is necessary to build a heart.

THE FUTURE OF 3D BIOPRINTING OF CARDIAC TISSUE

The research into 3D bioprinting of cardiac tissue has both short- and long-term goals. Researchers, as discussed earlier, have addressed the short-term goal to biofabricate the myocardium as a cutting edge treatment option for myocardial infarction.[9] In the long term, the goal of 3D bioprinting is to be able to fully print a functioning heart for humans in need of a human transplant, and researchers have begun to enter this realm. Therefore, despite exciting current techniques, there is still much more to look forward to and anticipate. Here, we will discuss some future ideas to consider. These future directions include bioprinting the whole human heart, heart valves, and early heart models. We will also discuss the ethical issues raised by these techniques.

Bioprinting A Whole Heart

The organ shortage dilemma continues. Each year, the number of people on the waiting list continues to grow much larger than the number of available transplants and the number of donors.[56] In the United States, there are 3979 patients currently waiting for a heart transplant[57] and as of July 1, 2018, 1370 individuals have received a transplant.[57] Through advocacy work and education, individuals have attempted to address this issue. Despite this work, the gap between supply and demand continues to exist.[58–60]

At the advent of 3D bioprinting, people recognized its potential to close this gap, but the idea of printing a functional heart seemed like science fiction. However, the significant printing advances discussed above lay a foundation of techniques, suggesting that the ability to print a heart is not necessarily so distant. In fact, the printing of the whole heart is of utmost interest in the field of cardiac tissue engineering.[58] In 2017, NASA launched a challenge offering a $500,000 prize to the first three teams successfully able to create a thick, metabolically functional humanized vascularized tissue able to survive for 30 days in laboratory conditions in vitro.[61]

What was initially a topic of discussion that seemed too impossible to be true has evolved to become a project on the cusp of success. This potential for revolutionizing healthcare has received considerable attention and the possibility of printing a heart has recruited many researchers. Notably, there are many leading research groups at academic institutions along with organ initiatives that are advancing current methods to enable printing of large-scale tissue. Some initiatives include the 3D organ initiative at the Wyss Institute of Harvard University[62] and the Bioengineered Organ Initiative at Carnegie Mellon University.[63] Furthermore, a startup called BIOLIFE4D has been of interest to many, as its ambitions align with many of the goals for bioprinting human cardiac tissue.[64,65] With many groups working toward the same goal, it is important to increase collaboration and create widely available biomedical research to allow other researchers to expand on current techniques that work.

However, even with the manpower and motivation to a build a heart, there are still several challenges to overcome. To successfully create a beating, vascularized human heart, it is important to understand past techniques for 3D bioprinting cardiac tissue and to continue adding to the successes thus far. Here, we will discuss several important traits that must improve. To build a large-scaled heart, future 3D bioprinters must address several key challenges: (1) resolution, (2) speed, (3) complexity and scaling, (4) biomaterial compatibility, and (5) cost. These challenges are similar to those that would apply to other organ systems as well.

Resolution

The future of 3D cardiac printing must involve printers that print at very high resolutions. Nutrients and oxygen can only diffuse through 150 µm of tissue, and without adequate vascularization, tissue necrosis will occur.[66] Thus, bulk tissue printing requires bioprinters to print single-cell-walled capillaries for vascular perfusion throughout the tissue. This is necessary to constantly feed the 3D tissue with oxygen and nutrients and remove the waste products from the microenvironment while limiting cell death.[66,67] There are several approaches to address this issue of vascularization. The bioink can be mixed with angiogenic factors or cells that are destined to create vasculature to construct a printed 3D complex with cells that can form vessels. The other way is to print a vascular structure within the tissue construct.

If addressing the issue with the latter method, bioprinters must operate at a high enough resolution to print the micrometer scale capillaries that supply the heart. Current technology allows for prints on the order of 50–15,000 µm in diameter, which is much higher than the average size of 5–10 µm of capillaries.[40,67] Without the capability to build such fine resolution capillaries and a functional vascular system, it would be difficult to create large tissues. Therefore, the future of 3D printers requires these technologies to print at the scale of a single cell (between 1 and 10 µm).[68,69] Through the popular extrusion-printing method of 3D cardiac printing, it is difficult to pattern high-resolution prints. High resolutions require a small diameter nozzle, increasing shear stress that directly correlates with decreased cell viability, which is why nozzle-free systems that avoid extrusion are being explored.[70] For example, personalized patches have been created using multiphoton 3D printing, which can achieve microresolution prints.[21]

Speed

With current bioprinting techniques, large tissue constructs may require many hours or days to complete. This is a concern because cells are fragile and sensitive to their environment, and thus require the strict maintenance of temperature and humidity of the printed construct.[71,72] Therefore, future research must enhance the ability to maintain physiological conditions in a printed construct, while also increasing the speed of the printer. However, this presents a challenge in cardiac tissue engineering when most successful techniques for 3D bioprinting rely on extrusion printing. Although extrusion printing is often used to produce large-scale scaffolds due to its fast deposition speed and its ability to dispense dense cellular material, this technique is known to worsen cell viability with increased pressures or smaller diameter nozzles, which takes a toll on both the print speed and print resolution.[73,74]

Furthermore, cells can only survive for a limited time without blood supply, which is why rapid printing is needed to return the tissue to physiologic environments. This is why current techniques for 3D bioprinting cardiac tissues are limited to printing several layer thick patches of cells, circumventing the vascularization challenge and allowing for easy perfusion throughout the printed tissue.[9]

Recently, Prellis Biologics developed a new technique to address these issues, and created a printing system that allows for the fast printing of high-resolution tissue that can be used to construct viable capillaries.[75] Their method uses a holographic printing technique that has a resolution of 0.5 μm and is 1000 times faster than conventional bioprinters. When the system is perfected, the company states that it will be able to print a block of issue with an entire vascular system in less than 12 hours.[76,77] This technology would be a key milestone in the quest to creating engineered organs.

Researchers must continue to address the challenge of improving the printing speed of bioprinters. Over the past several years, researchers have introduced various other techniques to print cardiac tissue, including the scaffold-free method that was previously described, which could be explored further to enhance the speed of 3D printing, and could cause less cell damage compared to the shear force from extrusion printing.

Complexity and scaling up

The heart is a large organ and is complex in its structural makeup. An immediate challenge is scaling up because an immense number of cells is necessary to print cardiac tissue. An average adult human heart is estimated to have around 2 billion heart muscle cells,[78] and a single standard confluent T-75 flask can hold up to 8.4 million cells, requiring about 238 T75 flasks. Of these cells, the heart is composed of three types of cardiac tissues: myocardium, endocardium, and pericardium. The cellular makeup consists of cardiomyocytes (30%−40%), cardiac fibroblasts, and endothelial cells.[79] The heart also includes specialized pacemaker cells in the right atrium necessary for generating electric pulses.[9,80] To create a functional heart, the printed construct must match the makeup of the heart in the functional subunits and structural alignments to be considered viable for transplantation.

Researchers have attempted to emulate the complexity of the heart by spatially patterning cells within the cardiac tissue. Jang et al.[35] created a patch by printing two separate bioinks composed of two different cells to create a layered organized structure, and Tijore et al.[36] tried printing a scaffold to guide cardiac cells to synchronously contract. These successful techniques both use extrusion methods, and thus may not be of high enough resolution to create the complexity needed for a bigger tissue. Multiphoton excitation, however, can create ultra-fine, 1-μm resolution.[21] By combining these two techniques, we can imagine a solution that satisfies both the complexity and resolution needed to scale up cardiac tissue. Thus, the future of 3D cardiac tissue bioprinting may lend itself to merging and combining successful existing printing technologies to utilize the benefits of each.

Biomaterial compatibility

The printing substrate used must be biocompatible with living cells and must not be toxic in vivo. It should ideally possess the proper mechanical, rheological, and biological properties of the target tissue.[81] Researchers have worked toward creating a microenvironment surrounding the cells by using synthetic and natural bioactive hydrogels such as gelatin, collagen, and fibrin as biomaterials.[82−84] Natural materials are isolated from natural sources and thus provide biochemical and physical stimuli to guide cellular behaviors. Compared to synthetic polymers however, natural materials are less mechanically stable and have higher variation in molecular weight and structure from batch to batch.[30] Synthetic polymers are robust, but due to their lack of active binding sites, allow for limited cell adhesion and thus can result in cell death.[5] Many of the early works in cardiac tissue engineering used natural bioactive hydrogels for the creation of the tissue patch and showed early successes. These hydrogel-based bioinks are biocompatible, biodegradable, readily cross-linked, and are highly tunable.[85] Nevertheless, researchers are still unable to make these synthetic and natural polymers emulate an ideal ECM for tissue engineering.[86]

Therefore, researchers began to explore bioinks made from natural dECM. ECM is an essential structural component of cells that contains the important signaling molecules for stem cell differentiation and survival,[87] and dECM preserves functional and structural proteins such as glycosaminoglycan and fibrous proteins found in ECM.[88] dECM has shown to induce higher expression of cardiac specific genes (Myh6 and Actn1) and higher expression of cardiac β-myosin heavy chain compared to a collagen-based construct,[87] and has also shown versatility and flexibility in the creation of cartilage, adipose, and liver tissue.[89] dECM is often combined with synthetic bioinks when used as bioink for cardiac tissue engineering because dECM is not otherwise sufficiently stiff.[86]

There have also been newer methods to completely eliminate the extracellular matrix itself, the so-called "scaffold-free methods."[29,90] An example of a scaffold-free method is to assemble cells using magnetic forces and to create a magnetic field to spatially control 3D culture.[91] Another method is using a microneedles approach, using the Japanese-built Regenova 3D bioprinter.[48] However, these scaffold-free techniques pose some challenges, especially since constructs that rely on the fusion of cells are not stable enough to maintain structure initially.[9,90] However, these techniques have the potential to transform the way cardiovascular disease is treated in the future, as this approach provides several advantages that scaffold-dependent bioprinting cannot, including improvements regarding cell damage, biocompatibility, and cellular interactions. Moreover, biomaterials can still be optionally added.

The development of the ideal biomaterials is by no means finished and will continue to be a topic of active research. It is also important to remember that a variety of bioinks is necessary to create structurally functional cardiac tissue. More specifically, bioinks can be categorized into five types, and all five are necessary to create functional tissue: structural, functional, sacrificial, supportive, and four-dimensional.[92] The deposition of structural bioinks allows for the fabrication of bioprinted constructs and can provide the correct mechanical, degradation, and cell-survivability properties. However, this does not provide the tissue with any functional capabilities. The incorporation of functional bioinks would allow for the capability to direct cell differentiation and guide cells toward specific phenotypes by containing growth factors and other biological cues. Sacrificial bioinks allow the creation of void regions that are highly important for the creation of vascular networks. Supportive bioinks include protective lattices that can be printed around softer bioprinted constructs to withstand forces if there is initially insufficient mechanical strength. Lastly, four-dimensional bioinks will be important as they are sensitive to external stimuli. These can be used in the application of electrical conduction, wherein the electrical stimulation results in simultaneous contraction of the bioink.[30,92–95]

The future of bioinks for 3D bioprinters is promising, but will require the continued development of novel biomaterials with molecular functionality and structural similar to native tissue.[81]

Cost

Cost is a big concern when trying to create large tissues. Many 3D bioprinters have starting prices between $10,000 and over $20,000, which is highly burdensome for research organizations with limited budgets. Moreover, these machines are often closed source and proprietary, making them difficult to modify.[96] Fortunately, researchers have slowly begun to address this issue, and we can continue to anticipate printers that are cheaper, faster, of higher resolution, and allow for scaling up compared to their predecessors.

Recently, researchers from Carnegie Mellon designed a syringe pump large volume extruder that can be built for under $500 that uses alginate, a common biomaterial for 3D bioprinting. Their technology aims to print human tissue on a larger scale at a higher resolution, allowing researchers to focus on other issues such as the biomaterial compatibility or the cells used for printing.[96] They hope to create more open-source research to allow others to expand upon their technology, which can quickly enhance and accelerate the creation of a functional 3D tissue. Although their printer has not been tested on live cells, this technology will significantly influence the field of cardiac tissue engineering. This is especially true because the currently successful techniques for printing cardiac tissue have been through extrusion printing, and further research can be done to leverage this cheaper printer for that purpose.

Aortic Heart Valve

Another area of focus to look forward to is the fabrication of engineered heart valves. An advantage of working with stem cells is their ability to remodel and grow. A lot of the conversation in 3D cardiac tissue printing has involved creating mature patches that are able to reconstruct fibrotic heart tissue or transplant a failed heart. However, there is a whole separate population of individuals that require attention who have conditions like aortic valve disease (AVD). AVD is a serious health condition and can affect people of all ages. The recommended treatment for aortic valve disease is surgical replacement of the defective valve with either a mechanical or chemically cross-linked tissue heart valve, which is a standard procedure for adults.[9] However, this does not make sense for children as they are growing and these will be inadequate for growing children.[97] Tissue engineering can thus create functional tissue that is able to remodel and grow with the patient. Tissue-engineered heart valves must have functional capabilities similar to those in vivo and include the natural geometry and performance of the valve root, cusps, and sinus walls.[71,98] Besides their ability to remodel with the patient, biological valves also present advantages over classical synthetic valves. Although synthetic valves are more mechanically robust and have a longer lifetime, biological valves do not require patients to take anticoagulants because they are made from an allogeneic or xenogeneic source.[99,100]

There have been several early studies in this field. Of the many valves in the heart, researchers have mainly focused on engineering the aortic valve, as it is involved with many cardiovascular diseases. Butcher et al. in 2013 implemented a method to fabricate a heterozygous (smooth muscle and valve interstitial cells) living trileaflet valve with anatomical resemblance to the native valve using an alginate/gelatin hydrogel with a dual-syringe system. They were aiming to print a structure of the valve root and leaflets and were able to fabricate a living aortic valve conduit with anatomical similarities to the native valve.[101] Although these results demonstrate that the aortic valve can be fabricated with 3D bioprinting, there were still limitations to their model: the hydrogel decreased in stiffness and strength, required a long print time, and has not been demonstrated to withstand the blood flow required in vivo.

Even with the advancements and successes of many bioprinting technologies in the field over the past several years, researchers are still unable to print a thin, cell-laden heart valve that is able to withstand physiologic pressures of a native heart.[97] Furthermore, there has been no functional testing of any printed valves. This will be an active area of research that can have many impactful applications to the future of cardiovascular disease treatment.

Heart Development

There is a separate future for tissue engineering aside from the goal of creating large-scale heart tissue. This is to engineer the developing heart. Although much interest has been given to repair damaged hearts and study the heart in vitro after it has finished differentiating into cardiomyocytes, less attention has been given to the beginning of life. The heart initially arises from the mesodermal tissues when the embryo is undergoing gastrulation and starts its life as a heart tube. By the fourth week, the tube begins to loop, and at this time, the primary heart tube within the pericardial cavity can be divided into atrial and ventricular components along with an outflow tract.[102,103] With congenital heart disease being one of the most common types of

birth defects, as well as beginning its damaging origin during the time of heart development, it would be powerful to understand and study the development of the heart in vitro in a 3D model.

In fact, Hoang et al.[104] created spatially patterned early-developing cardiac organoids using human pluripotent stem cells, demonstrating the potential to differentiate iPSCs into cells that resemble early heart development. These early-developing cardiac organoids can be translated to a cardiac model using 3D bioprinting, not just to analyze the complexities of early heart development in vitro, but also to further study specific CHD complications that arise in certain parts of the developing heart.[104,105] These can also be used to study treatments for the cardiac system on a patient's specific cells. 3D bioprinting may thus be able to create alternatives to animal testing, and is highly beneficial in pediatric patients.[106]

Ethics of Building a Heart

Future successes in 3D bioprinting would obviate the need for a long human organ transplant waiting list. It would make organs available to those who need them and by using the patient's own cells, would eliminate issues of transplant rejection. The multidecade issue of organ shortage would be solved. However, with tissue engineering comes many ethical issues worth considering, especially as genetic engineering improves, and researchers are able to create personalized, living heart tissues. The possibility of printing the heart does not seem so distant anymore and so the ethical ramifications of this technology are critical to begin considering now. These issues include equality of access for patients, safety, and human enhancement.[107–109]

Access for patients

The main motivation behind printing one's organs is for organ replacement. This is a critical issue that affects every nation in the world, including low- and middle-income nations, as cardiovascular disease is one of the most widespread causes of death around the world. Even within high-income nations, inconsistent access to advanced medical care through limited or privatized insurance systems means that not all individuals can reasonably expect to have the same access to advanced treatments.[110] This raises ethical concerns surrounding access: if this technology is capable of curing the primary drivers of death nationwide, must all people have access to it? And if not, and federal governments and insurance systems can limit who gets access, what are the ethical standards around who should have access? Should a child have equal access to a transplant as an older person who likely has fewer years left to live? Should the lifestyle choices of a patient be taken into account, such as eating a diet that makes cardiovascular disease more likely, or being a smoker that makes lung transplants more necessary? To some degree, societies have already started making such choices. For example, in the United States under the Affordable Care Act, insurance companies were barred from penalizing patients for preexisting conditions, *except* if they were smokers. In general, these are the same issues of access that ethicists grapple with for all medical technologies. However, it becomes particularly important in this case because of the extent of cardiovascular disease, and the particularly technical and expensive nature of transplantation. Moreover, highly technical transplant procedures mean that for the foreseeable future, they will largely be limited to nations (and cities within them) where there are highly trained surgeons and medical teams that can perform the operations and care for these complex patients. If one believes that this technology should be widely available to people across the world, it thus follows that it is necessary to significantly increase investment in support for surgical and highly specialized medical training around the world, which is needed to deliver this technology to all individuals.

Safety

Safety of 3D bioprinting treatments should also be considered.[111] Despite screening procedures to reduce the risk of organ rejection, a 3D bioprinted organ can still get rejected by the body.[112] Rejection occurs when there is an autoimmune reaction against a transplanted heart.[113] 3D bioprinting presents an advantage as tissue can specifically be engineered to reduce the risk of this happening, by using the patient's own stem cells to biofabricate the heart tissue. However, hiPSC-derived products have the risk of teratoma formation and also have the potential for chromosome instability and malignant transformation.[1,114,115] To limit the probability of this and to improve the safety of 3D bioprinted cardiac transplants, there must be a standardized way to test organ biofabrication. This is an important topic of concern in 3D bioprinting that will continue to be studied over the next several years as we enhance the ability to create safe bioinks for human implantation.

Human enhancement

The ability to use iPSCs as the cell source for 3D bioprinting of whole heart tissue presents a possibility for enhancing the heart. As iPSCs are used, researchers are able to avoid the destruction of human embryos for research by culturing differentiated tissues from human-induced pluripotent stem cells that are derivative of somatic cells and implanting them into a mouse to demonstrate functional abilities of the tissue. However, there have been ethical concerns raised regarding iPSCs, including the possibility of abnormal reprogramming in the induction of hiPSCs, and the generation of tumors in the process of stem cell therapy.[116] This can be used to create human hearts that are "better" than normal functioning hearts, such as creating heart tissue that does not fatigue as quickly as the predecessors and one that exceeds in performance and strength.[107]

In principle, hearts could be engineered that give humans otherwise impossible levels of strength, which raises numerous ethical questions. There is an often-hazy spectrum between what constitutes a "therapeutic" versus an "enhancement." A transplant is, in itself, an act of intervention that would not be possible without modern technology. In light of this, one could reasonably argue that it is equally reasonable to use modern technology to also improve heart function. As a broad policy though, this would pose several negative ramifications, principally in creating a slippery slope. Although individuals may feel comfortable getting small efficiency boosts in heart function relative to some baseline, using tissue engineering to improve organ function beyond ordinary levels would set a precedent for others to use the technology to enhance themselves for any organ in the body. Given that this technology is highly expensive, and the uneven distribution of wealth would force this use-case to be limited to those with higher incomes, a mandate to use organ transplantation for enhancement beyond ordinary human levels would allow society's wealthiest individuals the freedom to enhance their body functions and further this inequality. In light of this undesirable outcome, it is important to establish norms before developing surgical procedures with this technology that establish what constitutes a therapeutic result versus an enhancement.[109]

CONCLUSION

3D bioprinting will change the future of medicine, and the rapid pace of advancement in 3D bioprinting techniques for cardiac tissue engineering is remarkable. Just six years ago, the most primitive cardiac tissue construct was printed,[15] and as of 2019, researchers are able to manipulate various aspects of the printer to create a construct that is closer to mimicking the physiologic strength and electrical function of the native human heart. However, despite current technology, there are several challenges to tackle before researchers are able to print a functional human heart. The biggest challenge to printing the heart is that the organ is complex. It requires adequate vascularization, thickness, cellular composition, and biocompatibility to achieve clinically relevant function and the ability to survive within the host body. However, this is not to say that these hurdles are impossible to overcome. Researchers have been addressing these key issues through various printing techniques, using a multitude of cell types and experimenting with different bioinks.[7] We now have many developments to look forward to in cardiac tissue engineering: the ability to print the human heart, heart valves, and to study early heart development. At the same time, with this future, we should anticipate and welcome difficult discussions regarding the ethical implications of these technologies.

One of the most important changes to the field of 3D bioprinting has been the substantial increase in public attention. There are now dozens of published news articles on the successes of various groups and individuals. Moreover, individuals are beginning to invest in 3D bioprinting companies such as BIOLIFE4D and Prellis Biologics,[117] and even NASA, an agency responsible for aerospace and aeronautics, has created a challenge for researchers to create a thick, vascularized, metabolically functional tissue model.[61] This interest in the field is exciting and will help to accelerate the race to build an organ. With the support, technological capabilities, and rapid advancements thus far, 3D bioprinting of a heart is closer than ever before.

REFERENCES

1. Hirt MN, Hansen A, Eschenhagen T. Cardiac tissue engineering: state of the art. *Circ Res.* 2014;114(2):354–367.
2. Gaziano TA, Bitton A, Anand S, Abrahams-Gessel S, Murphy A. Growing epidemic of coronary heart disease in low- and middle-income countries. *Curr Probl Cardiol.* 2010;35(2):72–115.
3. Avolio E, Caputo M, Madeddu P. Stem cell therapy and tissue engineering for correction of congenital heart disease. *Front Cell Dev Biol.* 2015;3.
4. Talman V, Ruskoaho H. Cardiac fibrosis in myocardial infarction-from repair and remodeling to regeneration. *Cell Tissue Res.* 2016;365(3):563–581.
5. Jang J. 3D bioprinting and in vitro cardiovascular tissue modeling. *Bioengineering.* 2017;4.
6. Curtis MW, Russell B. Cardiac tissue engineering. *J Cardiovasc Nurs.* 2009;24(2):87–92.
7. Duan B. State-of-the-Art review of 3D bioprinting for cardiovascular tissue engineering. *Ann Biomed Eng.* 2017; 45(1):195–209.
8. Alrefai MT, Murali D, Paul A, Ridwan KM, Connell JM, Shum-Tim D. Cardiac tissue engineering and regeneration using cell-based therapy. *Stem Cells Cloning.* 2015; 8:81–101.
9. Borovjagin AV, Ogle BM, Berry JL, Zhang J. From microscale devices to 3D printing: advances in fabrication of 3D cardiovascular tissues. *Circ Res.* 2017;120(1): 150–165.
10. Bell A, Kofron M, Nistor V. Multiphoton crosslinking for biocompatible 3D printing of type I collagen. *Biofabrication.* 2015;7(3):035007.
11. Wolpert L. Evolution of the cell theory. *Philos Trans R Soc Lond B Biol Sci.* 1995;349(1329):227–233.
12. Partridge R, Conlisk N, Davies JA. In-lab three-dimensional printing: an inexpensive tool for experimentation and visualization for the field of organogenesis. *Organogenesis.* 2012;8:22–27.
13. Zhang X, Zhang Y. Tissue engineering applications of three-dimensional bioprinting. *Cell Biochem Biophys.* 2015;72(3):777–782.
14. Li J, Chen M, Fan X, Zhou H. Recent advances in bioprinting techniques: approaches, applications and future prospects. *J Transl Med.* 2016;14.
15. Gaetani R, Doevendans PA, Metz CH, et al. Cardiac tissue engineering using tissue printing technology and human cardiac progenitor cells. *Biomaterials.* 2012;33(6): 1782–1790.
16. Jia J, Richards DJ, Pollard S, et al. Engineering alginate as bioink for bioprinting. *Acta Biomater.* 2014;10(10): 4323–4331.
17. Le T, Chong J. Cardiac progenitor cells for heart repair. *Cell Death Dis.* 2016;2:16052.
18. Gaetani R, Feyen DA, Verhage V, et al. Epicardial application of cardiac progenitor cells in a 3D-printed gelatin/hyaluronic acid patch preserves cardiac function after myocardial infarction. *Biomaterials.* 2015;61: 339–348.
19. Smits AM, van Laake LW, den Ouden K, et al. Human cardiomyocyte progenitor cell transplantation preserves long-term function of the infarcted mouse myocardium. *Cardiovasc Res.* 2009;83(3):527–535.
20. Zhang YS, Arneri A, Bersini S, et al. Bioprinting 3D microfibrous scaffolds for engineering endothelialized myocardium and heart-on-a-chip. *Biomaterials.* 2016;110: 45–59.
21. Gao L, Kupfer ME, Jung JP, et al. Myocardial tissue engineering with cells derived from human-induced pluripotent stem cells and a native-like, high-resolution, 3-Dimensionally printed scaffold. *Circ Res.* 2017; 120(8):1318–1325.
22. Izadifar M, Chapman D, Babyn P, Chen X, Kelly ME. UV-assisted 3D bioprinting of nanoreinforced hybrid cardiac patch for myocardial tissue engineering. *Tissue Eng C Methods.* 2018;24(2):74–88.
23. Choudhury D, Tun HW, Wang T, Naing MW. Organ-derived decellularized extracellular matrix: a game changer for bioink manufacturing? *Trends Biotechnol.* 2018; 36(8):787–805.

24. Gasperini L, Mano JF, Reis RL. Natural polymers for the microencapsulation of cells. *J R Soc Interface.* 2014;11(100):20140817.

25. Whitford WG, Hoying JB. A bioink by any other name: terms, concepts and constructions related to 3D bioprinting. *Future Sci OA.* 2016;2(3).

26. Pati F, Cho DW. Bioprinting of 3D tissue models using decellularized extracellular matrix bioink. *Methods Mol Biol.* 2017;1612:381–390.

27. Jang J, Kim TG, Kim BS, Kim SW, Kwon SM, Cho DW. Tailoring mechanical properties of decellularized extracellular matrix bioink by vitamin B2-induced photo-crosslinking. *Acta Biomater.* 2016;33:88–95.

28. Norotte C, Marga FS, Niklason LE, Forgacs G. Scaffold-free vascular tissue engineering using bioprinting. *Biomaterials.* 2009;30(30):5910–5917.

29. Ong CS, Fukunishi T, Zhang H, et al. Biomaterial-free three-dimensional bioprinting of cardiac tissue using human induced pluripotent stem cell derived cardiomyocytes. *Sci Rep.* 2017;7(1):4566.

30. Gungor-Ozkerim PS, Inci I, Zhang YS, Khademhosseini A, Dokmeci MR. Bioinks for 3D bioprinting: an overview. *Biomater Sci.* 2018;6(5):915–946.

31. Forgacs G. Tissue engineering: perfusable vascular networks. *Nat Mater.* 2012;11:746–747. England.

32. Li YC, Zhang YS, Akpek A, Shin SR, Khademhosseini A. 4D bioprinting: the next-generation technology for biofabrication enabled by stimuli-responsive materials. *Biofabrication.* 2016;9(1):012001.

33. Moroni L, Burdick JA, Highley C, et al. Biofabrication strategies for 3D in vitro models and regenerative medicine. *Nature Reviews Materials.* 2018;3(5):21.

34. Gaebel R, Ma N, Liu J, et al. Patterning human stem cells and endothelial cells with laser printing for cardiac regeneration. *Biomaterials.* 2011;32(35):9218–9230.

35. Jang J, Park HJ, Kim SW, et al. 3D printed complex tissue construct using stem cell-laden decellularized extracellular matrix bioinks for cardiac repair. *Biomaterials.* 2017;112:264–274.

36. Tijore A, Irvine SA, Sarig U, Mhaisalkar P, Baisane V, Venkatraman S. Contact guidance for cardiac tissue engineering using 3D bioprinted gelatin patterned hydrogel. *Biofabrication.* 2018;10(2):025003.

37. Wang Z, Lee SJ, Cheng HJ, Yoo JJ, Atala A. 3D bioprinted functional and contractile cardiac tissue constructs. *Acta Biomater.* 2018;70:48–56.

38. Ong CS, Nam L, Ong K, et al. 3D and 4D bioprinting of the myocardium: current approaches, challenges, and future prospects. *BioMed Res Int.* 2018;2018:6497242.

39. Ozbolat IT, Hospodiuk M. Current advances and future perspectives in extrusion-based bioprinting. *Biomaterials.* 2016;76:321–343.

40. Datta P, Barui A, Wu Y, Ozbolat V, Moncal KK, Ozbolat IT. Essential steps in bioprinting: from pre- to post-bioprinting. *Biotechnol Adv.* 2018;36(5):1481–1504.

41. Ravnic DJ, Leberfinger AN, Koduru SV, et al. Transplantation of bioprinted tissues and organs: technical and

clinical challenges and future perspectives. *Ann Surg.* 2017;266(1):48–58.

42. Derakhshanfar S, Mbeleck R, Xu K, Zhang X, Zhong W, Xing M. 3D bioprinting for biomedical devices and tissue engineering: a review of recent trends and advances. *Bioact Mater.* 2018;3(2):144–156.

43. Hospodiuk M, Dey M, Sosnoski D, Ozbolat IT. The bio-ink: a comprehensive review on bioprintable materials. *Biotechnol Adv.* 2017;35(2):217–239.

44. Ozbolat IT, Yu Y. Bioprinting toward organ fabrication: challenges and future trends. *IEEE Trans Biomed Eng.* 2013;60(3):691–699.

45. Serpooshan V, Mahmoudi M, Hu DA, Hu JB, Wu SM. Bioengineering cardiac constructs using 3D printing. *J 3D Print Med.* 2017;1(2).

46. Ovsianikov A, Khademhosseini A, Mironov V. The synergy of scaffold-based and scaffold-free tissue engineering strategies. *Trends Biotechnol.* 2018;36(4):348–357.

47. Moldovan L, Barnard A, Gil CH, et al. iPSC-derived vascular cell spheroids as building blocks for scaffold-free biofabrication. *Biotechnol J.* 2017;12(12).

48. Moldovan NI, Hibino N, Nakayama K. Principles of the Kenzan method for robotic cell spheroid-based three-dimensional bioprinting. *Tissue Eng B Rev.* 2017;23(3):237–244.

49. Ong CS, Fukunishi T, Nashed A, et al. Creation of cardiac tissue exhibiting mechanical integration of spheroids using 3D bioprinting. *J Vis Exp.* 2017;125.

50. Mandrycky C, Wang Z, Kim K, Kim DH. 3D bioprinting for engineering complex tissues. *Biotechnol Adv.* 2016;34(4):422–434.

51. Hinton TJ, Jallerat Q, Palchesko RN, et al. Three-dimensional printing of complex biological structures by freeform reversible embedding of suspended hydrogels. *Sci Adv.* 2015;1(9):e1500758.

52. Taylor RE, Kim K, Sun N, et al. Sacrificial layer technique for axial force post assay of immature cardiomyocytes. *Biomed Microdevices.* 2013;15(1):171–181.

53. Kolesky DB, Truby RL, Gladman AS, Busbee TA, Homan KA, Lewis JA. 3D bioprinting of vascularized, heterogeneous cell-laden tissue constructs. *Adv Mater.* 2014;26(19):3124–3130.

54. Bertassoni LE, Cecconi M, Manoharan V, et al. Hydrogel bioprinted microchannel networks for vascularization of tissue engineering constructs. *Lab Chip.* 2014;14(13):2202–2211.

55. Miller JS, Stevens KR, Yang MT, et al. Rapid casting of patterned vascular networks for perfusable engineered 3D tissues. *Nat Mater.* 2012;11(9):768–774.

56. OPTN. *Organ Procurement and Transplantation Network - OPTN*; 2018. https://optn.transplant.hrsa.gov/.

57. *Transplant Trends | UNOS*; 2015. https://unos.org/data/transplant-trends/.

58. Morris S. Future of 3D printing: how 3D bioprinting technology can revolutionize healthcare? *Birth Defects Res.* 2018;110(13):1098–1101.

59. Buchholz S, Guenther SPW, Michel S, Schramm R, Hagl C. Ventricular assist device therapy and heart transplantation: benefits, drawbacks, and outlook. *Herz*. 2018; 43(5):406–414.

60. Truby LK, Garan AR, Givens RC, et al. Ventricular assist device utilization in heart transplant candidates: nationwide variability and impact on waitlist outcomes. *Circ Heart Fail*. 2018;11(4):e004586.

61. Harbaugh J. *About the Challenge. [Text]*; 2018. https://www.nasa.gov/directorates/spacetech/centennial_challenges/vascular_tissue/about.html.

62. *Focus Area: 3D Organ Engineering*; 2018. https://wyss.harvard.edu/focus-area/organ-engineering/.

63. *Advanced 3-D Bioprinting*; 2018. https://engineering.cmu.edu/organs/research/advanced-3d-bioprinting.html.

64. *3D Bioprinting — BIOLIFE4D*; 2018. https://biolife4d.com/.

65. Cui H, Nowicki M, Fisher JP, Zhang LG. 3D bioprinting for organ regeneration. *Adv Healthc Mater*. 2017;6(1).

66. Bishop ES, Mostafa S, Pakvasa M, et al. 3-D bioprinting technologies in tissue engineering and regenerative medicine: current and future trends. *Genes Dis*. 2017;4(4): 185–195.

67. Patra S, Young V. A review of 3D printing techniques and the future in biofabrication of bioprinted tissue. *Cell Biochem Biophys*. 2016;74(2):93–98.

68. Knight AD, Levick JR. The density and distribution of capillaries around a synovial cavity. *Q J Exp Physiol*. 1983; 68(4):629–644.

69. Vunjak-Novakovic G, Tandon N, Godier A, et al. Challenges in cardiac tissue engineering. *Tissue Eng B Rev*. 2010;16(2):169–187.

70. Graham AD, Olof SN, Burke MJ, et al. High-resolution patterned cellular constructs by droplet-based 3D printing. *Sci Rep*. 2017;7(1):7004.

71. Zhang J, Zhu W, Radisic M, Vunjak-Novakovic G. Can we engineer a human cardiac patch for therapy? *Circ Res*. 2018;123(2):244–265.

72. Zhao Y, Feric NT, Thavandiran N, Nunes SS, Radisic M. The role of tissue engineering and biomaterials in cardiac regenerative medicine. *Can J Cardiol*. 2014;30(11): 1307–1322.

73. Ning L, Chen X. A brief review of extrusion-based tissue scaffold bio-printing. *Biotechnol J*. 2017;12(8).

74. Tan Z, Parisi C, Di Silvio L, Dini D, Forte AE. Cryogenic 3D printing of super soft hydrogels. *Sci Rep*. 2017;7(1): 16293.

75. *HOME. Prellis Biologics*; 2018. https://www.prellisbiologics.co.

76. *Prellis Biologics Achieves Unprecedented Speed and Resolution in 3D Printing of Human Tissue with Capillaries*. Business Wire; 2018.

77. *Prellis Biologics Sets Out to Eliminate the Donor Waiting List with 3D Printed Organs*. 2017.

78. Adler CP, Costabel U. Cell number in human heart in atrophy, hypertrophy, and under the influence of cytostatics. *Recent Adv Stud Card Struct Metabol*. 1975;6:343–355.

79. Pinto AR, Ilinykh A, Ivey MJ, et al. Revisiting cardiac cellular composition. *Circ Res*. 2016;118(3):400–409.

80. Nag AC. Study of non-muscle cells of the adult mammalian heart: a fine structural analysis and distribution. *Cytobios*. 1980;28(109):41–61.

81. Gopinathan J, Noh I. Recent trends in bioinks for 3D printing. *Biomater Res*. 2018;22:11.

82. Bertassoni LE, Cardoso JC, Manoharan V, et al. Direct-write bioprinting of cell-laden methacrylated gelatin hydrogels. *Biofabrication*. 2014;6(2):024105.

83. Billiet T, Gevaert E, De Schryver T, Cornelissen M, Dubruel P. The 3D printing of gelatin methacrylamide cell-laden tissue-engineered constructs with high cell viability. *Biomaterials*. 2014;35(1):49–62.

84. Schmidt CE, Baier JM. Acellular vascular tissues: natural biomaterials for tissue repair and tissue engineering. *Biomaterials*. 2000;21(22):2215–2231.

85. Law N, Doney B, Glover H, et al. Characterisation of hyaluronic acid methylcellulose hydrogels for 3D bioprinting. *J Mech Behav Biomed Mater*. 2018;77: 389–399.

86. Kim BS, Kim H, Gao G, Jang J, Cho DW. Decellularized extracellular matrix: a step towards the next generation source for bioink manufacturing. *Biofabrication*. 2017; 9(3):034104.

87. Pati F, Jang J, Ha DH, et al. Printing three-dimensional tissue analogues with decellularized extracellular matrix bioink. *Nat Commun*. 2014;5:3935.

88. Fitzpatrick JC, Clark PM, Capaldi FM. Effect of decellularization protocol on the mechanical behavior of porcine descending aorta. *Int J Biom*. 2010;2010.

89. Skardal A, Devarasetty M, Kang HW, et al. A hydrogel bioink toolkit for mimicking native tissue biochemical and mechanical properties in bioprinted tissue constructs. *Acta Biomater*. 2015;25:24–34.

90. Moldovan NI. Progress in scaffold-free bioprinting for cardiovascular medicine. *J Cell Mol Med*. 2018;22(6): 2964–2969.

91. Souza GR. Three-dimensional tissue culture based on magnetic cell levitation. *Nat Nanotechnol*. 2018;5(4): 291–296.

92. @cellink3d. *A Look at Five Different Types of Bioink*. CELLINK; 2017.

93. Tarassoli SP, Jessop ZM, Kyle S, Whitaker IS. 8 - candidate bioinks for 3D bioprinting soft tissue. In: Thomas DJ, Jessop ZM, Whitaker IS, eds. *3D Bioprinting for Reconstructive Surgery*. Woodhead Publishing; 2018:145–172.

94. Gelinsky M. 6 — biopolymer hydrogel bioinks. In: Thomas DJ, Jessop ZM, Whitaker IS, eds. *3D Bioprinting for Reconstructive Surgery*. Woodhead Publishing; 2018: 125–136.

95. Holzl K, Lin S, Tytgat L, Van Vlierberghe S, Gu L, Ovsianikov A. Bioink properties before, during and after 3D bioprinting. *Biofabrication*. 2016;8(3):032002.

96. Pusch K, Hinton TJ, Feinberg AW. Large volume syringe pump extruder for desktop 3D printers. *HardwareX*. 2018;3:49–61.

97. Jana S, Lerman A. Bioprinting a cardiac valve. *Biotechnol Adv.* 2015;33(8):1503−1521.

98. Ong CS, Yesantharao P, Huang CY, et al. 3D bioprinting using stem cells. *Pediatr Res.* 2018;83(1−2):223−231.

99. Chambers J, Ely J. A comparison of the classical and modified forms of the continuity equation in the On-X prosthetic heart valve in the aortic position. *J Heart Valve Dis.* 2000;9(2):299−301. discussion 301-292.

100. Chambers JB. The echocardiography of replacement heart valves. *Echo Res Pract.* 2016;3(3):R35−r43.

101. Duan B, Hockaday LA, Kang KH, Butcher JT. 3D bioprinting of heterogeneous aortic valve conduits with alginate/gelatin hydrogels. *J Biomed Mater Res A.* 2013; 101(5):1255−1264.

102. Moorman A, Webb S, Brown NA, Lamers W, Anderson RH. Development of the heart: (1) formation of the cardiac chambers and arterial trunks. *Heart.* 2003;89:806−814.

103. Farraj KL, Zeltser R. Embryology, heart tube, formation. In: *StatPearls*. Treasure Island (FL): StatPearls Publishing-StatPearls Publishing LLC.; 2018.

104. Hoang P, Wang J, Conklin BR, Healy KE, Ma Z. Generation of spatial-patterned early-developing cardiac organoids using human pluripotent stem cells. *Nat Protoc.* 2018;13(4):723−737.

105. Ma Z, Wang J, Loskill P, et al. Self-organizing human cardiac microchambers mediated by geometric confinement. *Nat Commun.* 2015;6:7413.

106. Vijayavenkataraman S, Fuh JYH, Lu WF. 3D printing and 3D bioprinting in pediatrics. *Bioengineering.* 2017;4(3).

107. Vermeulen N, Haddow G, Seymour T, Faulkner-Jones A, Shu W. 3D bioprint me: a socioethical view of bioprinting human organs and tissues. *J Med Ethics.* 2017;43(9):618−624.

108. Michalski MH, Ross JS. The shape of things to come: 3D printing in medicine. *Jama.* 2014;312(21): 2213−2214.

109. Vijayavenkataraman S, Lu WF, Fuh JYH. 3D bioprinting − an ethical, legal and social aspects (ELSA) framework. *Bioprinting.* 2016;1−2:11−21.

110. Corporation AB. *3D Printing Raises Ethical Issues in Medicine. [current]*; 2015. http://www.abc.net.au/science/articles/2015/02/11/4161675.htm.

111. Gilbert F, O'Connell CD, Mladenovska T, Dodds S. Print me an organ? Ethical and regulatory issues emerging from 3D bioprinting in medicine. *Sci Eng Ethics.* 2018; 24(1):73−91.

112. Ingulli E. Mechanism of cellular rejection in transplantation. *Pediatr Nephrol.* 2010;25:61−74.

113. Wood KJ. Regulatory T cells in transplantation. *Transplant Proc.* 2011;43(6):2135−2136.

114. Lee MO, Moon SH, Jeong HC, et al. Inhibition of pluripotent stem cell-derived teratoma formation by small molecules. *Proc Natl Acad Sci U S A.* 2013;110(35): E3281−E3290.

115. Bedel A, Beliveau F, Lamrissi-Garcia I, et al. Preventing pluripotent cell teratoma in regenerative medicine applied to hematology disorders. *Stem Cells Transl Med.* 2017;6(2):382−393.

116. Zheng YL. Some ethical concerns about human induced pluripotent stem cells. *Sci Eng Ethics.* 2016;22(5): 1277−1284.

117. *Investment in 3D Bioprinting and Tech Demo Centers Advances.* 2018.

Index

Note: Page numbers followed by "t" indicate tables and "f" indicate figures.

Printed and bound by CPI Group (UK) Ltd, Croydon, CR0 4YY

08/05/2025

01864761-0003